Review of
CLINICAL ANESTHESIA

FOURTH EDITION

Review of
CLINICAL ANESTHESIA

FOURTH EDITION

Edited By

Neil Roy Connelly, M.D.

Professor of Anesthesiology
Tufts University School of Medicine
Director of Anesthesia Research
Department of Anesthesiology
Baystate Medical Center
Springfield, Massachusetts

David G. Silverman, M.D.

Professor and Director of Clinical Research
Department of Anesthesiology
Yale University School of Medicine
Medical Director of Pre-Admission Testing
Yale–New Haven Hospital
New Haven, Connecticut

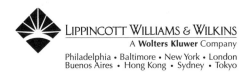

LIPPINCOTT WILLIAMS & WILKINS
A **Wolters Kluwer** Company
Philadelphia • Baltimore • New York • London
Buenos Aires • Hong Kong • Sydney • Tokyo

Acquisitions Editor: Brian Brown
Managing Editor: Franny Murphy
Developmental Editor: Grace R. Caputo, Dovetail Content Solutions
Production Editor: Dave Murphy
Manufacturing Manager: Ben Rivera
Marketing Manager: Angela Panetta
Design Manager: Doug Smock
Compositor: TechBooks
Printer: Edwards Brothers

Printed in the USA

Library of Congress Cataloging-in-Publication Data

Review of clinical anesthesia / edited by Neil Roy Connelly, David G.
  Silverman.— 4th ed.
    p. ; cm.
  ISBN 0-7817-8299-6 (alk. paper)
  1. Anesthesiology—Examinations, questions, etc.   2. Anesthesia—Examinations,
questions, etc.   I. Connelly, Neil Roy.   II. Silverman, David G.
  [DNLM: 1. Anesthesia—Examination Questions.   2. Anesthesiology—Examination
Questions.   WO 218.2 R454 2005]
  RD82.3.R48   2005
  617.9′6′076–dc22

                                                                2005022797

Care has been taken to confirm the accuracy of the information presented and to describe generally accepted practices. However, the authors, editors, and publisher are not responsible for errors or omissions or for any consequences from application of the information in this book and make no warranty, expressed or implied, with respect to the currency, completeness, or accuracy of the contents of the publication. Application of this information in a particular situation remains the professional responsibility of the practitioner.

The authors, editors, and publisher have exerted every effort to ensure that drug selection and dosage set forth in this text are in accordance with current recommendations and practice at the time of publication. However, in view of ongoing research, changes in government regulations, and the constant flow of information relating to drug therapy and drug reactions, the reader is urged to check the package insert for each drug for any change in indications and dosage and for added warnings and precautions. This is particularly important when the recommended agent is a new or infrequently employed drug.

Some drugs and medical devices presented in this publication have Food and Drug Administration (FDA) clearance for limited use in restricted research settings. It is the responsibility of the health care provider to ascertain the FDA status of each drug or device planned for use in their clinical practice.

To purchase additional copies of this book, call our customer service department at (800) 638-3030 or fax orders to (301) 824-7390. International customers should call (301) 714-2324.

Visit Lippincott Williams & Wilkins on the Internet: at LWW.com. Lippincott Williams & Wilkins customer service representatives are available from 8:30 am to 6 pm, EST.

10 9 8 7 6 5 4 3

THIS BOOK IS DEDICATED TO OUR WIVES—
ANN GIANCASPRO CONNELLY AND SALLY KNIFFIN.
AND TO OUR CHILDREN—
KEVIN MATTHEW AND ELLEN ALEKSANDRA CONNELLY
AND TYLER AND CHARLOTTE SILVERMAN.
AND TO MARY M. CONNELLY.
AND TO THE LATE ARTHUR SILVERMAN.

CONTRIBUTORS

Neil Roy Connelly, M.D.
Professor of Anesthesiology
Tufts University School of Medicine
Director of Anesthesia Research
Department of Anesthesiology
Baystate Medical Center
Springfield, Massachusetts

Katharine O. Freeman, M.D.
Assistant Professor
Tufts University School of Medicine
Department of Anesthesiology
Baystate Medical Center
Springfield, Massachusetts

Kamel H. Ghandour, M.D.
Resident in Anesthesiology
Department of Anesthesiology
Baystate Medical Center
Springfield, Massachusetts

Natalie F. Holt, M.D., M.P.H.
Resident in Anesthesiology
Yale University School of Medicine
Yale–New Haven Hospital
New Haven, Connecticut

Wandana Joshi, D.O.
Assistant Professor
Tufts University School of Medicine
Department of Anesthesiology
Baystate Medical Center
Springfield, Massachusetts

Brian Kiessling, M.D.
Chief of Anesthesia
Northwest Michigan Surgery
  Center
Traverse City, Michigan

Timothy L. Lacy, M.D.
Resident in Anesthesiology
Department of Anesthesiology
Baystate Medical Center
Springfield, Massachusetts

Tanya P. Lucas, M.D.
Assistant Professor
Tufts University School
  of Medicine
Department of Anesthesiology
Baystate Medical Center
Springfield, Massachusetts

Thomas S. Pedersen, M.D.
Attending Anesthesiologist
Concord Hospital
Concord, New Hampshire

Armin Rahimi, D.O.
Pain Management Services
South County Anesthesia
St. Anthony's Medical
  Center
St. Louis, Missouri

Stelian Serban, M.D.
Fellow in Anesthesiology
Department of Anesthesiology
Memorial Sloan-Kettering
  Cancer Center
New York, New York

G. Brent Shulman, M.D.
Cheif of Anesthesia
Department of Anesthesiology
Marshfield, Wisconsin

David G. Silverman, M.D.
Professor and Director of
  Clinical Research
Department of Anesthesiology
Yale University School of
  Medicine
Medical Director of Pre-Admission
  Testing
Yale–New Haven Hospital
New Haven, Connecticut

John F. Vullo, M.D.
Resident in Anesthesiology
Department of Anesthesiology
Baystate Medical Center
Springfield, Massachusetts

One of the best ways to judge a book is by the company it keeps. Thus, even before it hits the bookstore shelves, *Review of Clinical Anesthesia* is a "winner." This totally revised work, which parallels the new (fifth) edition of *Clinical Anesthesia,* enjoys a distinguished position on a CDROM along with *Clinical Anesthesia* and other significant texts in the field of anesthesiology.

As stated in the introductions to the previous editions of this review book, the amount of information related to our specialty appears to be growing exponentially; even a carefully honed text such as *Clinical Anesthesia* can seem quite imposing. At times, the reader would like to pause and see what he or she has learned or should learn. These factors were the impetus behind the development of *Review of Clinical Anesthesia.* In its simplest form, the multiple-choice questions in this text can be used as a means of self-assessment before taking a written examination. However, we feel that this book may be of even greater benefit if it is incorporated throughout one's studies: a pretest will help the novice as well as the expert focus his or her reading; a posttest will allow one to assess self-mastery of most relevant material.

The fourth edition of this text has benefited from the extensive updating of the parent text, *Clinical Anesthesia.* This has led to our revision of the material in virtually every chapter, as well as to the addition of several new chapters. As was the case in the third edition, a heading and a page number appear at the end of each answer that refer the reader to a section in *Clinical Anesthesia.* This information can be used to direct the reader to a more extensive discussion of the subject matter addressed in the question.

Neil Roy Connelly, M.D.
David G. Silverman, M.D.

ACKNOWLEDGMENTS

The generation of the questions in this text could not have been accomplished without the dedicated efforts of Ms. Lynda Paglia at Baystate and Ms. Jacki Fitzpatrick at Yale. The entire secretarial staffs of our respective institutions walked the extra mile and typed the extra question to bring this book to fruition. We appreciate the efforts of the members of the staff at Lippincott Williams & Wilkins Publishers who were vital to the organization and completion of this text. We would like to acknowledge the assistance of Grace Caputo and the previous help of Craig Percy. We also wish to thank the editors (Drs. Paul Barash, Bruce Cullen, and Robert Stoelting) and authors of *Clinical Anesthesia* for, once again, providing us with such a fine source of material. Their careful attention to detail and relevance have facilitated our efforts. We also would like to express our appreciation to our coauthors, whose assiduous efforts have enabled us to assemble a detailed yet cohesive series of questions and answers. Mostly, we would like to thank our families, who waited patiently as we waded through pages of text in search of the perfect questions.

CONTENTS

SECTION VI ■ POSTANESTHESIA AND CONSULTANT PRACTICE

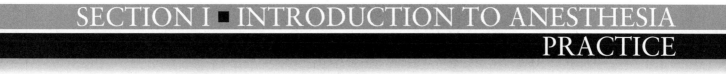

SECTION I ▪ INTRODUCTION TO ANESTHESIA PRACTICE

CHAPTER 1 ■ THE HISTORY OF ANESTHESIA

1. Nitrous oxide was first prepared by:

   A. Thomas Beddoes
   B. Joseph Priestley
   C. Humphry Davy
   D. Horace Wells
   E. Valerius Cordus

2. The man credited with the earliest documented use of diethyl ether for painless surgery is:

   A. Crawford W. Long
   B. Henry Hill Hickman
   C. William T.G. Morton
   D. Horace Wells
   E. Charles T. Jackson

3. Who published the use of chloroform for anesthesia during labor and childbirth in the *Lancet* in 1847?

   A. James Young Simpson
   B. Virginia Apgar
   C. William Morton
   D. Joseph Clover
   E. Queen Victoria

4. Who first described the technique of intravenous regional anesthesia in 1908?

   A. Harvey Cushing
   B. August Bier
   C. Carl Koller
   D. Leonard Corning
   E. Heinrich Braun

5. Elmer McKesson is credited with the innovation of which of the following features of modern-day anesthesia machines?

   A. Oxygen fail-safe valve
   B. Flow-ratio system
   C. Oxygen flush valve
   D. Variable bypass vaporizers
   E. Partial rebreathing circuits

6. According to Severinghaus, "the most important technological advance ever made in monitoring the well-being and safety of patients during anesthesia" is the advent of which monitoring system?

   A. Continuous capnography
   B. Electrocardiography
   C. Mass spectrometry
   D. Oxygen sensors
   E. Pulse oximetry

7. Which notable advancement in the field of anesthesiology can be credited primarily to work done by American surgeon Joseph O'Dwyer in the mid-1880s?

   A. Tracheal intubation
   B. Central venous cannulation
   C. Direct laryngoscopy
   D. Brachial plexus conduction block
   E. Anesthetic record

8. Which pioneer in the field of anesthesiology can be credited with the development of the cuffed endotracheal tube?

   A. Ralph Waters
   B. Joseph O'Dwyer
   C. Arthur Guedel
   D. Elmer McKesson
   E. Ivan Magill

9. The cardiovascular effects of which drug became widely appreciated only after a series of fatalities among military casualties during World War II?

   A. Curare
   B. Thiopental
   C. Fentanyl
   D. Halothane
   E. Cyclopropane

10. Who committed suicide in 1848 after being discouraged when nitrous oxide failed to act predictably as a dental anesthetic in front of a hostile audience in 1845?

    A. William Morton
    B. Charles Jackson
    C. Horace Wells
    D. Gardner Quincy Colton
    E. Crawford Long

11. Trichloroethylene, a nonexplosive volatile anesthetic, releases what compound when it is warmed in the presence of soda lime?

    A. Compound X
    B. Compound A
    C. Factor X
    D. Phosgene
    E. Ethyl chloride

12. What anesthetic, although popular in the mid-twentieth century, was abandoned after it was learned that dose-related nephrotoxicity was associated with its prolonged use?

    A. Chloroform
    B. Methoxyflurane
    C. Ether
    D. Enflurane
    E. Halothane

13. Drs. Bier and Hildebrandt performed a successful spinal anesthetic when Dr. Hildebrandt did not feel pain after his legs were hit with a hammer and his testicles were pulled; how did these physicians celebrate?

    A. Wine and cigars
    B. Going out to the opera and then a cabaret
    C. Visiting an opium den in Kiel, Germany
    D. Repeating the spinal anesthetic
    E. With more hammers

14. Who described a continuous spinal anesthetic technique on or about 1940?

    A. Heinrich Quincke
    B. August Bier
    C. Theodor Tuffier
    D. William Lemmon
    E. Richard Hall

15. Achille Dogliott described what anesthetic technique in 1931?

    A. Intravenous regional anesthesia of the arm
    B. Loss of resistance to identify the epidural space
    C. Blind nasotracheal intubation
    D. Cervical spinal anesthesia
    E. Regional block of the ankle

16. Who created the first clinic for the treatment of chronic pain in the United States?

    A. Emery Rovenstine

    B. Frederick Cotton
    C. John Snow
    D. John Booka
    E. Ambrose Bierce

17. What medication introduced in the late twentieth century suppressed pharyngeal reflexes, produced anesthesia rapidly, had antiemetic properties, allowed patients to wake promptly, and popularized total intravenous anesthetic techniques?

    A. Ketamine
    B. Propofol
    C. Meperidine
    D. Chlorpromazine
    E. Droperidol

18. Oncologists identified the antiemetic properties of what medication(s) when dealing with intracranial edema from tumors?

    A. Antihistamines
    B. Propofol
    C. Droperidol
    D. Corticosteroids
    E. Promethazine

19. Dr. Archie Brain made what contribution to airway management by his radical thinking?

    A. Patil face mask
    B. Laryngeal mask airway
    C. Wu-scope
    D. Flexible fiberoptic bronchoscope
    E. Bullard laryngoscope

For questions 20 to 23, choose A if 1, 2, and 3 are correct; B if 1 and 3; C if 2 and 4; D if 4; E if all.

20. In the late nineteenth century and early twentieth century, which of the following explosive volatile anesthetics were in use?

    1. Chloroform
    2. Ether
    3. Cyclopropane
    4. Nitrous oxide

21. Lenard Corning performed and described what block(s) using cocaine in the late nineteenth century?

    1. Spinal
    2. Intravenous regional of the arm
    3. Epidural
    4. Brachial plexus

22. Which of the following statements regarding the history of cocaine as an anesthetic is/are TRUE?

    1. Cocaine was the first effective local anesthetic.
    2. Its utility as a local anesthetic was first introduced to the medical community by Carl Koller in 1884.

3. Cocaine was the agent used in the first successful spinal anesthetic.
4. Although its local anesthetic actions were well recognized, cocaine was not used in surgical procedures until 1911.

23. Which of the following statements regarding the "to-and-fro" device for carbon dioxide absorption developed by Ralph Waters in 1924 is/are TRUE?

1. It was the first simplistic device utilizing soda lime as a carbon dioxide absorbent.
2. It was developed primarily for physician cost savings.
3. It was based on the pioneering work of pharmacologist Dennis Jackson in 1915.
4. The device was incompatible with inflammable anesthetics.

ANSWERS

1. **B.** Nitrous oxide was first prepared in 1773 by the British clergyman and scientist Joseph Priestley. Priestley prepared several other gases during his investigations, the most notable being isolated oxygen. Davy and Wells performed later experiments with nitrous oxide, whereas Valerius Cordus is credited with having distilled diethyl ether in the sixteenth century. (See page 5: Inhaled Anesthesia.)

2. **A.** Although William Morton has been credited with having first introduced diethyl ether as a successful anesthetic in the public arena on October 16, 1846, it is Dr. Crawford W. Long of Athens, GA, who has the distinction of the first documented successful use of ether in the surgical setting. Long first administered ether preoperatively on March 30, 1842, but he neglected to make his findings known until 1849, well after Morton's demonstration. (See page 5: Almost Discovery.)

3. **A.** Although Simpson, an accomplished obstetrician in Edinburgh, Scotland, had been a champion of the use of ether and chloroform anesthesia for labor and childbirth, the relief of obstetric pain had long been discouraged on prevailing religious grounds. It was not until John Snow, an English contemporary of Simpson, administered chloroform to a laboring Queen Victoria that widespread acceptance of obstetric anesthesia came into being. As head of the Church of England, the Queen's endorsement of the practice ended the debate as to the appropriateness of such anesthetics. (See page 7: Chloroform and Obstetrics.)

4. **B.** Intravenous regional anesthesia was first reported in 1908 by August Bier, who used a technique in which procaine was injected into a vein of the upper limb between two tourniquets. The technique was not widely used in the clinical setting until 1963, when Mackinnon Holmes modified the block by exsanguination before applying a single proximal cuff. (See page 10: Spinal Anesthesia)

5. **C.** Elmer McKesson, one of the first specialists in anesthesiology in the United States, developed a series of gas machines. Because of concerns over inflammable anesthetics, McKesson popularized anesthetic inductions with 100% nitrous oxide, with titration of small volumes of oxygen as the anesthetic progressed. McKesson developed the oxygen flush valve to add oxygen quickly to the system in the event that the resultant cyanosis became too profound. (See page 11: Early Anesthesia Delivery Systems.)

6. **E.** Pulse oximetry, described by Severinghaus as the most important technologic monitoring advance in the history of anesthesia, was developed by Takuo Aoyagi, a Japanese engineer. His work was a refinement of earlier investigations performed by Glen Millikan, an American physiologist, which pertained to oximetric sensors for fighter pilots during World War II. (See page 17: Electrocardiography, Pulse Oximetry, and Capnography.)

7. **A.** Although elective oral tracheal intubation was first performed by William Macewen in 1878, it was the work of American surgeon Joseph O'Dwyer that popularized the technique. In 1885, O'Dwyer developed a set of metal laryngeal tubes, which he inserted blindly between the vocal cords of children suffering diphtheritic crises as an alternative to hasty tracheotomies. Three years later, he developed a rigid endotracheal tube with a conical tip, which allowed positive-pressure endotracheal ventilation to be used during thoracic procedures. (See page 14: Tracheal Intubation in Anesthesia.)

8. **C.** In 1926, Arthur Guedel began a series of experiments that led to the introduction of the cuffed endotracheal tube. His goal was to combine tracheal anesthesia with the closed-circuit technique recently refined by Waters. To showcase the utility of these new tubes, Guedel performed a series of demonstrations with his own dog "Airway," whom he anesthetized and submerged underwater while using the cuffed endotracheal tube. (See page 15: Anesthesiologists Inspired Laryngoscopes.)

9. **B.**   Thiopental was synthesized in 1932 by Tabern and Volwiler of the Abbott Company and was first administered to a patient at the University of Wisconsin in March, 1934. The cardiovascular depressive effects of thiopental were widely appreciated only after its use led to fatalities among civilian and military casualties of World War II. After these experiences, fluid replacement therapy was used more aggressively, and thiopental was administered with greater caution. (See page 18: Intravenous Medications in Anesthetics.)

10. **C.**   Although the failure of Dr. Wells that day may have been multifactorial (e.g., an uncooperative patient, hostile audience, beginning the dental extraction before a sufficient anesthetic level) the principal reason may have been the need for adjunct anesthesia when using nitrous oxide in order for it to act predictably. (See page 5: Almost Discovery.)

11. **D.**   Trichloroethylene was a widely used nonexplosive volatile anesthetic. It was found to be toxic to multiple organ systems when it was administered for prolonged periods or at high concentrations. When the gas is exposed to heated soda lime carbon dioxide absorbent, it produces phosgene as a byproduct. When phosgene is inhaled, it reacts with water in the lungs to form hydrochloric acid and carbon monoxide, with resultant pulmonary edema. Phosgene was used extensively during World War I as a choking agent. Among the chemicals used in the war, phosgene was responsible for the majority of deaths. (See page 7: The Second Generation of Inhaled Anesthetics.)

12. **B.**   Methoxyflurane use over a protracted period led to increased serum fluoride concentrations and nephrotoxicity. Before this was discovered, methoxyflurane was a very popular volatile anesthetic during the 1960s. (See page 7: The Second Generation of Inhaled Anesthetics.)

13. **A.**   The first clearly defined spinal anesthetic involved the release of cerebrospinal fluid, an end point still used, and this led to the first described postdural puncture headache. Drs. Bier and Hildebrandt erroneously attributed the headache to the celebratory wine and cigars. (See page 10: Spinal Anesthesia.)

14. **D.**   Dr. Lemmon described the use of a malleable silver needle to puncture the dura, and local anesthetic was introduced as needed through a hole in the operating table mattress. Later, the same technique was described by Waldo Edwards and Robert Hingson for continuous caudal anesthesia in obstetric patients. (See page 10: Spinal Anesthesia.)

15. **B.**   Achille M. Dogliotti of Turin, Italy, wrote a classic study that made the epidural technique well known. Dogliotti identified it by the loss-of-resistance technique. (See page 10: Epidural Anesthesia.)

16. **A.**   Emery Rovenstine and his colleagues used invasive techniques to lyse sensory nerves and to inject local anesthetics in an attempt to treat chronic pain. This association of physicians focused on pain management was the first of its kind in North America. (See page 10: Spinal Anesthesia.)

17. **B.**   Propofol combined with variable-duration paralytics and faster-acting narcotics made total intravenous anesthesia techniques more accessible. Propofol's antiemetic property, along with a ceiling context-sensitive half-life, makes it a popular anesthetic agent to this day. (See page 18: Intravenous Medications in Anesthesia.)

18. **D.**   Corticosteroids acted to decrease intracranial edema in patients with mass lesions and tumors. They also had the side effect of reducing nausea. This antiemetic effect was quickly recognized by anesthesiologists. (See page 18: Intravenous Medications.)

19. **B.**   Archie Brain produced and made popular the laryngeal mask airway after he realized that it was an effective means to ventilate and deliver anesthetics to a patient. Shigeto Ikeda developed the first flexible fiberoptic bronchoscope. Roger Bullard developed the Bullard laryngoscope to "see around the corner" of the airway. The Wu-scope was later developed to improve on the idea of the Bullard laryngoscope. The Patil Face Mask, developed by Vijay Patil, was developed to oxygenate the anesthetized patient while a flexible fiberoptic bronchoscope is used to intubate the airway. All these innovations were prompted by the need to manage patients with challenging, difficult airways. (See page 16: Airway Management Devices.)

20. **A.**   Both ether and chloroform were known to be flammable gases and to be explosion hazards. Cyclopropane (also called trimethylene) is an explosive, colorless gas first used in 1934 as a volatile general anesthetic. Both induction and emergence from cyclopropane anesthesia were reported to be usually rapid and smooth, but because it is flammable and could be a source of explosion in the operating area, cyclopropane was replaced by nonflammable gases. Nitrous oxide can support combustion, but it is not explosive. (See page 8: Fluorinated Anesthetics.)

21. **B.**   Dr. Lenard Corning performed successful neuraxial blocks in his practice; it is not clear whether he differentiated between the two types. (See page 10: Spinal Anesthesia.)

22. **A.**   The anesthetic properties of cocaine, an extract of the coca leaf, had been known for centuries before its formal introduction in 1884 by Carl Koller. Soon thereafter, cocaine gained widespread acceptance as an anesthetic agent for surgical procedures involving mucous membranes, such as the eye, mouth, nose,

larynx, trachea, and rectum. Cocaine also was the agent used by Leonard Corning for the first successful spinal anesthetic in 1885. (See page 9: Regional Anesthesia.)

23. **A.** Waters developed his "to-and-fro" apparatus for carbon dioxide absorption based on work done by Dennis Jackson (using solutions of sodium and calcium hydroxide). Waters fashioned a simplified absorber (using soda lime granules placed in a canister) between a facemask and an adjacent breathing bag to which the fresh gas flow was attached. The device originally was designed as a cost-saving measure, at a time when private patients and insurance companies were reluctant to pay for a specialist's services, including drugs and supplies. (See page 11: Early Anesthesia Delivery Systems.)

CHAPTER 2 ■ PRACTICE AND OPERATING ROOM MANAGEMENT

1. Full Joint Commission on Accreditation of Healthcare Organizations (JCAHO) accreditation lasts for how many years?

    A. 1
    B. 2
    C. 3
    D. 4
    E. 5

2. The main goal of a managed care organization (MCO) is to attempt to manage what aspects of the health care system?

    A. Number of facilities in a geographic area
    B. Utilization of services within a patient population
    C. Outline of the best management for each particular condition
    D. Ensuring that physicians are managed to improve physician income
    E. Being a division of the National Institutes of Health whose goal is the development of universal coverage

For questions 3 to 8, choose A if 1, 2, and 3 are correct; B if 1 and 3; C if 2 and 4; D if 4; E if all.

3. Which of the following statements regarding claims-made insurance is/are TRUE?

    1. Policies cover all malpractice claims made while the insurance is being paid.
    2. Policies are very expensive during the first year of practice.
    3. Tail coverage is a hidden expense with claims-made policies.
    4. Claims-made policies are more expensive for insurance companies because they have a longer period in which they are exposed to possible claims.

4. Establishing standards of care, practice parameters, and guidelines in anesthesia practice affords individuals with which of the following benefits?

    1. Improvement in quality of care
    2. Providing the basis for legal defense in malpractice cases
    3. Guiding thought processes through difficult clinical scenarios
    4. Fulfilling legal mandates

5. Following a critical adverse event, which of the following should be implemented?

    1. Obtain appropriate help immediately.
    2. The risk management department in the hospital should be involved only if a suit is filed.
    3. Any additions or alterations of the facts in the chart should be recorded as amendments.
    4. Charting of the event should include the facts of the events and speculations regarding the cause of the incident.

6. Computer scheduling of cases has advantages over handwritten systems in which of the following ways?

    1. Historical precedents of time for procedures can prevent overbooking.
    2. It can result in a decrease of staff overtime costs.
    3. It can easily generate reports and statistics for future use.
    4. It can reduce personal bias in scheduling of cases.

7. Which of the following regarding the Health Insurance Portability and Accountability Act of 1996 (HIPAA) is/are TRUE?

    1. Attention is focused on protected health information.
    2. A "privacy officer" must be appointed for each practice group.
    3. Patient charts must be locked away overnight.

4. A fax containing patient information does not need any special handling.

8. Which of the following regarding antitrust considerations is/are TRUE?

1. Antitrust laws involve the rights of individuals to engage in business.

2. The Sherman Antitrust Act is approximately 50 years old.

3. The per se rule is the most frequently applied rule when judging violations.

4. Antitrust laws are concerned with the preservation of competition in a defined marketplace.

ANSWERS

1. C. Full JCAHO accreditation lasts for 3 years. (See page 31: Establishing Standards of Practice and Understanding Standard of Care.)

2. B. MCOs are companies that provide health care for large populations. Their main goal is to attempt to control costs through providing appropriate care, negotiating for lowest price on services, and restricting access to more expensive services such as operative procedures. (See page 49: Managed Care and New Practice Arrangements.)

3. B. There are two primary types of malpractice insurance: occurrence and claims-made. Occurrence insurance covers claims while the insurance was in effect (i.e., if the policy was in effect during 1990 to 1995, a claim made during 1993 would be covered, but a claim made in 1989 would not). Claims-made policies only cover claims filed while the insurance is in effect (i.e., policyholders will be covered for malpractice while they are paying for the insurance regardless of the date of injury). With termination of a claims-made policy, no coverage will then exist. Claims-made policies are favored by insurance companies because they limit exposure to claims filed during the period in which the insured is actually paying for the insurance. When the insured stops coverage, the individual must purchase tail coverage to cover any malpractice claims made following cancellation of the policy. A benefit of claims-made policies is that, during the first year, the cost of insurance is the lowest. The cost increases for the next 5 years and then plateaus. (See page 40: Malpractice Insurance.)

4. A. Standards of care, practice guidelines, and parameters have been increasingly used over the past couple of decades. The impetus for their increased use centers primarily on the improvement of quality of care for patients. American Society of Anesthesiologists (ASA) Monitoring Standards of Care is an excellent example of standard of care guidelines. The ASA Difficult Airway Algorithm is an outstanding example of practice guidelines. These guidelines, if followed, typically improve patient outcome and cost-effectiveness by reducing unnecessary tests and ineffective treatments. Because these standards usually are developed by experts in the field, they constitute a powerful legal defense in light of a malpractice suit. Practicing outside the standards of the specialty would require one to justify one's actions and decisions. Standards of care, practice parameters, and practice guidelines are not legally mandated. (See page 31: Establishing Standards of Practice and Understanding Standard of Care.)

5. B. Following the identification of a critical event, help should be called to minimize the sequelae of the event. Should permanent injury occur, early involvement of the anesthesia department, hospital administration, risk management department, and insurance company is essential. Charting of the event is critical. Only facts should be included in the chart. No speculation regarding the cause or who is to blame should be recorded. Any change to the chart's original documentation should be recorded as an amendment and labeled as such, with an indication regarding why such an amendment was necessary. (See page 40: Malpractice Insurance.)

6. E. Computer scheduling programs are powerful tools in operating room management. By inputting historical times for procedures, the program can prevent optimistic bookings by surgeons and can prevent operating room time from running long and thus requiring payment of overtime. Inputting this type of data can allow the program to generate reports and statistics that will aid in future planning. The program can examine the schedule and determine whether any staff or equipment double booking has occurred, which may not be obvious on a standard ledger schedule. Computer programs require a large commitment to training and data entry. Computerization can eliminate personal bias in the scheduling of case time. (See page 56: Computerization.)

7. A. HIPAA requires that attention is focused on protected health information. Each practice group must designate and appoint a "privacy officer." HIPAA provisions require that patient charts must be locked

away overnight. Telephone calls and faxes must be handled specially if they contain identifiable patient information. (See page 51: HIPAA.)

8. **D.**   The Sherman Antitrust Act is more than 100 years old. Antitrust laws do not involve the right of individuals to engage in business, but rather are solely concerned with the preservation of competition within a defined marketplace. The per se rule, which is rarely applied, makes conduct that obviously limits competition illegal. (See page 46: Antitrust Considerations.)

CHAPTER 3 ■ EXPERIMENTAL DESIGN AND STATISTICS

1. If a target population contains several strata of importance, the best method of obtaining a representative population sample is:

   A. limit sampling
   B. convenience sampling
   C. crossover sampling
   D. random sampling
   E. double blind

2. An example of a contemporaneous-parallel control would be:

   A. Each patient could receive the standard drug under identical experimental circumstances at another time.
   B. A group of patients could have been studied previously with the standard drug under similar circumstances.
   C. Another group of patients receiving the standard drug could be studied simultaneously.
   D. Literature reports show the effects of the drug under related but not necessarily identical circumstances.
   E. Each patient could receive the standard drug under nonexperimental conditions simultaneously with the test group.

3. The best method for random allocation of treatment groups is:

   A. based on the day of the week
   B. based on assignment of a previous patient
   C. using hospital chart numbers
   D. patient preference
   E. computer-generated random numbering

4. The most potent scientific tool for evaluating medical treatment is:

   A. a longitudinal, prospective study, of deliberate intervention, with historical controls
   B. a longitudinal, prospective study, of deliberate intervention, with concurrent controls
   C. a longitudinal, retrospective study, with concurrent case controls
   D. a longitudinal, retrospective study, with historical controls
   E. a cross-sectional, prospective study without controls

5. The error of failing to reject a false null hypothesis is called a:

   A. false-positive
   B. type II error
   C. alpha error
   D. zero-order error
   E. parameter

6. Variance is the:

   A. statistical average
   B. average deviation
   C. average squared deviation
   D. square root of the average deviation
   E. square of the standard error

7. The mean ± 3 standard deviations will encompass what percent of the sample population?

   A. 50
   B. 68
   C. 75
   D. 95
   E. 99

8. A study is performed looking at the difference in postoperative nausea in males and females undergoing laparoscopic cholecystectomy. The category male or female is an example of:

   A. ordinal data
   B. dichotomous data
   C. nominal data
   D. discrete interval data
   E. continuous interval data

For questions 9 to 12, choose A if 1, 2, and 3 are correct; B if 1 and 3; C if 2 and 4; D if 4; E if all.

9. The probability of a type II error increases with which of the following?

    1. Small alpha value
    2. Larger variability in populations being compared
    3. Small difference between experimental conditions
    4. Large sample size

10. Which of the following are summary statistics?

    1. Mean
    2. F ratio
    3. Mode
    4. *P* Value

11. Nonparametric statistics:

    1. are used whenever there are serious concerns about the shape of the data
    2. do not require any assumptions about probability distributions of the populations
    3. are less able than parametric tests to distinguish between the null and alternative hypotheses if the data are normally distributed
    4. are also called "order statistics"

12. Which of the following statements is/are TRUE?

    1. A confidence interval describes how likely it is that the population parameter is estimated by any particular sample statistic such as the mean.
    2. SE is used to describe the dispersion of the sample.
    3. Sample size planning is important because this is the main mechanism for increasing statistical power.
    4. Studies using historical controls will obtain the same results as studies with concurrent controls if appropriate strata are selected.

ANSWERS

---

1. **D.** A sample is a subset of the target population. The best hope for a representative sample of the population would be realized if every subject in the population had the same chance of being in the experiment; this is called random sampling. If there are several strata of importance, random sampling from each stratum would be appropriate. Convenience sampling is subject to the nuances of the surgical schedule, the goodwill of the referring physician and attending surgeon, and the willingness of the patient to cooperate. At best, the convenience sample is representative of patients at that institution, with no assurance that these patients are similar to those elsewhere. Convenience sampling is also the rule in studying new anesthetic drugs in volunteers; such studies typically are performed on "healthy, young students." (See page 64: Sampling.)

2. **C.** A researcher can obtain comparative data in several ways: (1) each patient could receive the standard drug under identical experimental circumstances at another time; (2) another group of patients receiving the standard drug could be studied simultaneously; (3) a group of patients could have been studied previously with the standard drug under similar circumstances; and (4) literature reports of the effects of the drug under related, but not necessarily identical, circumstances could be used. Under the first two possibilities, the control group is contemporaneous: either self-control (crossover) or a parallel control group. The second two possibilities are examples of the use of historical controls. (See page 64: Control Groups.)

3. **E.** The experimental groups should be as similar to each other as possible in reflecting the target population; if the groups are different, this introduces a bias into the experiment. Although randomly allocating subjects of a sample to one or another of the experimental groups requires additional work, this principle prevents selection bias by the researcher, minimizes (but cannot always prevent) the possibility that important differences exist among the experimental groups, and disarms the critics' complaints about research methods. Random allocation most commonly is accomplished by computer-generated random numbers. (See page 64: Random Allocation of Treatment Groups.)

4. **B.** The randomized, controlled clinical trial is the most potent scientific tool for evaluating medical treatment. Randomization into treatment groups is relied on to equally weight the subjects' baseline attributes that could predispose or protect the subjects from the outcome of interest. (See page 65: Types of Research Design.)

5. **B.** Because the statistics deal with probabilities and not certainties, there is a chance that the decision concerning the null hypothesis is erroneous. The error of wrongly rejecting the null hypothesis (false-positive) is called the type I or alpha error. The error of failing to reject a false null hypothesis (false-negative) is called a type II or beta error. A parameter is a number describing a variable of a population. (See page 66: Logic of Proof.)

6. **C.**   The concept of describing the spread of a set of numbers by calculating the average distance from each number to the center of the numbers applies to both a sample and a population; this average squared distance is called the variance. (See page 68: Spread or Variability.)

7. **E.**   Most biological observations appear to come from populations with normal or gaussian distributions. By accepting this assumption of a normal distribution, further meaning can be given to the sample summary statistics that have been calculated. This involves the use of the expression $\bar{x} \pm \kappa \times s$, where k = 1, 2, 3, etc. If the population from which the sample is taken is unimodal and roughly symmetric, then the bounds for 1, 2, and 3 encompasses roughly 68%, 95%, and 99% of the sample and population members. (See page 68: Spread or Variability.)

8. **B.**   Dichotomous data allow only two possible variables. Ordinal data have three or more categories that can be logically ranked or ordered. Discrete interval data can have only integer values (e.g., age in years), whereas continuous interval data can be decimal fractions (e.g., temperature of 37.1°C). A nominal variable can be placed into a category that has no logical ordering (e.g., eye color). (See page 67: Data Structure, and Table 3-4 Data Types.)

9. **A.**   The error of failing to reject a false null hypothesis (false-negative) is called a type II or beta error. The power of a test is 1-beta. The probability of a type II error depends on four factors. Unfortunately, the smaller the alpha, the greater the chance of a false-negative conclusion; this fact keeps the experimenter from automatically choosing a very small alpha. Second, the more variability there is in the populations being compared, the greater the chance of a type II error. This is analogous to listening to a noisy radio broadcast; the more static there is, the harder it will be to discriminate between words. Third, increasing the number of subjects will lower the probability of a type II error. The fourth and most important factor is the magnitude of the difference between the two experimental conditions. The probability of a type II error goes from very high, when only a small difference exists, to extremely low, when the two conditions produce large differences in population parameters. (See page 66: Logic of Proof.)

10. **B.**   Although the results of a particular experiment may be presented by repeatedly showing the entire set of numbers, there are concise ways of summarizing the information content of the set into a few numbers. These numbers are called sample or summary statistics. The three most common summary statistics are the mean, the median, and the mode. (See page 68: Central Location.)

11. **E.**   Statistical tests that do not require any assumptions about probability distributions of the populations are known as nonparametric tests; they can be used whenever there is very serious concern about the shape of the data. Nonparametric statistics are also the tests of choice for ordinal data. The basic concept behind nonparametric statistics is the ability to rank or order the observations; nonparametric tests are also called order statistics. The currently available nonparametric tests are not used more commonly because they do not adapt well to complex statistical models and because they are less able than parametric tests to distinguish between the null and alternative hypotheses if the data are, in fact, normally distributed. (See page 72: Robustness and Nonparametric Tests.)

12. **B.**   The four options for decreasing type II error (increasing statistical power) are to (1) raise alpha, (2) reduce population variability, (3) make the sample bigger, and (4) make the difference between the conditions greater. Under most circumstances, only the sample size can be varied; thus, sample size planning has become an important part of research design for controlled clinical trials. When describing the spread, scatter, or dispersion of the sample, one should use standard deviation; when describing the precision with which the population center is known, one should use the SE. A confidence interval describes how likely it is that the population parameter is estimated by any particular sample statistic such as the mean.

Historical controls usually show a favorable outcome for a new therapy, whereas studies with concurrent controls (i.e., parallel control group or self-control) less often reveal a benefit. If the outcome with an old treatment is not studied simultaneously with the outcome of a new treatment, one cannot know whether any differences in results are a consequence of the two treatments, or of unsuspected and unknowable differences between the patients, or of other changes over time in the general medical environment. (See page 66: Sample Size Calculations, and page 69: Confidence Intervals.)

CHAPTER 4 ■ OCCUPATIONAL HEALTH

1. Which of the following substances found in latex gloves is responsible for the majority of generalized allergic reactions?

   A. Preservatives
   B. Polyisoprenes
   C. Protein
   D. Talc
   E. Lipids

2. Which of the following statements concerning tuberculosis (TB) is FALSE?

   A. It is transmitted by bacilli carried on airborne particles.
   B. Using any facemask will prevent infection.
   C. Patients with HIV are at increased risk of infection.
   D. Examining sputum for bacilli is an accurate means of testing.
   E. Elective surgery should be postponed for infected patients.

3. Airborne precautions would be an effective preventative measure against which of the following infectious agents?

   A. Cytomegalovirus (CMV)
   B. Tuberculosis (TB)
   C. Herpes simplex
   D. Herpetic whitlow
   E. All of the above

4. Signs of substance abuse inside the hospital include:

   A. signing out large quantities of narcotics
   B. refusing breaks
   C. volunteering to relieve others and taking extra calls
   D. disappearing between cases
   E. all of the above

For questions 5 to 14, choose A if 1, 2, and 3 are correct; B if 1 and 3; C if 2 and 4; D if 4; E if all.

5. Which of the following statements are TRUE regarding studies of anesthetic trends in the operating room and effects on fertility and childbearing?

   1. Scavenging anesthetic lowers levels in operating rooms.
   2. It is difficult to quantify the levels of anesthetic in an operating room.
   3. There is a slight increase in the relative risk of congenital anomalies in the children of female physicians who work in the operating room.
   4. Levels of anesthetic exposure are correlated with reproductive outcome.

6. Which of the following statements about methylmethacrylate is/are TRUE?

   1. Methylmethacrylate causes cardiovascular effects but no respiratory effects.
   2. The Occupational Safety and Health Administration (OSHA) has established an 8-hour, time-weighted allowable exposure of 100 ppm of methylmethacrylate.
   3. Below OSHA's established limits for methylmethacrylate, cutaneous and genitourinary problems are not seen.
   4. Scavenging devices for venting methylmethacrylate vapor, when used properly, decrease the peak environmental concentration of vapor by 75%.

7. Which of the following statements regarding latex allergy is/are TRUE?

   1. The prevalence in anesthesia personnel is about 13%.
   2. Sensitivity to latex can be reversed by avoiding latex-containing compounds.

3. Contact dermatitis accounts for approximately 80% of allergic reactions.
4. Type IV reaction (T-cell mediated) is the more severe allergic reaction seen with latex allergy.

8. Which of the following statements concerning influenza viruses is/are TRUE?

1. They are spread by coughing, sneezing, or talking via small particle aerosols.
2. Vaccination with inactivated virus confers immunity for life.
3. General anesthesia results in no increase of respiratory morbidity in asymptomatic patients infected with influenza virus.
4. Influenza virus vaccine contains two viral strains: one type A and one type B.

9. Which of the following forms of hepatitis primarily is/are transmitted by blood?

1. B
2. D
3. C
4. E

10. Which of the following form(s) of hepatitis can lead to a chronic carrier state?

1. C
2. D
3. B
4. A

11. Which of the following statements is/are TRUE?

1. Respiratory syncytial virus (RSV) can be recovered for up to 6 hours on contaminated environmental surfaces.
2. Severe acute respiratory syndrome (SARS) is spread by close person-to-person contact.

3. Transmission of CMV occurs through person-to-person contact and contact with contaminated urine or blood.
4. Rubella infection can be associated with congenital malformations and fetal death if it is contracted during the first trimester of pregnancy.

12. Which of the following statements concerning hepatitis B is/are TRUE?

1. Contaminated dry blood on an environmental surface may be infectious for more than 1 week.
2. Routine vaccination has reduced the risk of occupationally acquired hepatitis B virus (HBV) infection.
3. The presence of hepatitis B surface antigen in serum is indicative of active viral replication in hepatocytes.
4. The rate of transmission is significantly less after mucosal contact with infected oral secretions than after percutaneous blood exposure.

13. Human immunodeficiency virus (HIV) spread has been implicated in transmission by which of the following routes?

1. Sexual contact
2. Blood
3. Perinatal transmission
4. Saliva and tears

14. Which of the following statements is/are TRUE?

1. The magnitude of radiation absorbed is a function of total exposure intensity, distance from the source of radiation, and the use of radiation shielding.
2. Radiation exposure is proportional to the square of the distance from the source.
3. Radiation exposure becomes minimal at a distance greater than 36 inches from the source.
4. Wearing a thyroid collar in addition to a lead apron protects most vulnerable sites.

ANSWERS

1. **C.** Latex is a complex substance containing polyisoprenes, lipids, phospholipids, and proteins. Numerous additional substances, including preservatives, accelerators, antioxidants, vulcanizing compounds, and lubricating agents, are added to latex gloves. The protein content is responsible for causing the majority of allergic reactions. (See page 80: Physical Hazards-Latex.)

2. **B.** A special mask that is fitted to the person wearing it, and that is capable of filtering particles 1 to 5 mm in diameter, is required to protect a health

care worker from a patient with active TB. (See page 84: Infection Hazards.)

3. **B.** Preventive measures for the listed infectious agents are as follows: CMV, standard precautions; TB, airborne precautions and isoniazid and/or ethambutol for purified protein derivative (PPD) conversion; herpes simplex, standard precautions and contact precautions if disseminated disease; influenza, vaccine, prophylactic antiretrovirals, and droplet precautions. (See page 85: Table 4-4, Prevention of Occupationally Acquired Infections.)

4. **E.**   Signing out large quantities of narcotics, refusing breaks, volunteering to relieve others, disappearing between cases, weight loss, pale skin, pinpoint pupils, and taking extra calls are all signs of substance abuse. Addicts also have unusual changes of behavior, have sloppy charts, and want to work alone in order to divert narcotics for personal use. They are difficult to find between cases. Their patients often complain of pain in the recovery room. (See page 93: Table 4-6, Signs of Substance Abuse and Dependence)

5. **B.**   The use of scavenging techniques lowers the environmental anesthetic levels in operating rooms. Review of existing epidemiologic studies suggest a slight increase in the relative risk of spontaneous abortion and congenital anomalies in the children of female physicians working in the operating room. Although it is easy to quantify the levels of anesthetic in an operating room, it is harder to assess the effects of other factors such as stress, fatigue, and alterations in work schedule. Levels of anesthetic exposure have not correlated with reproductive outcome. (See page 76: Physical Hazards.)

6. **C.**   When methylmethacrylate is prepared in the operating room to cement prostheses to bone, concentrations up to 280 ppm have been measured. Scavenging devices for venting the vapor can decrease peak concentrations by 75%. OSHA has established an 8-hour, time-weighted average allowable exposure of 100 ppm. Reported risks from occupational exposure include allergic reactions and asthma, dermatitis, eye irritation, headache, and neurologic signs. These may occur at levels below the OSHA cutoffs. (See page 80: Physical Hazards: Methyl Methacrylate.)

7. **B.**   Contact dermatitis accounts for 80% of allergic reactions from latex-containing gloves. True allergic reactions present as type IV (T-cell–mediated contact dermatitis) and the more severe type I (immunoglobulin E–mediated anaphylactic reaction). Sensitivity cannot be reversed. (See page 80: Physical Hazards: Latex Allergy.)

8. **B.**   Influenza viruses are easily transmitted by small particle aerosols (sneezing, coughing, or talking). General anesthesia results in no increase in respiratory morbidity in asymptomatic patients infected with influenza virus. Antigenic variation of influenza viruses occurs over time, so new viral strains (usually two type A and one type B) are selected for inclusion in each year's vaccine. Because the virus has antigenic variation from year to year, immunity is not for life. (See page 84: Infection Hazards.)

9. **A.**   Hepatitis A is primarily transmitted by the fecal-oral route. Hepatitis B, C, and D are transmitted by blood. Hepatitis E is enterically transmitted. (See page 84: Infection Hazards.)

10. **A.**   Hepatitis B, C, and D can progress to chronic hepatitis and a chronic carrier state. (See page 84: Infection Hazards.)

11. **E.**   RSV can be recovered for up to 6 hours on contaminated environmental surfaces. SARS is spread by close person-to-person contact, large respiratory droplets, and possibly airborne transmission. Transmission of CMV occurs through person-to-person contact and contact with contaminated urine or blood. Rubella infection can be associated with congenital malformations and fetal death if it is contracted during the first trimester of pregnancy. (See page 84: Infection Hazards.)

12. **E.**   HBV may be infectious for at least 1 week in dried blood on environmental surfaces. The rate of transmission is less after mucosal contact with infected oral secretions than after percutaneous blood exposure. Routine vaccinations, use of safety devices, and postexposure prophylaxis have significantly reduced the risk of occupationally acquired HBV infection. The presence of hepatitis B surface antigen in serum is indicative of active viral replication in hepatocytes and increases the risk of transmission. (See page 84: Infection Hazards.)

13. **A.**   HIV may be transmitted by sexual contact, exposure to contaminated blood, and perinatally. It can be found in saliva, tears, and urine, but these body fluids have not been implicated in viral transmission. (See page 84: Infection Hazards.)

14. **B.**   Radiation exposure is inversely proportional to the square of the distance from the source. Lead aprons and thyroid collars leave many vulnerable sites exposed, such as the long bones of the extremities, the cranium, the skin on the face, and the eyes. The magnitude of radiation absorbed by operating room personnel is a function of total exposure intensity, distance from the source of radiation, and the use of radiation shielding. Radiation exposure becomes minimal at a distance of greater than 36 inches from the source. (See page 81: Radation: Physical Hazards.)

CHAPTER 5 ■ PROFESSIONAL LIABILITY, QUALITY IMPROVEMENT, AND ANESTHETIC RISK

1. All the following statements are true EXCEPT:

   A. The duty that the anesthesiologist owes the patient is to be a prudent and reasonable physician.
   B. Obtaining informed consent is a responsibility that all physicians have to their patients.
   C. It is not the responsibility of the physician to disclose limitless risk to the patient in the discussion of informed consent.
   D. Causation refers to the fact that a reasonably close causal relation exists between the anesthesiologist's acts and the resultant injury.
   E. General damages are those actual damages that are a consequence of the injury, such as medical expenses.

2. The court establishes "standard of care" through all EXCEPT:

   A. factual witness
   B. expert witness
   C. published societal guidelines
   D. textbooks
   E. written hospital policies

3. Which of the following statements concerning risk management and quality improvement is TRUE?

   A. Quality improvement is broadly oriented toward reducing liability exposure of the organization.
   B. Quality improvement is concerned with patient safety, but risk management is not.
   C. Risk management's main goal is the maintenance and improvement of patient care.
   D. Risk management involves professional liability, contracts, employee safety, and public safety.
   E. Quality improvement concerns itself primarily with liability exposure of the institution.

4. All of the following statements concerning record keeping are true EXCEPT:

   A. Good records can form a strong defense in the face of malpractice litigation.
   B. Change of anesthetic personnel should be documented.
   C. The anesthesiologist's report of a catastrophic event need not be consistent with concurrent records because inconsistencies are easy to defend.
   D. A record-keeping error should be crossed out yet remain legible.
   E. Catastrophic events should be documented in narrative form in the patient's progress notes.

5. The National Practitioner Data Bank (NPDB) requires input from all of the following EXCEPT:

   A. medical malpractice payment
   B. licensing actions by medical boards
   C. peer review outcomes by departments
   D. clinical privilege actions by hospitals
   E. actions taken by the Drug Enforcement Agency

6. Considering continuous quality improvement (CQI), which statement is FALSE?

   A. The focus of CQI is not on blame but rather on identification of the causes of undesirable outcomes.
   B. CQI continually tries to identify random errors and prevent them from recurring.
   C. Peer review is critical to the CQI process.
   D. Once areas in need of improvement are identified by CQI programs, outcomes are measured and documented.
   E. Total quality management (TQM) is an extension of CQI that extends beyond patient care.

7. Which of the following is a TRUE flaw of the peer review process?

   A. It is performed by one individual, so personal bias is prevalent.
   B. It is outside the realm of CQI.
   C. There is a tendency to judge the quality of care based on the severity of outcome.

D. Only critical incidents resulting in bad outcomes are reviewed.

E. There is a high degree of agreement between anesthesiologists reviewing the case on whether the management was appropriate.

For questions 8 to 15, choose A if 1, 2, and 3 are correct; B if 1 and 3; C if 2 and 4; D if 4; E if all.

8. In order for a malpractice suit against a physician to succeed, the patient/plaintiff must prove:

    1. breach of duty
    2. damages
    3. causation
    4. duty

9. Considering the cause of lawsuits against anesthesiologists, which of the following statements is/are TRUE?

    1. The leading causes of death and brain damage injury are airway management problems.
    2. Ulnar nerve injury often occurs despite apparently adequate positioning.
    3. Anesthesia is a high-risk endeavor because of the use of complex equipment and potent drugs.
    4. The leading injury for suits against anesthesiologists is brain damage.

10. When the plaintiff's attorney files a complaint, the anesthetist should take certain actions, including which of the following?

    1. Review records, but do not alter.
    2. Cooperate fully with the attorney provided by the insurer.
    3. Make a detailed account of all events.
    4. Discuss the case with all involved operating room personnel.

11. If a physician is deposed by the plaintiff's attorney, the physician should do which of the following?

    1. Never attempt to change his or her image by dressing conservatively.
    2. Volunteer all information he or she has about the case.

3. Not spend too much time preparing so the responses do not seem to be rehearsed.
4. Feel free to qualify leading questions made during the deposition.

12. Concerning Jehovah's Witnesses and blood transfusions, which of the following statements is/are TRUE?

    1. Physicians are obligated to treat all patients who apply for treatment, even if they refuse to have a blood transfusion.
    2. Jehovah's Witnesses who are the sole support of children may *not* refuse blood products for themselves, because the interests of the state supersede the rights of the patients in this situation.
    3. If a Jehovah's Witness consents to a blood transfusion, the physician needs to obtain a court order before giving the transfusion.
    4. Some Jehovah's Witnesses will not accept an autotransfusion even if their blood remains in constant contact with their body via tubing.

13. When considering the NPDB, which of the following statements is/are TRUE?

    1. Once a report is submitted to the NPDB, the physician has 60 days to dispute the input.
    2. Creation of the NPDB has allowed physicians to settle nuisance suits because their names are not added to the database.
    3. A practitioner may query the NPDB about his or her file at any time.
    4. NPDB is a statewide information system.

14. Considering quality improvement programs, which of the following statements is/are TRUE?

    1. Peer review falls outside the domain of quality improvement.
    2. Quality improvement outcome studies are easily applied to the field of anesthesia because it has a high rate of catastrophic outcomes.
    3. Sentinel events are events with poor outcomes that are directly related to operator actions.
    4. Critical incidents are events that cause or have the potential to cause patient injury if they are not noticed and corrected in a timely manner.

ANSWERS

1. **E.** In most general terms, the duty that the anesthesiologist owes to the patient is to adhere to the "standard of care" for the treatment of the patient. Because it is virtually impossible to delineate specific standards for all aspects of medical practice, the courts have created the concept of the reasonable and prudent physician. One of the general duties of the

physician is obtaining informed consent for a procedure. The requirement that the consent be "informed" is somewhat more opaque. The patient must have received a fair and reasonable account of the proposed procedure and risks inherent to these procedures. The duty to disclose risk is not limitless. The definition of "causation" is that a reasonably close causal relation exists between the anesthesiologist's acts and the resultant injury. "Breach of duty" is defined as the the failure of the anesthesiologist to fulfill his or her duty. The court will try to find that the anesthesiologist either did something that should not have been done or failed to do something that should have been done by a prudent and reasonable physician. "General damages" are those such as pain and suffering that directly result from the injury. "Special damages" are those actual damages that are a consequence of the injury, such as medical expenses, loss of income, and funeral expenses. (See page 99: Professional Liability.)

2. **A.** In the most general terms, the duty that the anesthesiologist owes to the patient is to adhere to the "standard of care" for the treatment of the patient. Because medical practice usually includes issues beyond the comprehension of the lay jurors and judges, the court establishes a standard of care for a particular case by the testimony of "expert witnesses." These witnesses differ from factual witnesses mainly in that they are allowed to give opinions. When a physician is called to court as the defendant in a malpractice suit, he or she becomes a factual witness. The standard of care also may be determined from published societal guidelines, written policies of a hospital or department, or textbooks and monographs. (See page 100: Standard of Care.)

3. **D.** Risk management and quality improvement programs work hand in hand to minimize liability and to maximize quality of patient care. The two programs overlap their focus on patient safety. A hospital risk management program is broadly oriented toward reducing the liability exposure of the organization. This includes not only professional liability and therefore patient safety, but also contracts, employee safety, public safety, and any other liability exposure of the institution. Quality improvement programs have as their main goals the maintenance and improvement of the quality of patient care. (See page 102: Risk Management and Quality Improvement.)

4. **C.** Good records can form a strong defense if they are adequate, and inadequate records can be disastrous. The anesthetic record itself should be accurate, complete, and as neat as possible. In addition to the patient's vital signs recorded every 5 minutes, special attention should be paid to ensure that the American Society of Anesthesiologists classification, monitors utilized, fluid administered, and doses and times of drugs given are accurately charted. All respiratory variables that are monitored should be documented. It is important to note when a change of anesthesia personnel occurs during the conduct of a case. If a critical incident occurs during the conduct of an anesthetic regimen, the anesthesiologist should document in *narrative form* in the patient's progress notes what happened, which drugs were used, the time sequence, and who was present. A catastrophic intra-anesthetic event cannot be summarized adequately in a small amount of space on the usual anesthetic record. The report should be as consistent as possible with concurrent records such as those pertaining to the anesthetic, the operating room, the recovery room, and cardiac arrest. (See page 102: Risk Management.)

5. **C.** The NPDB is a nationwide information system that theoretically allows licensing boards and hospitals a means of detecting adverse information about physicians. The NPDB requires input from five sources: medical malpractice payments, licensing actions by medical boards, clinical privilege actions by hospitals and professional societies, actions by the Drug Enforcement Agency, and Medicare/Medicaid exclusions. There is no requirement for departments that have peer review studies to report their outcome data. (See page 103: National Practitioner Data Bank.)

6. **B.** CQI takes a system approach to identifying and improving quality. A CQI program may focus on undesirable outcomes as a way to identify opportunities for improvement in the structure and process of care. The focus is not on blame but rather on identification of the causes of undesirable outcomes. Peer review and input are critical to this process. Random errors are inherently difficult to prevent, and programs focused in this direction are misguided. System errors, however, should be controllable, and strategies to minimize them should be within reach. Once areas are identified for improvement, their current status is measured and documented. If a change is identified that should lead to improvement, it is implemented. An extension of the CQI method is TQM. A TQM program would extend beyond patient care to apply CQI methods to all aspects of patient care delivery system. (See page 104: Structure, Process and Outcome: The Building Blocks of Quality.)

7. **C.** Peer review is a part of quality improvement programs and refers to the review of cases by members of one's specialty. It provides the basis for analysis of trends and incidents and suggests hypotheses for their causes and changes in the system that could improve the structure, process, and outcome of care. Peer review is subject to biases that may not be recognized by participants. There is a tendency for anesthesiologists to judge care as less than appropriate when severe patient injury occurs. Only a moderate level of agreement exists among anesthesiologists' assessments of cases. Different anesthesiologists may not always agree on whether or not the care was appropriate. Incorporation of multiple anesthesiologists into the process of case review will compensate for this lack of agreement. Peer review is not to be reserved for critical incidences resulting in bad outcomes; any case that had a

potential for a bad outcome is appropriate for review. (See page 105: Peer Review.)

8. **E.** "Malpractice" is a lay term that refers to professional negligence pursued in the legal system of civil laws. A successful malpractice suit must prove four things: (1) duty: that the anesthesiologist owed the patient a duty; (2) breach of duty: that the anesthesiologist failed to fulfill his or her duty; (3) causation: that a reasonably close causal relationship exists between the anesthesiologist's acts and the resultant injury; and (4) damages: that actual damage resulted because of a breach in the standard of care. (See page 99: Tort System.)

9. **A.** The principal cause of lawsuits against anesthesiologists is patient injury. Leading injuries for which suits were filed were death (22%), nerve damage (21%), and brain damage (10%). The causes of death and brain damage were predominantly problems in airway management. In the past, ulnar nerve injury was the most common cause of nerve damage claims, and it often occurs despite apparently adequate positioning. In the 1990s, spinal cord injury led the list. Anesthesia is a high-risk endeavor for many reasons, including the fact that death and brain damage are high-cost injuries, and anesthesiologists use complex equipment (which can fail or be used incorrectly) and potent drugs (mistakes in dosage or labeling can have disastrous consequences). (See page 101: Causes of Suit.)

10. **A.** A lawsuit begins when the patient/plaintiff's attorney files a complaint. The anesthesiologist will need assistance in answering the complaint. Specific actions that should be taken at this point include the following: (1) do not discuss the case with anyone, including colleagues who may have been involved, operating personnel, or friends; (2) never alter any records; (3) gather all pertinent records, including a copy of the anesthetic record, billing statements, and any correspondence concerning the case; (4) make notes recording all events recalled about the case; (5) cooperate fully with the attorneys provided by the insurer. (See page 101: What To Do When Sued.)

11. **D.** After a complaint has been filed, the malpractice suit will move on to the discovery phase. A deposition is the second mechanism of discovery. The plaintiff's attorney will depose the anesthesiologist, and the anesthesiologist must be constantly aware that what is said during the deposition carries as much weight as what is said in court. It is important to be factually prepared for the deposition. Review of notes, anesthetic records, and medical records is necessary. The physician should dress conservatively and professionally. Information should never be volunteered. The physician may be asked leading questions that are not possible to answer without

qualification. In this case, the physician may qualify his or her answer but should avoid giving lengthy opinion answers. (See page 101: What To Do When Sued.)

12. **C.** The religious beliefs of Jehovah's Witnesses preclude them from receiving blood or blood products. Physicians are not obligated to treat all patients who apply for treatment. The physician has the right to refuse to care for a patient in an elective situation if the patient unacceptably limits the physician's ability to provide optimal care. The physician and patient together may decide to limit the physician's obligation to adhere to the patient's religious beliefs. Any agreement should be documented clearly in the medical record. It is true that some patients will not allow any blood that has left the body to be infused, but others will accept transfusion if the blood remains in constant contact with the body via tubing. There are two exceptions to a patient's rights to refuse blood transfusions: pregnant women and adults who are the sole supporters of minor children. The interests of the fetus surviving supersede the rights of the mother, and, in the case of an adult who is the sole support of minor children, the interests of the state in not being obligated to provide for the welfare of the dependent children may supersede the patient's right to refuse blood products. (See page 103: Jehovah's Witnesses and Other Treatment Obligations.)

13. **B.** The NPDB is a nationwide information system that theoretically allows licensing boards and hospitals a means of detecting adverse information about physicians. A practitioner may query the NPDB any time about his or her file. Once a report has been submitted, the physician is notified and has 60 days to dispute the input. The existence of the NPDB reporting requirements has made physicians reluctant to allow settlement of nuisance suits because it will cause their names to be added to the data bank. (See page 103: National Practitioner Data Bank.)

14. **D.** It is generally accepted that attention to quality will improve patient safety and satisfaction. Quality improvement programs are generally guided by requirements of the Joint Commission on Accreditation of Healthcare Organizations (JCAHO). However, adverse outcomes are relatively rare in anesthesia, thus making measurement of improvement difficult. To complement outcome measurements, anesthesia quality improvement programs can focus on critical incidents and sentinel events. Critical incidents are events that cause or have the potential to cause patient injury if they are not noticed and corrected in a timely manner. Sentinel events are single isolated events that may indicate a systematic problem. Peer review is an integral part of quality improvement programs. (See page 104: Difficulty of Outcome Measurement in Anesthesia.)

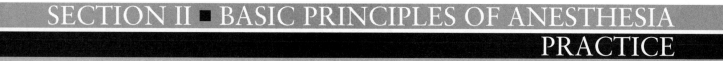

SECTION II ■ BASIC PRINCIPLES OF ANESTHESIA PRACTICE

CHAPTER 6 ■ CELLULAR AND MOLECULAR MECHANISMS OF ANESTHESIA

1. For volatile anesthetics, potency is proportional to:

   A. lipid solubility
   B. vapor pressure
   C. critical temperature
   D. minimum alveolar concentration (MAC)
   E. none of the above

2. The Meyer-Overton rule:

   A. correlates the potency of anesthetic gases with their solubility in oil
   B. suggests the anesthetic target site to be hydrophilic in nature
   C. is contradicted by the Unitary Theory of Anesthesia
   D. applies only to liquids
   E. applies only to gases

3. In humans, the definition of MAC is:

   A. the alveolar partial pressure of a gas at which 50% of humans will not mount a sympathetic response
   B. the alveolar partial pressure of a gas at which 50% of humans will not respond to a surgical incision
   C. the alveolar partial pressure of a gas at which 30% of humans will not respond to a surgical incision
   D. the alveolar partial pressure of a gas at which 50% of subjects remain unresponsive to verbal stimuli
   E. the alveolar partial pressure of a gas at which 50% of subjects will follow a simple command

For questions 4 to 6, choose A if 1, 2, and 3 are correct; B if 1 and 3; C if 2 and 4; D if 4; E if all.

4. General anesthesia results from interruption of nervous system activity at which of the following levels?

   1. Cerebral cortex
   2. Spinal cord
   3. Brainstem
   4. Peripheral sensory receptors

5. Which of the following statements is/are TRUE?

   1. Gamma-Aminobutyric acid (GABA) is an excitatory neurotransmitter.
   2. Volatile anesthetics modulate GABA receptor function.
   3. Benzodiazepines have no effect on GABA receptors.
   4. Barbiturates and etomidate act at GABA receptors.

6. General anesthetics have been shown to inhibit excitatory synaptic transmission in:

   1. sympathetic ganglia
   2. olfactory cortex
   3. hippocampus
   4. spinal cord

ANSWERS

1. **A.** Anesthetic potency is proportional to lipid solubility. (See page 121: What Is the Chemical Nature of Anesthetic Target Sites?)

2. **A.** The Meyer-Overton rule states that the potency of anesthetic gases is proportional to their lipid solubility. Because many different structurally unrelated anesthetics obey this rule, it has been speculated that all anesthetics act at the same molecular site. This concept is known as the Unitary Theory of Anesthesia. The Meyer-Overton rule applies only to gases and volatile liquids, because an oil/gas partition coefficient cannot

be determined for liquid anesthetics. (See page 121: What Is the Chemical Nature of Anesthetic Target Sites?)

3. B.   MAC is the alveolar partial pressure of a gas at which 50% of subjects will respond to a surgical incision. The use of end-tidal gas concentration provides an index of the "free" concentration of drug required to produce anesthesia. (See page 112: How Is Anesthesia Measured?)

4. A.   Anesthetics are able to produce effects on a variety of anatomic structures in the central nervous system, including the cerebral cortex, brainstem, and spinal cord. Anesthetics clearly alter cortical electrical activity, as evidenced by the consistent changes (increased latency, decreased amplitude) in surface electroencephalographic patterns recorded during anesthesia. A role for the brainstem in anesthetic action is supported by studies examining somatosensory evoked potentials. The actions of volatile anesthetics in the spinal cord are mediated, at least in part, by direct effects on the excitability of spinal motor neurons. This is supported by several electrophysiologic studies showing inhibition of excitatory synaptic transmission in the spinal cord. Animal studies have shown that volatile anesthetics have no significant effects on peripheral sensory receptors. (See page 113: Where in the Central Nervous System Do Anesthetics Work?)

5. C.   GABA receptors mediate the postsynaptic response to synaptically released GABA, an important inhibitory neurotransmitter. Barbiturates, benzodiazepines, propofol, etomidate, and volatile anesthetics all have been shown to modulate GABA receptor function. (See page 117: Anesthetic Effects on Ligand-Gated Ion Channels.)

6. E.   General anesthetics have been shown to inhibit excitatory synaptic transmission in sympathetic ganglia, and in the olfactory cortex, hippocampus, and spinal cord. (See page 114: How Do Anesthetics Interfere with the Electrophysiologic Function of the Nervous System?)

CHAPTER 7 ■ GENOMIC BASIS OF PERIOPERATIVE MEDICINE

1. The term used to refer to nearby single nucleoside polymorphisms on a chromosome that are inherited in blocks is:

   A. alleles
   B. haplotypes
   C. polymorphic mutations
   D. indels
   E. phenotype

2. One of the most common inherited prothrombotic risk factors is a point mutation in which factor?

   A. Factor II
   B. Factor V
   C. Factor VII
   D. Factor XI
   E. Factor XII

3. Following cardiac surgery, what is the incidence of significant neurologic morbidity (ranging from focal stroke to coma)?

   A. 0.6%
   B. 2%
   C. 6%
   D. 20%
   E. 40%

4. Malignant hyperthermia follows what pattern of inheritance?

   A. Autosomal dominant
   B. Autosomal recessive
   C. X-linked dominant
   D. X-linked recessive
   E. It is not an inherited disease.

5. In classical genetics, what is meant by "wild-type" individual?

   A. Individual with individual gene mutations
   B. Individual with traits controlled by multiple genes

   C. Individual with genes acutely affected by the environment
   D. Individual with nonmutant individual genes
   E. Your uncontrollable 3-year-old nephew

6. What is a "knockout" animal?

   A. Animals that misexpress an additional gene
   B. Animals that overexpress an additional gene
   C. A kangaroo with boxing gloves
   D. An animal with a nonfunctional gene
   E. An animal with a gene predisposing to sleep

7. Our understanding of pain has been increased by mice with knockout genes for:

   A. substance P
   B. opioid transmitters
   C. nerve growth factors
   D. all of the above
   E. none of the above

8. Numerous clinical trials attempting to block single inflammatory mediators in sepsis have been largely unsuccessful. Which of the following best explains the lack of success?

   A. Large tertiary care centers have a low incidence of septic shock.
   B. There is a lack of clinical investigators having an interest in septic shock.
   C. Septic shock is unimportant as a disease syndrome.
   D. Cascades of biological pathways that interact in complex and redundant ways are triggered by stressful stimuli.
   E. Sepsis has a negligible worldwide economic impact and thus receives a small percentage of funds for investigation.

ANSWERS

1. **B.** Haplotypes are inherited in blocks, and an analysis of these can be useful in discovering diseased genes. An indel is an insertion or deletion of one or more nucleotides. (See page 134: Genetic Basis of Disease.)

2. **B.** A point mutation in coagulation factor V results in resistance to activated protein C and is commonly known as factor V Leiden. This factor has been associated with thromboses in the postoperative setting. (See page 137: Genomics and Perioperative Risk Profiling.)

3. **C.** The incidence of significant neurologic morbidity postcardiac surgery is approximately 6%. More subtle deficits occur in up to 69% of patients. This variability in neurologic deficit is poorly explained by risk factors related to the procedure. The role of apolipoprotein E genotypes in relation to modulating the inflammatory response, extent of aortic atheroma, and cerebral blood flow and autoregulation may explain observed associations with poor neurologic outcomes. (See page 137: Genetic Susceptibility and Adverse Perioperative Neurologic Outcomes.)

4. **A.** Malignant hyperthermia is a rare autosomal dominant genetic disease of skeletal muscle calcium metabolism. Susceptibility to malignant hyperthermia has been linked to the ryanodine receptor gene locus on chromosome 19. (See page 139: Pharmacogenomics and Anesthesia.)

5. **D.** In classical genetics, single gene traits were identified and studied. Phenotypic differences attributed by individual genes were observed, and the genes were isolated. The nonmutant or original phenotype expressed by a single gene was termed "wild-type" and was compared with the new phenotypes or "mutants." (See page 140: Genetic Variability and Response to Anesthetic Agents.)

6. **D.** "Knockout" animals are created by inserting a vector with a disrupted gene into an animal. Typically, a mouse is used. The goal is to achieve two nonfunctioning alleles so a gene is not expressed. This is done to study specific functions of specific genes. Animals that misexpress or overexpress a gene are termed "transgenic." (See page 140: Genetic Variability and Response to Anesthetic Agents.)

7. **D.** Multiple genes appear to mediate sensitivity to noxious stimuli and chronically painful exposure. Various knockout mice missing functional genes for neurotrophins, nerve growth factors, substance P, opioid transmitters, and nonopioid transmitters, and their receptors have significantly contributed to our knowledge of pain processing. (See page 142: Genetic Variability and Response to Pain.)

8. **D.** At the cell level, various cascades and pathways are triggered when an organism is stressed. These pathways are often times interrelated and work to both increase and suppress gene expression. Because negative and positive feedback occurs in a complex manner, attempts to study how the expression of a single gene (products such as tumor necrosis factor alpha) have been difficult. (See page 143: Genomics and Critical Care.)

CHAPTER 8 ■ ELECTRICAL AND FIRE SAFETY

*For questions 1 to 8, choose A if 1, 2, and 3 are correct;
B if 1 and 3; C if 2 and 4; D if 4; E if all.*

1. Electrical contact can produce which of the following
types of injuries?

   1. Disruption of normal electrical function of the cells
   2. Respiratory paralysis
   3. Muscle contraction
   4. Cardiac arrhythmias

2. Injury from macroshock is affected by which of the
following?

   1. Skin resistance
   2. Duration of contact with the electrical source
   3. Current density
   4. Capacitance

3. Which of the following statements regarding grounded
electrical systems is/are TRUE?

   1. The hot wire (black) carries a voltage of 120 V
above ground.
   2. A ground wire (green or bare) is necessary to
complete a circuit.
   3. The white wire is neutral.
   4. The circuit breaker prevents macroshock by
preventing current flow.

4. An ungrounded electrical system has which of the
following properties?

   1. It makes obsolete the use of a ground wire.
   2. The 120-V potential exists only between the two
wires in the system.
   3. It eliminates the potential for microshock.
   4. It requires the presence of an isolation transformer.

5. Which of the following statements regarding the line
isolation monitor (LIM) is/are TRUE?

   1. The LIM measures the impedance of current flow to
ground that exists in the system.

2. The LIM is set to alarm at 2 to 5 mA.
3. The LIM is necessary to identify faulty
equipment, which, despite a contact to ground,
will function normally in an ungrounded
system.
4. The value on the LIM display indicates that current
is actively flowing to ground.

6. Which of the following statements regarding fires in the
operating room is/are TRUE?

   1. Fires in the operating room present much less
danger compared with 100 years ago, when patients
were anesthetized with flammable anesthetic
agents.
   2. A combination of 50% oxygen and 50% nitrous
oxide would support combustion as well as 100%
oxygen.
   3. An ignition source and an oxidizer are enough to
start a fire.
   4. Paper drapes are much easier to ignite and can
burn with greater intensity compared with cloth
drapes.

7. Regarding fires in the operating room, which of the
following is/are TRUE?

   1. Major ignition sources for operating room fires are
the electrosurgical unit and the laser.
   2. The ends of some fiber-optic light cords can become
hot enough to start a fire.
   3. Fires on a patient occur most often during surgery
in and around the head and neck where the patient
is receiving monitored anesthesia care.
   4. Fires in or on the patient represent an unlikely
although possible type of operating room fire.

8. Regarding the response to an operating room fire,
which is/are TRUE?

   1. The operating room sprinkler systems effectively
respond to the majority of fires.

2. If an endotracheal tube is on fire, it should be removed immediately and then extinguished.
3. If the paper drapes are burning, water or saline will likely douse the fire effectively.

4. Common acronyms for responding to a fire include "RACE" and "PASS."

ANSWERS

1. **E.** Electrical contact can result in flow of current through an individual. First, the electrical current can disrupt the normal electrical function of cells. Depending on magnitude, it can cause muscle contraction, changes in brain function, respiratory paralysis, and disruption of normal heart function leading to ventricular fibrillation. Depending on the path taken, the flow of current through tissue will produce heat if the resistance to flow is high. (See page 151: Source of Shocks.)

2. **A.** Injury from electricity is influenced by skin resistance, duration of contact with the electrical source, and current density. High skin resistance decreases the transfer of electricity and thus is protective. Contact time results in more current flow and thus more energy transferred, which will produce more tissue damage in high-resistance tissues. Furthermore, prolonging the exposure to current flow increases the risk of inducing ventricular fibrillation during a vulnerable period of the cardiac cycle. Current density describes the surface area onto which the current is transferred. The quantity of injury is inversely related to the surface area and is directly related to the quantity of current transferred through that surface area. This is the reason that small voltages applied to a small surface area of a vulnerable tissue result in injury (i.e., ventricular fibrillation with current down a central line). Capacitance refers to the storage of current in two conductive materials separated by an insulatory layer. It does not play a role in the magnitude of injury, although capacitance can store current, which can result in injury even when an item is unplugged. (See page 150: Capacitance and page 151: Source of Shocks.)

3. **B.** In a normal grounded circuit, the power company delivers a hot wire with a voltage above ground. Within a house, it will be carried by a black wire. The power company also supplies a neutral wire for the current to return to the earth. This is usually a white wire. These two wires are all that are needed to produce the path for the current to flow through a resistance and perform work. A circuit breaker between the hot supply and the receptacle prevents current flow in excess of the wire's capabilities. Exceeding the wire's capabilities will result in heat production and a possible fire hazard. Circuit breakers do not prevent macroshock. The ground wire, which is bare or green, acts as a safety feature to prevent shock in the event that the object containing

the electricity comes in contact with the hot wire. In these malfunctioning devices, the casing of the object becomes hot and carries the same potential as the hot wire. Should someone come into contact with the case (and if he or she is grounded), the individual will provide a path for current to flow and be electrocuted. The ground wire acts as a low-resistance pathway for electrical potentials within the case and thus reduces the flow in the individual. A ground wire is a safety feature but is not necessary to complete a circuit. (See page 153: Electrical Power Grounded.)

4. **C.** An ungrounded power supply uses an isolation transformer to separate itself from the power company. The isolation transformer creates a power gradient of 120 V between the two wires within the system but no gradient between any of the two wires and ground. Thus, individuals can contact either wire of an ungrounded system and not complete a circuit. An individual who contacts both wires within the isolated system will complete a circuit and be electrocuted. Isolation transformer systems thus significantly reduce the risk of macroshock in the operating room environment, but they do not reduce the risk of microshock. The use of a ground wire within an isolation transformer system is still used because it constitutes an additional, alternative safety system. The ground wire is attached to the device's case to provide a low-resistance pathway should the case of the device become electrically hot. (See page 157: Electrical Power Ungrounded.)

5. **A.** The LIM is a device that monitors the integrity of the isolation of the ungrounded electrical system. Such monitoring is essential in that a first fault to ground in an isolated system will result in normal function of an electrical device (but will alert that the isolation of the power has been breached). The typical cause of loss of isolation is that the case and the ground wire have become connected. Because the ground is not in the path of the isolated power, no short circuit exists, and the equipment is safe to use and will continue to function. However, should an individual come into contact with the other limb of the isolated circuit, he or she would then be in contact with both sides of the isolated power (through the ground and the ground wire) and will thus receive a shock. The LIM monitors the impedance to ground of each side of the isolated power. The value measured on the LIM does not mean that current is actually flowing; rather, it indicates how

much current would flow in the event of a fault. Normally, the LIM is set to alarm at 2 to 5 mA. In a perfect system, the impedance to ground is infinite, but because alternating current creates capacitance (and this can leak to ground even with perfect isolation), a buffer of acceptable leak is permitted to prevent alarming secondary to capacitance leakage. (See page 159: The Line Isolation Monitor.)

6. **C.** Fires in the operating room are just as much a danger today as they were 100 years ago, when patients were anesthetized with flammable anesthetic agents. Today, the risk of an operating room fire is probably as great as or greater than the days when ether and cyclopropane were used. This is because of the routine use of potential sources of ignition in an environment rich in flammable materials. For a fire to start, three elements are necessary. The first part of the triad is a heat or ignition source, the second part is fuel, and the third part is an oxidizer. The main oxidizers in the operating room are air, oxygen, and nitrous oxide. Oxygen and nitrous oxide function equally well as oxidizers, so a combination of 50% oxygen and 50% nitrous oxide would support combustion as well as 100% oxygen. Fuel for a fire can be found everywhere in the operating room. Paper drapes have largely replaced cloth drapes, and these are much easier to ignite and can burn with greater intensity. Other sources of fuel include gauze dressings, endotracheal tubes, gel mattress pads, and even facial or body hair. (See page 169: Fire Safety.)

7. **A.** Major ignition sources for operating room fires are the electrosurgical unit and the laser. However, the ends of some fiber-optic light cords can also become hot enough to start a fire if they are placed on paper drapes. Operating room fires can be divided into two different types. The more common type of fire occurs in or on the patient. These include endotracheal tube fires, fires during laparoscopy or bronchoscopy, or a fire in the oropharynx, which may occur during a tonsillectomy.

The other type of operating room fire is one that is remote from the patient. This includes an electrical fire in a piece of equipment. Fires on the patient seem to have become the most frequent type of operating room fire. These cases most often occur during surgery in and around the head and neck where the patient is receiving monitored anesthesia care and supplemental oxygen is being administered by either a facemask or a nasal cannula. (See page 169: Fire Safety.)

8. **D.** If a fire does occur, it is important to extinguish it as soon as possible. This is best accomplished by removing the oxidizer from the fire. Therefore, if an endotracheal tube is on fire, disconnecting the anesthetic circuit from the tube or disconnecting the inspiratory limb of the circuit will usually put the fire out immediately. It is not recommended to remove a burning endotracheal tube because this may cause even greater harm to the patient. Once the fire is extinguished, the endotracheal tube can be safely removed, the airway inspected via bronchoscopy, and the patient's trachea reintubated. If the drapes are burning, particularly if they are paper drapes, they must be removed and placed on the floor. Paper drapes are impervious to water, so throwing water or saline on them will do little to extinguish the fire. Once the burning drapes are removed from the patient, the fire can then be extinguished with a fire extinguisher. In most operating room fires, the sprinkler system is not activated. This is because sprinklers are usually not located directly over the operating room table, and operating room fires seldom are hot enough to activate the sprinklers. To use a fire extinguisher effectively, the acronym "PASS" can be helpful. This stands for Pull the pin to activate the fire extinguisher, Aim at the base of the fire, Squeeze the trigger, and Sweep the extinguisher back and forth across the base of the fire. When responding to a fire, the acronym RACE is useful. This stands for Rescue, Alarm, Confine, Extinguish. (See page 169: Fire Safety.)

CHAPTER 9 ■ ACID-BASE, FLUIDS, AND ELECTROLYTES

For questions 1 to 22, choose the best answer.

1. A previously healthy patient acutely develops metabolic alkalosis resulting from intravenous diuretic administration. The measured [HCO_3] is 36 mEq/L. An arterial blood gas analysis would show:

   A. pH 7.51, $Paco_2$ 47, Po_2 90
   B. pH 7.42, $Paco_2$ 52, Po_2 90
   C. pH 7.51, $Paco_2$ 47, Po_2 110
   D. pH 7.61, $Paco_2$ 52, Po_2 90
   E. pH 7.51, $Paco_2$ 40, Po_2 100

2. Metabolic acidosis with a normal anion gap may be caused by:

   A. aspirin toxicity
   B. diabetic ketoacidosis
   C. chronic diarrhea
   D. uremia
   E. lactic acidosis

3. The best interpretation of this arterial blood gas (pH 7.35, $Paco_2$ 60, Po_2 80, HCO_3 32) is:

   A. acute respiratory acidosis
   B. chronic respiratory acidosis with metabolic compensation
   C. chronic respiratory acidosis without metabolic compensation
   D. chronic metabolic alkalosis with respiratory compensation
   E. acute metabolic alkalosis

4. The best interpretation of this arterial blood gas analysis (pH 7.24, $Paco_2$ 60, Po_2 80, HCO_3 26) is:

   A. acute respiratory acidosis
   B. chronic respiratory acidosis with appropriate metabolic compensation
   C. chronic respiratory acidosis with inappropriate metabolic compensation

   D. chronic metabolic alkalosis with respiratory compensation
   E. acute metabolic alkalosis

5. The best interpretation of this arterial blood gas (pH 7.50, $Paco_2$ 30, Po_2 110, HCO_3 22) is:

   A. acute respiratory alkalosis
   B. chronic respiratory alkalosis with metabolic compensation
   C. acute metabolic acidosis with respiratory compensation
   D. chronic metabolic alkalosis with respiratory compensation
   E. chronic metabolic acidosis

6. Total body water is approximately ___ % of total body weight.

   A. 10
   B. 20
   C. 40
   D. 60
   E. 80

7. Intracellular volume (ICV) is ___ % of total body weight.

   A. 10
   B. 20
   C. 40
   D. 60
   E. 80

8. Plasma volume is approximately ___ % of the extracellular volume (ECV).

   A. 10
   B. 20
   C. 30
   D. 40
   E. 50

9. The extracellular concentrations of sodium (Na) is approximately ___ mEq/L

A. 150
B. 130
C. 140
D. 120
E. 110

10. The intracellular concentration of potassium (K) is approximately ___ mEq/L

A. 110
B. 130
C. 150
D. 4
E. 10

11. An acute blood loss of 2,000 mL represents ___ % of the predicted blood volume in a previously healthy 70-kg man.

A. 10
B. 20
C. 30
D. 40
E. 50

12. To achieve more than transient 2,000 mL restoration of plasma volume would require infusion of ___ mL of D5W solution.

A. 2,000
B. 4,500
C. 7,000
D. 14,000
E. 28,000

13. To achieve more than transient 2-L restoration of plasma volume using lactated Ringer's solution would require infusion of approximately ___ L.

A. 10
B. 15
C. 30
D. 45
E. 50

14. To achieve more than transient 2-L restoration of plasma volume using 5% albumin would require infusion of ___ L.

A. 1
B. 2
C. 5
D. 7
E. 10

15. To achieve more than transient 2-L restoration of plasma volume using 6% hetastarch would require infusion of ___ L.

A. 1
B. 2
C. 5

D. 7
E. 10

16. Chronic gastric losses tend to cause:

A. hypochloremic alkalosis
B. hyperchloremic alkalosis
C. hypochloremic acidosis
D. hyperchloremic acidosis
E. alkalosis with a normal chloride value

17. Chronic diarrhea tends to produce:

A. hypochloremic acidosis
B. hyperchloremic alkalosis
C. hyperchloremic acidosis
D. hyperchloremic alkalosis
E. alkalosis with a normal chloride value

18. What is the osmolality (mOsm/kg) of plasma that contains 140 mEq/L of Na, 90 mg/dL of glucose, and a blood urea nitrogen (BUN) of 11.5 mg/dL?

A. 280
B. 290
C. 300
D. 310
E. 320

19. Which of the following formulas accurately expresses Starling law of capillary filtration?

A. $Q = kA[(Pc - Pi) + k(\pi_i - \pi_c)]$
B. $Q = kA[(Pc - Pi) - k(\pi_i - \pi_c)]$
C. $Q = kA[(Pc - Pi) - \sigma(\pi_i - \pi_c)]$
D. $Q = kA[(Pc - Pi) + \sigma(\pi_i - \pi_c)]$
E. $Q = kA[(Pc - Pi) + (\pi_i - \pi_c)]$

20. Which of the following is NOT a typical finding during hypovolemia?

A. BUN >20 mg/dL
B. BUN/serum creatinine >20
C. Urinary Na 20 < mEq/L
D. Urinary osmolality >400 mOsm/kg
E. Serum/urine creatine ratio >1:40

21. What is the typical daily fluid requirement for a 30-kg child?

A. 300
B. 3,000
C. 1,100
D. 1,400
E. 1,700

22. Which of the following statements concerning Na regulation is FALSE?

A. Aldosterone promotes reabsorption of Na in the kidney.
B. Aldosterone promotes exchange of Na for K and hydrogen.
C. Stretching of the atria promotes release of atrial natriuretic peptide.

D. Antidiuretic hormone (ADH) affects serum Na concentration.

E. Excess ADH results in increased free water excretion.

For questions 23 to 41, choose A if 1, 2, and 3 are correct; B if 1 and 3; C if 2 and 4; D if 4; E if all.

23. Physiologic consequences of metabolic alkalosis include:

    1. rightward shift of the oxyhemoglobin dissociation curve
    2. hyperkalemia
    3. hypercalcemia
    4. hypercarbia

24. TRUE statements concerning the treatment of metabolic acidosis with HCO_3 include:

    1. It improves cardiovascular response to catecholamines.
    2. It is clearly effective in improving outcome.
    3. The appropriate dose is $0.7 \times$ (body weight in kg) $(24 - [HCO_3])$.
    4. It reduces plasma ionized calcium.

25. Respiratory alkalosis and metabolic alkalosis both:

    1. produce hypokalemia
    2. decrease cerebral blood flow
    3. potentiate digoxin toxicity
    4. may be appropriately treated with HCl

26. Renal adaptation to hypovolemia and decreased cardiac output includes:

    1. decreased renal vascular resistance
    2. redistribution of blood flow from outer cortical to inner cortical nephrons
    3. increased reabsorption of water and Na resulting from increased atrial natriuretic hormone
    4. increased reabsorption of water from medullary collecting ducts

27. TRUE statements concerning fluid resuscitation and the brain include:

    1. The cerebral capillary membrane is highly impermeable to protein.
    2. Hyperglycemia may aggravate ischemic brain injuries.
    3. Normal saline is superior to lactated Ringer's solution in the context of brain injury.
    4. Cerebral edema is an early sign of reduced plasma protein.

28. Which of the following statements concerning abnormal Na^+ concentrations is/are TRUE?

    1. A decrease in plasma Na^+ leads to a decrease in intracellular brain water.
    2. Hyponatremia may result from inappropriate ADH secretion.

    3. Mannitol may result in hypernatremia in the presence of a high serum osmolality.
    4. Absorption of irrigant solution during transurethral resection of the prostate may result in hyponatremia in the presence of a high serum osmolality.

29. TRUE statements concerning hypermagnesemia include:

    1. The therapeutic range for treatment of pre-eclampsia is between 15 and 18 mg/dL.
    2. Heart block commonly is noted at 18 mg/dL.
    3. Hypotension is not noted until concentrations are 13 mg/dL.
    4. Areflexia often is noted by 12 mg/dL.

30. Which of the following statements concerning diabetes insipidus is/are TRUE?

    1. It is more common after pituitary surgery.
    2. Central diabetes insipidus is exacerbated by desmopressin.
    3. In nephrogenic diabetes insipidus, the collecting ducts are resistant to ADH.
    4. It often results in hyponatremia.

31. Which of the following statements concerning regulation of serum K levels is/are TRUE?

    1. Aldosterone increases K excretion.
    2. K excretion is increased in the presence of nonreabsorbable anions in the renal luminal fluid.
    3. Insulin causes an intracellular shift of K.
    4. Epinephrine and exogenous beta$_2$-agonists cause an extracellular shift of K.

32. Which of the following statements concerning hypokalemia is/are TRUE?

    1. The ratio of intracellular to extracellular K remains relatively stable with chronic K loss.
    2. As a general rule, a decrease of 1.0 mEq/L represents a total body deficit of 200 to 300 mEq.
    3. Both metabolic and respiratory alkalosis lead to decreases in plasma K concentration.
    4. Hypothermia may cause acute hypokalemia.

33. Changes associated with hypokalemia include:

    1. hyperpolarization of cardiac cells
    2. ST segment depression
    3. re-entrant arrhythmias
    4. exacerbation of digitalis toxicity

34. Which of the following statements concerning hyperkalemia is/are TRUE?

    1. It may be treated with triamterene.
    2. It may result from mineralocorticoid deficiency.
    3. It may be treated with angiotensin-converting enzyme (ACE) inhibitors.
    4. Furosemide promotes kaliuresis.

35. Effects of hyperkalemia include:
    1. tall, peaked T waves
    2. shortened P-R interval
    3. widened QRS complex
    4. peaked P waves

36. Symptomatic hyperkalemia may be treated with:
    1. calcium chloride
    2. $NaHCO_3$
    3. regular insulin
    4. beta$_2$-agonists

37. TRUE statements about ionized calcium include:
    1. The ionized calcium concentration in the extracellular fluid is approximately 1.0 mM.
    2. Its concentration is increased by increased parathyroid hormone activity.
    3. Its concentration may be decreased by hyperphosphatemia.
    4. Its concentration is decreased by acidemia.

38. TRUE statements concerning hypocalcemia include:
    1. It may cause increased sensitivity to digitalis.
    2. It does not necessarily occur after transfussion, even if 20 units of blood are infused within 1 hour.
    3. It may cause Q-T shortening.
    4. It may cause laryngeal spasm.

39. TRUE statements about hypercalcemia include:
    1. Severe symptoms generally are noted when the total serum calcium concentration is >13 mg/dL
    2. Symptoms include lethargy, anorexia, nausea, and polyuria.
    3. Cardiovascular effects include hypertension, heart block, and cardiac arrest.
    4. The patient with hypercalcemia typically is helped by infusion of NaCl.

40. TRUE statements about altered phosphate concentrations include:
    1. High concentrations promote deposition of calcium in the bone, soft tissues, and kidneys.
    2. Hypophosphatemia leads to muscle weakness, which may lead to decreased ventilatory strength.
    3. The serum concentration of phosphate decreases in response to acute alkalemia.
    4. Rapid administration of phosphate to a patient with hypocalcemia may precipitate more severe hypocalcemia.

41. TRUE statements concerning hypomagnesemia include:
    1. Symptoms generally develop when the serum magnesium (Mg^{2+}) concentration is <1.0 mg/dL.
    2. It predisposes to digitalis toxicity.
    3. Rapid correction of hypermagnesemia may cause symptoms consistent with hypocalcemia.
    4. It predisposes to coronary artery spasm.

ANSWERS

1. **A.** This represents metabolic alkalosis with partial respiratory compensation. The rules of thumb for calculating the expected response to metabolic alkalosis are as follows: (1) Paco$_2$ increases approximately 0.5 to 0.6 mm Hg for each 1.0 mEq/L increase in [HCO$_3$]; and (2) the last two digits of the pH should equal the [HCO$_3$] + 15. Hypercarbia will be accompanied by a reduced Pao$_2$ as given by the alveolar gas equation. (See page 176: Metabolic Alkalosis.)

2. **C.** Metabolic acidosis may be characterized by a high anion gap or a normal anion gap. Metabolic acidosis with a high anion gap results from excess anions such as lactate, ketoacetate, sulfate, and salicylate. Metabolic acidosis with a normal anion gap is caused by loss of HCO$_3$ resulting from diarrhea, biliary drainage, or renal tubular acidosis. (See page 177: Metabolic Acidosis.)

3. **B.** The pH <7.40 suggests acidosis as the primary event, and the Paco$_2$ 46 shows it to be respiratory acidosis. The appropriate chronic metabolic compensation is that [HCO$_3$] will increase 4 mEq/L

for each 10 mm Hg increase in Paco$_2$, thus bringing the [HCO$_3$] to 32 mEq/L. The pH will return toward normal. (See page 179: Practical Approach to Acid-Base Interpretation.)

4. **A.** The pH 7.24 suggests acidosis as the primary event, and the Paco$_2$ 60 shows it to be respiratory acidosis. (See page 179: Practical Approach to Acid-Base Interpretation.)

5. **A.** The pH 7.50 suggests alkalosis as the primary event, and the Paco$_2$ 30 shows it to be respiratory alkalosis. (See page 179: Practical Approach to Acid-Base Interpretation.)

6. **D.** Total body water (in liters) is equal to approximately 60% of total body weight (in kilograms). ICV constitutes 40% of total body weight, and ECV constitutes 20% of body weight. (See page 181: Body Fluid Compartments.)

7. **C.** Total body water consists of ICV, which constitutes 40% of total body weight (28 L in a 70-kg person), and ECV, which constitutes 20% of body

weight (14 L). (See page 181: Body Fluid Compartments.)

8. **B.** Plasma volume, approximately 3 L, equals about one-fifth (20%) of the ECV. The remainder of the ECV is interstitial fluid. Red cell volume, approximately 2 L, is part of the ICV. Total blood volume is approximately 5 L (3 L of plasma + 2 L of red blood cell mass). (See page 181: Body Fluid Compartments.)

9. **C.** The extracellular fluid contains most of the Na in the body, with equal Na concentrations (~140 mEq/L) in the plasma and interstitium. (See page 181: Body Fluid Compartments.)

10. **C.** The predominant intracellular cation is K^+, with an intracellular concentration of approximately 150 mEq/L. (See page 181: Body Fluid Compartments.)

11. **D.** A 2,000-mL blood loss represents approximately 40% of the predicted 5-L blood volume in a previously healthy 70-kg patient. The normal blood volume is approximately 70 mL/kg; the normal plasma volume is three-fifths of this value, or approximately 3 L. (See page 181: Body Fluid Compartments.)

12. **E.** The volume that is to be infused to achieve a 2-L increase in plasma volume (PV) is equal to: (expected PV increment) (distribution volume of infusate)/(normal PV). The normal plasma volume is 3 L; the distribution volume for D5W is the total body water, which is 42 L (60% of 70 kg). Hence, the equation becomes: $(2 L)(42 L)/(3 L) = 28$ L. If one wanted to achieve a 2-L increase in overall intravascular volume, then, theoretically, 28 L of D5W would be required. (See page 181: Body Fluid Compartments.)

13. **A.** The distribution volume for lactated Ringer's solution is the extracellular fluid, which is 14 L (20% of 70 kg). Hence the equation for plasma expansion becomes: $(2 L)(14 L)/3 L = 9.3$ L. (See page 181: Distribution of Infused Fluids.)

14. **B.** The distribution volume of 5% albumin is approximately equal to that of the plasma. Hence, the replacement volume would be equal to the volume lost. (See page 181: Distribution of Infused Fluids.)

15. **B.** The distribution volume of 6% hetastarch is approximately equal to that of the plasma. Hence the replacement volume would be equal to the volume lost. (See page 181: Distribution of Infused Fluids.)

16. **A.** Chronic gastric losses tend to produce hypochloremic metabolic alkalosis; K also may be

lost. (See page 184: Surgical Fluid Requirements.)

17. **C.** Chronic diarrhea may produce hyperchloremic metabolic acidosis. (See page 184: Surgical Fluid Requirements.)

18. **B.** The osmotic activity of body fluids represents the number of osmotically active particles per kilogram of solvent. It is conventionally reported as osmolality (mmol/kg) and can be estimated as follows: Osmolality = $([Na^+] \times 2) + (Glucose/18) + (BUN/2.3)$, where $[Na^+]$ is expressed in mEq/L, serum glucose is expressed in mEq/dL, and BUN is expressed in mg/dL. Hence, plasma, which contains 140 mEq/L of Na^+, 90 mg/dL of glucose, and a BUN of 11.5 mg/L, has $280 + 5 + 5$ for a total of 290 mmol/kg. The $[Na^+]$ is doubled to account for "matching" anions (e.g., Cl). (See page 185: Colloids, Crystalloids, and Hypertonic Solutions.)

19. **D.** The filtration rate of fluid from the capillaries into the interstitial space is the net result of a combination of forces, including the gradient between intravascular and interstitial hydrostatic pressures and the gradient between interstitial and intravascular colloid oncotic pressures. The net filtration from capillary to interstitium may be expressed by the following equation: $Q = kA [(P_c - P_i) + \sigma(\pi_i - \pi_c)]$ where Q is fluid filtration, k is the capillary filtration coefficient (conductivity of water), A is the area of the capillary membrane, $P_c - P_i$ is the difference between capillary and interstitial hydrostatic pressures, $\pi_i - \pi_c$ is the difference between interstitial and capillary oncotic pressures. (See page 185: Colloids, Crystalloids, and Hypertonic Solutions.)

20. **E.** If the ratio of BUN to serum creatinine exceeds the normal range (10–20), one should suspect dehydration or one of the individual factors that alter the serum concentration of the two metabolites. In prerenal oliguria, enhanced Na reabsorption should reduce urinary Na <20 mEq/L, and enhanced water reabsorption should increase urinary concentration (i.e., urinary osmolality >400 mOsm/kg; urine/plasma creatinine ratio >40:1). (See page 187: Assessment of Hypovolemia and Tissue Hypoperfusion.)

21. **E.** Typical maintenance requirements may be calculated according to formulas for hourly or daily administration. For the first 10 kg of weight, administer 4 mL/kg per hour or 100 mL/kg per day. For the eleventh to twentieth kg, administer 2 mL/kg per hour (or 50 mL/kg per day). For each additional kilogram, administer 1 mL/kg per hour (or 20 mL/kg per day). Thus, for a 30-kg child, $1000 + 500 + 200 = 1,700$ mL. (See page 184: Fluid Replacement Therapy.)

22. **E.** Increased secretion of ADH results in reabsorption of water by the kidneys and subsequent

dilution of the plasma [Na^+]; inadequate ADH secretion results in renal free water excretion that, in the absence of adequate water intake, results in hypernatremia. Total body Na also is regulated by aldosterone, which is responsible for renal Na reabsorption in exchange for K and hydrogen. Alternatively, stretching of the cardiac atria causes secretion of atrial natriuretic peptide, which increases renal Na excretion. (See page 188: Sodium.)

23. **D.**   Metabolic alkalosis is associated with decreased serum K and ionized calcium. There is a compensatory respiratory acidosis leading to hypercarbia. The oxyhemoglobin curve is shifted to the left, thereby impairing oxygen delivery to tissues. Bronchial tone is increased and may lead to atelectasis. (See page 176: Metabolic Alkalosis.)

24. **D.**   Although many clinicians administer $NaHCO_3$ to patients with persistent lactic acidosis, there is little evidence that it is efficacious or improves outcome. $NaHCO_3$ does not improve cardiovascular response to catecholamines and reduces plasma ionized calcium. The initial dose of HCO_3 may be calculated as:

$$NaHCO_3(mEq/L) = \frac{Wt(kg) \times 0.3 \times (24 mEq/L - Actual\,HCO_3^-)}{2}$$

where 0.3 is the assumed distribution space of the HCO_3. (See page 177: Metabolic Acidosis.)

25. **B.**   Alkalosis regardless of origin may produce hypokalemia, hypocalcemia, cardiac dysrhythmias, bronchoconstriction, and hypotension, and it may potentiate the toxicity of digoxin. Cerebral blood flow is reduced by acute hypocapnia; metabolic alkalosis may be compensated by hypercapnia, causing increased cerebral blood flow. Only metabolic alkalosis may be appropriately treated with an acid. (See page 175: Acid-Base Interpretation and Treatment.)

26. **C.**   The renal response to hypovolemia and decreased cardiac output is to increase renal vascular resistance and decrease loss of Na and water. Blood is redistributed to inner cortical nephrons, which have longer loops of Henle that penetrate more deeply into the hypertonic renal medulla. Increased ADH release promotes water reabsorption through medullary collecting ducts and cortical collecting tubules. Aldosterone promotes Na reabsorption, primarily in the distal tubules. The response to hypovolemia also includes suppression of the release of atrial natriuretic hormone. The increased release of renin promotes conversion of angiotensinogen to angiotensin I. (See page 182: Regulation of Extracellular Fluid Volume.)

27. **A.**   The osmolality of replacement fluid is very important in the presence of brain injury. Lactated Ringer's solution is slightly hypo-osmotic relative to serum and thus may be associated with increased cortical water content. Hypertonic solutions may exert favorable effects on cerebral hemodynamics. The benefit usually is transient, and hypertonic therapy may be associated with complications including subdural hematoma. The cerebral capillary membrane (the blood–brain barrier) is highly impermeable to protein, and oncotic pressure exerts little if any effect on brain water accumulation. Hyperglycemia may aggravate ischemic brain injury. (See page 186: Implications of Crystalloid and Colloid Infusions on Intracranial Pressure.)

28. **C.**   Although the blood–brain barrier is poorly permeable to Na, water equilibrates rapidly. Thus, acute hyponatremia causes a prompt increase in intracellular brain water. An acute lowering of serum Na^+ concentration may be induced by mannitol, sorbitol, and other non-Na solutes, which do not diffuse freely across cell membranes and may cause an increase in ECV. Hyponatremia likewise may result from high levels of ADH. (See page 188: Sodium.)

29. **C.**   Normal serum Mg^{2+} ranges between 1.8 and 2.4 mg/dL (0.8–1.2 mmol/L; 1.6–2.4 mEq/L). The therapeutic range for treatment of pre-eclampsia is between 5 and 8 mg/dL. Symptoms develop above 3 mg/dL: hypotension (>3), hyporeflexia (>5), somnolence (>8.5), areflexia and respiratory insufficiency (>12), heart block and respiratory paralysis (>18), and cardiac arrest (>24). (See page 202: Magnesium.)

30. **B.**   Diabetes insipidus is associated with a loss of free water. It may be central in origin, with decreased ADH secretion; this has an increased incidence after pituitary surgery. It also may be peripheral in origin (nephrogenic), with the collecting ducts being resistant to ADH. Both the central and peripheral forms lead to hypernatremia. Treatments include water replacement, desmopressin (DDAVP), vasopressin, and drugs that stimulate ADH release (chlorpropamide, clofibrate, thiazide diuretics). (See page 188: Sodium.)

31. **A.**   Aldosterone increases renal reabsorption of Na^+ and excretion of K^+. Renal excretion of K^+ also is increased by high urinary flow rates and the presence in the renal tubular fluid of nonreabsorbable anions such as carbenicillin and phosphates. An intracellular shift of K^+ is caused by insulin, alkalosis, and $beta_2$-agonists. (See page 194: Potassium.)

32. **E.**   A chronic K loss that causes a 1.0 mEq/L decrease of plasma [K^+] typically is associated with a total body deficit of 200 to 300 mEq. However, in contrast to the hyperpolarization that accompanies an acute loss, the ratio of intracellular to extracellular K^+ remains relatively stable during a chronic loss. An intracellular shift of K^+ (and hypokalemia) may accompany respiratory and metabolic alkalosis and severe hypothermia; the changes resolve upon

correction of the alkalosis and rewarming. (See page 194: Potassium.)

33. **E.**   Acute hypokalemia causes hyperpolarization of the cardiac cell. This may lead to ventricular escape activity, re-entrant arrhythmias, and delayed conduction, with potentiation of digitalis-induced effects. Common signs include first-degree atrioventricular block and ST segment depression. (See page 194: Potassium.)

34. **C.**   A mineralocorticoid deficiency may lead to hyperkalemia. Likewise, administration of a drug that reduces the release of aldosterone (e.g., ACE inhibitors) or opposes the effects of aldosterone (e.g., triamterene or spironolactone) will cause an increase in K^+ levels. These effects may be offset by a drug that promotes kaliuresis (e.g., furosemide). They also may be treated with mineralocorticoid supplementation. (See page 194: Potassium.)

35. **B.**   With progressive hyperkalemia, the electrocardiogram shows tall, peaked T waves, followed by a prolonged P-R interval and then a decrease in P-wave height. These changes may progress to widening of the QRS complex and asystole. The effects are exacerbated by hyponatremia, hypocalcemia, acidosis, and digitalis toxicity. (See page 194: Potassium.)

36. **E.**   Serum K^+ concentrations may be acutely lowered by administration of $NaHCO_3$ (50–100 mEq); 5 to 10 units of regular insulin administered intravenously with 50 mL of 50% glucose; $beta_2$-adrenergic agonists; and/or furosemide (or related diuretics). Acute therapy also may include calcium chloride; this depresses the membrane threshold potential. More delayed forms of therapy include Na polystyrene sulfonate resin (Kayexalate) exchanges. (See page 194: Potassium.)

37. **A.**   The concentration of free calcium in the extracellular fluid normally is 1 to 1.25 mM. Because calcium is divalent, this corresponds to 2 to 2.5 mEq/L. The remaining 50% of extracellular calcium is protein bound (40%) or chelated (10%). Parathyroid hormone helps regulate the concentration of the physiologically active (ionized) form; it increases calcium plasma levels. Calcium may be lowered by increased phosphate. Hyperphosphatemic hypocalcemia results from calcium precipitation and suppression of calcitriol synthesis. Acute acidemia decreases protein-bound calcium (i.e., increases ionized calcium), whereas acute alkalemia increases protein-bound calcium (i.e., decreases ionized calcium). (See page 198: Calcium.)

38. **C.**   Hypocalcemia causes increased neuronal membrane irritability and tetany, as demonstrated by eliciting the Chvostek or Trousseau sign. It causes Q-T and ST prolongation and T-wave inversion.

Hypocalcemia may cause laryngeal spasm after parathyroid removal. In massive transfusion, citrate may produce hypocalcemia by chelating calcium. However, a healthy, normothermic adult with intact hepatic and renal function can adequately metabolize the citrate provided (without becoming hypocalcemic) when 20 units of blood are infused in 1 hour. When citrate clearance is decreased and/or when blood transfusion rates are rapid (e.g., 0.5–2 mL/kg per minute), severe hypocalcemia can occur. (See page 198: Calcium.)

39. **E.**   Patients with moderate hypercalcemia (total serum calcium 11.5–13 mg/dL) may show symptoms of lethargy, anorexia, nausea, and polyuria. Severe hypercalcemia (total serum calcium >13 mg/dL) is associated with severe neuromyopathic symptoms (including muscle weakness, depression, impaired memory, emotional lability, lethargy, stupor, and coma), renal calcium salt precipitation (nephrocalcinosis), and cardiovascular changes (hypertension, arrhythmias, heart block, cardiac arrest, and digitalis sensitivity). General supportive treatment includes hydration, correction of associated electrolyte abnormalities, removal of offending drugs, and dietary calcium restriction. Infusion of 0.9% saline will dilute serum calcium, reverse Na and water depletion, and promote renal excretion. Other treatments include calcitonin, mithramycin, and etidronate disodium (a diphosphonate). (See page 198: Calcium.)

40. **E.**   The clinical features of hyperphosphatemia relate primarily to the development of hypocalcemia and ectopic calcification. Hyperphosphatemia can promote calcification in vital organs such as the kidneys and myocardium. Neurologic manifestations include paresthesias, encephalopathy, delirium, seizures, and coma. Hematologic abnormalities include dysfunction of erythrocytes, platelets, and leukocytes. Muscle changes include myopathies, with respiratory muscle failure and myocardial dysfunction. Phosphate should be administered cautiously to hypocalcemic patients because of the risk of precipitating more severe hypocalcemia. (See page 201: Phosphate.)

41. **E.**   Normal Mg^{2+} levels in the plasma are approximately 1.7 mg/dL. Symptoms of hypomagnesemia occur at levels <1.0 mg/dL. The clinical features of hypomagnesemia, like those of hypocalcemia, are characterized by increased neuronal irritability, tetany, weakness, lethargy, muscle spasms, paresthesias, and depression. Severe hypomagnesemia may induce cardiovascular abnormalities, including coronary artery spasm, cardiac failure, dysrhythmias, hypotension, and increased myocardial sensitivity to digitalis. Rapid correction of hypomagnesemia may cause symptoms consistent with hypocalcemia. (See page 202: Magnesium.)

CHAPTER 10 ■ HEMOTHERAPY AND HEMOSTASIS

For questions 1 to 5, choose the best answer.

1. Which organ has the highest risk of ischemia under the conditions of isovolemic hemodilution?

   A. Bowel
   B. Heart
   C. Lung
   D. Liver
   E. Kidney

2. Which of the following is the most common infection associated with red blood cell (RBC) transfusion?

   A. Hepatitis A
   B. Human T-cell lymphotropic virus (HTLV-1 and HTLV-2)
   C. Hepatitis C
   D. Human immunodeficiency virus (HIV)
   E. Hepatitis B

3. Which of the following is true regarding coagulation?

   A. Most clotting factors circulate in an active form.
   B. Most clotting factors are synthesized extrahepatically.
   C. von Willebrand factor and coagulation factor VIII combine to form factor IX.
   D. Factors V and VIII have short storage half-lives.
   E. Seven clotting factors are vitamin K dependent.

4. Which of the following is not a vitamin K–dependent factor?

   A. II
   B. V
   C. VII
   D. IX
   E. X

5. Which of the following is not a common cause of platelet dysfunction?

   A. Dialysis

B. Nonsteroidal anti-inflammatory drugs (NSAIDs)
C. Chronic liver disease
D. Disseminated intravascular coagulopathy (DIC)
E. Cardiopulmonary bypass (CPB)

For questions 6 to 20, choose A if 1, 2, and 3 are correct; B if 1 and 3; C if 2 and 4; D if 4; E if all.

6. Which of the following conditions may decrease the tolerance for anemia and influence the RBC transfusion threshold?

   1. Hyperthermia
   2. Hypothermia
   3. Myocardial dysfunction
   4. High altitude

7. Which of the following is/are important factors in a patient's ability to compensate for the anemia associated with isovolemic hemodilution?

   1. Leftward shift in the oxyhemoglobin dissociation curve
   2. Decrease in systemic vascular resistance
   3. Decrease in oxygen extraction ratio
   4. Increase in cardiac stroke volume

8. The principal factor(s) affecting hemoglobin's P_{50} is/are:

   1. pH
   2. temperature
   3. 2,3-diphosphoglycerate (2,3-DPG) levels
   4. oxygen extraction ratio

9. Which of the following statements regarding compatibility testing is/are TRUE?

   1. Patients with Rh-negative blood will have anti-D antibodies in serum.
   2. Antibody screening is a check for anti-A and anti-B antibodies in donor serum.

3. Rh-negative patients given Rh-positive blood will always have hemolytic reactions.
4. Cross matching of blood involves simulation of actual anticipated transfusion by mixing of recipient and donor blood.

10. Which of the following statements regarding citrate intoxication is/are TRUE?

   1. It occurs with multiple transfusions of packed RBCs over long periods of time.
   2. It may result in electrocardiographic (ECG) changes.
   3. It may result in hypertension secondary to increased SVR.
   4. The citrate causes a temporary reduction of ionized calcium levels.

11. Immediate-type hemolytic transfusion reactions:

   1. may result from incompatibility in the Kell, Kidd, Lewis, or Duffy systems
   2. may be treated with sodium bicarbonate and mannitol
   3. are immune mediated and occur more commonly with antibodies that fix complement
   4. can be confirmed by haptoglobin, plasma and urine hemoglobin, and bilirubin assays

12. Delayed hemolytic transfusion reactions:

   1. usually follow an apparently compatible transfusion
   2. can be confirmed by an indirect Coombs' test
   3. require previous exposure
   4. generally result in hemolysis and have the same symptoms as immediate hemolytic transfusion reactions

13. Transfusion reactions resulting from white cell antigens:

   1. are immediate and life-threatening
   2. result from antibodies to human leukocyte antigens (HLAs) on transfused leukocytes
   3. may produce transfusion-related acute lung injury, which is a form of pulmonary edema associated with cardiogenic causes following blood transfusion
   4. often result in fever

14. Which of the following statements regarding antithrombin III (ATIII) is/are TRUE?

   1. It is inactivated by heparin.
   2. It is a naturally occurring anticoagulant.
   3. It is nonfunctional without the heparin cofactor.
   4. In the presence of heparin, it can bind activated factors IX, X, and XII to accelerate anticoagulation.

15. Which of the following statements regarding fibrinolysis is/are TRUE?

1. Tissue plasminogen activator (t-PA) is produced by vascular endothelial cells.
2. The primary fibrinolytic enzyme is t-PA.
3. t-PA differs from streptokinase in that its action is more localized.
4. Fibrin degradation products are produced by the action of t-PA on plasminogen.

16. Which of the following statements regarding the laboratory evaluation of coagulation is/are TRUE?

   1. The prothrombin time (PT) tests the extrinsic pathway of coagulation by adding tissue factors to whole blood.
   2. The thrombin time will be prolonged by low amounts of any of the factors that prolong the PT.
   3. The international normalized ratio (INR) standardizes the PT results obtained from varying thromboplastin reagents.
   4. The reptilase test uses snake venoms to confirm abnormal INR numbers.

17. Which of the following statements regarding von Willebrand disease is/are TRUE?

   1. It is a rare hereditary bleeding disorder.
   2. The activated partial thromboplastin time (aPTT) is commonly prolonged because of the diminished half-life of factor VIII in von Willebrand disease.
   3. Desmopressin (DDAVP) helps all types of von Willebrand disease to some extent.
   4. Patients have a prolonged bleeding time (BT) and normal platelet count.

18. Which of the following statements regarding hemophilia is/are TRUE?

   1. Hemophilia A is caused by a deficiency of factor VIII activity.
   2. Hemophilia B is an autosomal recessive disorder that occurs almost exclusively in Ashkenazi Jews.
   3. Hemophilia A may be treated with DDAVP.
   4. Patients with hemophilia A usually have an abnormal PT and BT.

19. Which of the following statements regarding DIC is/are TRUE?

   1. It is triggered by the appearance of excessive procoagulant material (tissue factor or equivalent) in the circulation
   2. PT and aPTT may remain normal.
   3. Activated protein C should be considered in any sustained episode of DIC.
   4. Heparin has been advocated in those situations in which thrombosis is clinically problematic.

20. Which of the following statements regarding low molecular weight heparins is/are TRUE?

   1. They are associated with a lesser incidence of heparin-induced thrombocytopenia.
   2. Protamine successfully neutralizes low molecular weight heparin.

3. Their half-life is longer than that of standard heparin.

4. They cause more platelet inhibition than standard heparin.

ANSWERS

1. **B.** With isovolemic hemodilution, blood flow to the tissues increases, but this increased blood flow is not distributed equally to all tissue beds. Organs with higher extraction ratios (brain and heart) receive disproportionately more of the increase in blood flow than organs with low extraction ratios (muscle, skin, viscera). The redistribution of blood flow to the coronary circulation is the principal means by which the healthy heart compensates for anemia. Because the heart under basal conditions already has a high extraction ratio (between 50–70% versus 30% in most tissues) and the primary compensation for anemia involves cardiac work (increasing cardiac output), the heart must rely upon redistributing blood flow to increase oxygen supply. These factors make the heart the organ at greatest risk under conditions of isovolemic hemodilution. When the heart can no longer increase either cardiac output or coronary blood flow, the limits of isovolemic hemodilution are reached. Further decreases in oxygen delivery will result in myocardial injury. (See page 215: Compensatory Mechanisms during Anemia.)

2. **E.** The rate of viral infectivity has decreased dramatically in the last 2 decades. It is in particular the advent of universal (in the United States) nucleic acid testing (NAT) for HIV and the hepatitis C virus (HCV) that has reduced the frequency of transmission of those agents to very low levels, i.e., 1 in two million. Hepatitis B remains the greatest risk, currently about one in 350,000 donor exposures. Transmission of hepatitis A virus (HAV) by transfusion has been very rare. Blood banks screen for HAV by history only, and there is no carrier state for this virus. HTLV-1 and HTLV-2 belong to the same retrovirus family as HIV. The incidence of clinical disease resulting from transmitted virus appears to be very low, and the transmission rate is very low, around one in 2.9 million. (See page 209: Infectious Risks Associated with Blood Product Administration.)

3. **D.** Most of the clotting factors circulate as inactive proenzymes. Most clotting factors are synthesized by the liver. Factor VIII is actually a large, two molecule complex (von Willebrand factor and coagulant factor VIII). Four clotting factors are vitamin K dependent. Factors V and VIII have short storage half-lives. Factors V and VIII are also referred to as the "labile factors" because their coagulant activity is not durable in stored blood.

Although packed RBCs contain residual plasma with clotting factors, massive transfusion with stored blood will nonetheless lead to a dilutional coagulopathy because of diminished activity of factors V and VII. (See page 222: The Coagulation Mechanism.)

4. **B.** Most of the coagulation proteins are synthesized by the liver. Four of the clotting factors, II, VII, IX, and X, require vitamin K for proper synthesis. (See page 222: The Coagulation Mechanism.)

5. **A.** The causes of thrombocytopenia may be categorized as follows: (1) inadequate production by the bone marrow, (2) increased peripheral consumption or destruction (non–immune-mediated), (3) increased peripheral destruction (immune-mediated), (4) dilution of circulating platelets, and (5) sequestration. Bone marrow production of platelets can be impaired in many ways. Chronic disease states such as uremia and liver disease can cause bone marrow suppression. The many conditions that cause DIC will also cause platelets to be consumed or destroyed faster than they can be produced. Numerous medications are administered expressly for the purpose of platelet inhibition to reduce the risk of myocardial infarction, stroke, and other thromboembolic complications. These medications induce platelet dysfunction by several mechanisms, which include inhibition of cyclo-oxygenase, inhibition of phosphodiesterase, adenosine diphosphate (ADP) receptor antagonism, and blockade of the glycoprotein IIb/IIIa receptor. Indomethacin, phenylbutazone, and all the NSAIDs similarly inhibit cyclo-oxygenase. Platelets are subject to contact activation by the CPB circuit, thus causing their numbers to decline. Platelet dysfunction is common in uremic patients. The accumulation of guanidinosuccinic acid and hydroxyphenolic acid is thought to contribute to this dysfunction through interference with the platelet's ability to expose the PF3 phospholipid surface. These compounds are dialyzable, and, accordingly, dialysis frequently improves the hemostatic defect associated with uremia. (See page 234: Thrombocytopenia.)

6. **E.** Ultimately, the decision to transfuse RBCs should be made based on the clinical judgment that the oxygen-carrying capacity of the blood must be increased to prevent oxygen consumption from outstripping oxygen delivery. Conditions that may decrease the tolerance for anemia and influence the

RBC transfusion threshold include factors that increase oxygen demand, limit the ability to increase cardiac output, cause a left shift of the oxyhemoglobin, and impair oxygenation. These factors include a wide range of states including hyperthermia, coronary artery disease and myocardial dysfunction, hypothermia, and high altitude. (See page 214: Red blood cells, Table 10-5: Conditions that may decrease tolerance for anemia and influence the RBC transfusion threshold.)

7. **C.**   When anemia develops but blood volume is maintained (isovolemic hemodilution), four compensatory mechanisms serve to maintain oxygen delivery: an increase in cardiac output, a redistribution of blood flow to organs with greater oxygen requirements, increases in the extraction ratios of some vascular beds, and alteration of oxygen-hemoglobin binding to allow the hemoglobin to deliver oxygen at lower oxygen tensions. With isovolemic hemodilution, cardiac output increases primarily because of an increase in stroke volume brought about by reductions in SVR. Organs with higher extraction ratios (brain and heart) receive disproportionately more of the increase in blood flow than organs with low extraction ratios (muscle, skin, viscera). Increasing oxygen extraction ratio (ER) is thought to play an important adaptive role when the normovolemic hematocrit drops below 25%. The oxyhemoglobin dissociation curve can be shifted to the left or right. When the curve is shifted to the left, the hemoglobin molecule is more "stingy" and requires lower oxygen partial pressures to release oxygen to the tissues. By contrast, right shifting of the oxyhemoglobin dissociation curve decreases hemoglobin affinity for the oxygen molecule and release of oxygen to tissues at higher partial pressures of oxygen. (See page 215: Compensatory Mechanisms during Anemia.)

8. **A.**   The partial pressure of oxygen at which the hemoglobin molecule is 50% saturated is termed the P_{50}. Changes in pH, temperature, and 2,3-DPG levels can shift the oxyhemoglobin dissociation curve and can thus raise or lower the P_{50} value. Changes in P_{50} determine how tightly oxygen and hemoglobin bind and ultimately affect oxygen extraction ratios. (See page 215: Compensatory Mechanisms during Anemia.)

9. **D.**   Unlike the ABO system, patients who have Rh-negative blood will not necessarily have Rh antibodies or D antibodies in their serum. Therefore, patients who have Rh-negative blood initially may receive Rh-positive blood without risk of hemolysis. Antibody screening checks for unexpected antibodies in the serum (excluding the ABO and Rh systems). The final phase of compatibility testing is called cross matching and actually does simulate anticipated transfusion by mixing donor RBCs with recipient serum. (See page 219: Compatibility Testing.)

10. **C.**   Commonly used additive solutions contain citrate, which anticoagulates by chelation of ionized calcium. When large volumes of stored blood (>1 blood volume) are administered rapidly, the citrate can cause a temporary reduction in ionized calcium levels. Decreased ionized calcium levels should not occur unless the rate of transfusion exceeds 1 mL/kg per minute or about 1 unit of blood per 5 minutes in an average-sized adult. Signs of citrate intoxication (hypocalcemia) include hypotension, narrow pulse pressure, and elevated intraventricular end-diastolic pressure and central venous pressure, prolonged Q-T interval, widened QRS complexes, and flattened T waves. (See page 214: Citrate Intoxication.)

11. **A.**   Immediate hemolytic transfusion reactions are the result of incompatibility in antibodies that fix complement and commonly produce immediate intravascular hemolysis. This would include anti-A, anti-B, anti-Kell, anti-Kidd, anti-Lewis, and anti-Duffy antibodies. Although serum haptoglobin, plasma and urine hemoglobin, and bilirubin tests give evidence of hemolysis, they are not specific for an immune reaction. The confirmatory test for an immune reaction is a direct antiglobulin or direct Coombs' test. Clinical management of patients centers on three main goals: maintenance of systemic blood pressure, preservation of renal function, and prevention of DIC. Urine output should be promoted by administration of fluids and the use of diuretics, either mannitol or furosemide, or both. Sodium bicarbonate can be administered to alkalinize the urine. (See page 210: Reactions to RBC Antigens.)

12. **B.**   Delayed hemolytic transfusion reactions occur when the donor RBCs possess an antigen that the recipient at some time has been exposed to (either by previous transfusion or pregnancy) and thus has been immunized. Over time, the recipient antibodies fall to levels too low to be detected by subsequent compatibility testing. Thus, these reactions appear in patients who have an apparently compatible transfusion. Because the recipient experiences an anamnestic response, it will require time for reaction to develop. These reactions occur outside of the vascular tree, resulting in a less severe and less likely fatal reaction. Confirmatory evidence is based on direct antiglobulin or direct Coombs' testing. (See page 211: Delayed Hemolytic Transfusion Reactions.)

13. **C.**   Patients who receive multiple transfusions of RBCs or platelets often develop antibodies to the HLA antigens on the passenger leukocytes in these products. During subsequent RBC transfusions, febrile reactions may occur as a result of antibody attack on donor leukocytes. Patients may experience fever only, but they may also develop chills, respiratory distress, anxiety, headache, myalgias, nausea, and a nonproductive cough. Transfusion-related acute lung

injury is a noncardiogenic form of pulmonary edema associated with blood product administration. It occurs when agents present in the plasma phase of donor blood activate leukocytes in the host. (See page 212: White Cell–Related Transfusion Reactions.)

14. **C.** ATIII is a circulating serine protease inhibitor that binds to thrombin and thereby inactivates it. It can bind and inactivate each of the activated clotting factors of the classical "intrinsic" coagulation cascade—factors XIIa, XIa, IXa, and Xa. In the absence of heparin, ATIII has a relatively low affinity for thrombin. However, when heparin is bound to ATIII, the efficiency of binding of ATIII to thrombin and the other factors increases dramatically. (See page 227: Thrombin and Antithrombin III.)

15. **B.** The process of fibrinolysis leads to dissolution of fibrin clots. Fibrinolysis serves to remodel fibrin clots and "recanalize" vessels that have been occluded by thrombosis. The primary fibrinolytic enzyme is plasmin, which is derived by the conversion of plasminogen to plasmin in the presence of t-PA and fibrin. Fibrin split products or fibrin degradation products are produced by the action of plasmin on fibrin clots. The therapeutic fibrinolytic agents, streptokinase and urokinase, differ from t-PA in that they will activate circulating plasminogen, leading to more widespread fibrinolysis. (See page 225: Fibrinolysis.)

16. **B.** The PT is measured by adding tissue thromboplastin or tissue factor to the blood and measuring the time until clot formation occurs. PT will be prolonged if deficiencies, abnormalities, or inhibitors of factors I, II, V, VII, or X exist. This tests the classical extrinsic pathway. Because different thromboplastin reagents produce values with different normal ranges, comparison of PT results among laboratories is difficult. The INR value takes into account the different sensitivities of varying reagents and allows INR results to be directly compared from one laboratory to another. The thrombin time measures the ability of thrombin to convert fibrinogen to fibrin. This test bypasses all other preceding reactions and will not necessarily be prolonged by abnormalities of many of the factors of the extrinsic pathway. Reptilase, a snake venom, converts fibrinogen to fibrin; this is unaffected by the presence of heparin. The reptilase test is used to differentiate a prolonged thrombin time as a result of heparin versus fibrin degradation products. (See page 228: Laboratory Evaluation of Coagulation.)

17. **D.** von Willebrand disease is the most common hereditary bleeding disorder in humans. When von Willebrand factor is deficient, platelet function is impaired, leading to an abnormal BT in the presence of normal platelet count. The aPTT and the PT may be normal in the patient with von Willebrand disease. Although the half-life of factor VIII:C is diminished in von Willebrand disease, there is usually sufficient VIII:C to yield a normal aPTT in basal conditions. DDAVP is effective first-line therapy for most (~80%) patients with von Willebrand disease, including those with type 1 and type 2A disease. However, the recognition of subtype 2B is important because DDAVP will cause thrombocytopenia in these patients. (See page 232: Von Willebrand Disease.)

18. **B.** Hemophilia A is caused by a deficiency of factor VIII activity, whereas hemophilia B (Christmas disease) is caused by a deficiency of factor IX. Both hemophilia A and B are sex-linked recessive disorders, which therefore occur almost exclusively in boys and men. Hemophilia C is an autosomal recessive disorder that occurs almost exclusively in Ashkenazi Jews. Hemophilia A generally is treated with factor VIII concentrates. However, DDAVP is helpful in increasing plasma factor VIII and von Willebrand factor concentrations; it is most effective in patients with factor VIII:C levels >5%. Laboratory diagnosis of hemophilia A is based on the finding of a prolonged aPTT and a specific factor assay demonstrating deficiency of factor VIII. The patient will have a normal PT and a normal BT. (See page 233: The Hemophilias.)

19. **E.** DIC is triggered by the appearance of procoagulant material (tissue factor or equivalent) in the circulation in amounts sufficient to overwhelm the mechanisms that normally restrain and localize clot formation. PT and aPTT may remain normal in spite of decreasing factor levels because of the presence of high levels of activated factors including thrombin and Xa. Heparin has been advocated. However, the contemporary practice is to restrict its use to only those situations in which thrombosis is clinically problematic. An insufficiency in the protein C endogenous coagulation inhibition system is thought to contribute to the prothrombotic state in DIC. Activated protein C has been shown to decrease mortality and organ failure in patients with sepsis, and that improvement is also evident among patients with sepsis with overt DIC. The use of this agent should be considered in any sustained episode of DIC. (See page 237: Disseminated Intravascular Coagulation.)

20. **B.** Protamine neutralization of low molecular weight heparin is reported to be incomplete. The half-life is longer than that of standard heparin, allowing for once per day dosing. It appears to cause less platelet inhibition and is associated with a lower incidence of heparin-induced thrombocytopenia than standard heparin. (See page 235: Acquired Disorders of Clotting Factors.)

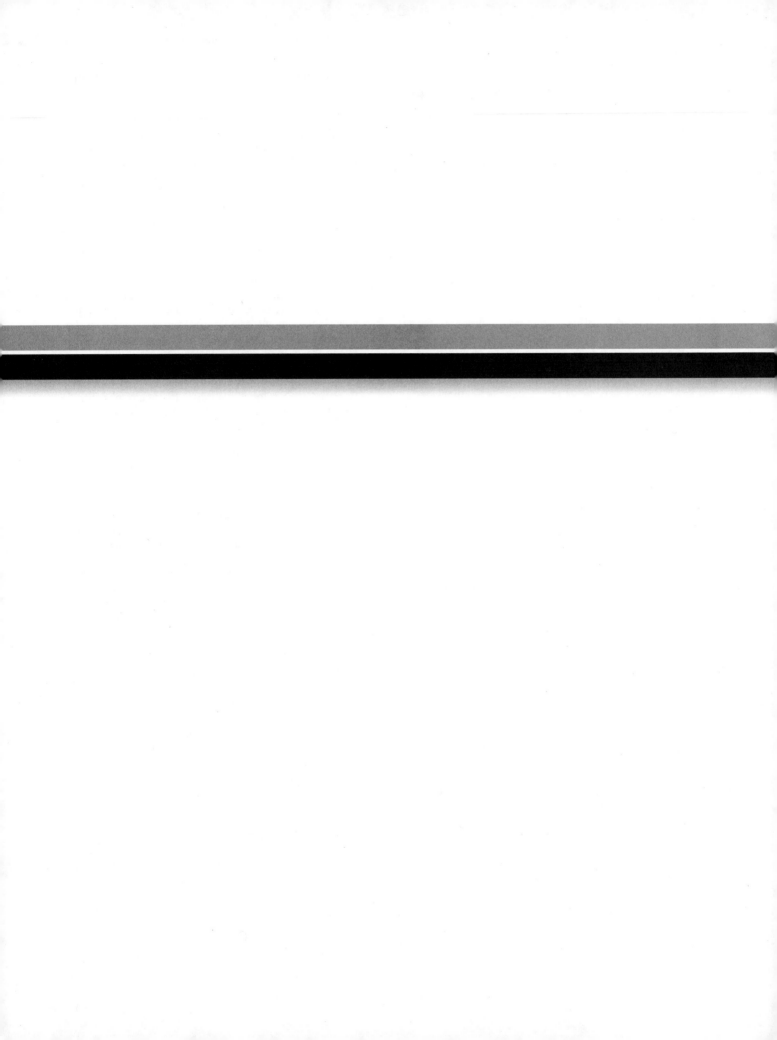

SECTION III ■ BASIC PRINCIPLES OF
PHARMACOLOGY IN ANESTHESIA PRACTICE

CHAPTER 11 ■ BASIC PRINCIPLES OF CLINICAL PHARMACOLOGY

For questions 1 to 21, choose the best answer.

1. Which of the following statements concerning passage of drugs across membranes is FALSE?

   A. The distribution of neuromuscular blockers essentially is limited to the extracellular fluid.
   B. The walls of most capillaries do not allow passage of water-soluble drugs.
   C. Reabsorption of drugs from the renal tubules is increased for lipid-soluble compounds.
   D. Thiopental easily crosses cell membranes.
   E. Reabsorption of drugs from the intestines (e.g., after excretion in bile) is increased for lipid-soluble compounds.

2. Which of the following statements concerning acid-base balance is FALSE?

   A. The pKa of an acid is inversely proportional to the pH.
   B. The closer the pKa is to the ambient pH, the greater the change in the degree of ionization for a given change in pH.
   C. The nonionized fraction of weak acids, such as salicylates, is greater at low pH values.
   D. The nonionized fraction of opioids increases as the pH increases above the drug's pKa.
   E. The nonionized fraction of local anesthetics increases as the pH increases above the drug's pKa.

3. Which of the following statements concerning routes of administration is TRUE?

   A. The relatively high molecular weight and high water solubility of volatile anesthetics facilitate their passage across alveolar membranes.
   B. Nitroglycerin is absorbed after sublingual administration because it is highly water soluble.
   C. Dissolving diazepam in propylene glycol does not ensure its reliable uptake after intramuscular injection.

   D. Lipid-soluble drugs are more readily absorbed after intramuscular injection than are drugs in aqueous solutions.
   E. Water-soluble drugs can more effectively penetrate intact skin than their lipid-soluble counterparts.

4. Which of the following statements about drug distribution to the central nervous system (CNS) is FALSE?

   A. Equilibration in the brain and muscle do not occur simultaneously.
   B. Diffusion of water-soluble drugs into the brain is severely restricted.
   C. For more polar compounds, the rate of entry into the brain is proportional to their lipid solubility.
   D. Distribution of highly lipid-soluble drugs into the CNS is directly proportional to cerebral blood flow.
   E. Recovery from a single dose of thiopental is dependent primarily on hepatic elimination.

5. How many minutes after an intravenous injection does the brain concentration of thiopental peak?

   A. 1
   B. 4
   C. 6
   D. 8
   E. 11

6. You are about to induce general anesthesia for an elective cesarean section. Which of the following statements is TRUE?

   A. Most drugs cross the placenta by active transport.
   B. Fetal pH typically is higher than maternal pH.
   C. The maternal-fetal pH gradient causes the ionized fraction of opioids to be higher in the mother.
   D. At equilibrium, the concentration of free nonionized drug will be greater on the fetal side of the placenta.

E. The maternal-fetal pH gradient causes the ionized fraction of local anesthetics to be higher in the fetus.

7. The FALSE statement about drug elimination is:

    A. Elimination can occur by excretion of unchanged drug.
    B. Metabolism is a step in some drug elimination.
    C. The liver and kidney are the most important organs in drug elimination.
    D. The liver eliminates drugs primarily by excretion.
    E. The kidney primarily excretes water-soluble, polar compounds.

8. Which of the following indicates the units for drug clearance?

    A. mL/minute
    B. mL/kg/min
    C. %/kg
    D. mL/ kg
    E. kg/%

9. Which of the following statements concerning the volume of drug distribution and clearance is TRUE?

    A. The smaller the volume of distribution, the longer the half-time of elimination.
    B. The calculated volume of steady-state distribution can exceed the actual volume of the body.
    C. The volume of distribution is equal to the total amount of drug present divided by plasma volume and vessel-rich group volume.
    D. The volume of distribution provides information regarding the tissues into which the drug distributes and the concentration in those tissues.
    E. The volume of distribution cannot be as small as the plasma volume.

10. If 10 mg of drug is present and the plasma concentration is 2 mg/L, then the volume of distribution is _____ L.

    A. 5
    B. 50
    C. 500
    D. 20
    E. 0.2

11. The average glomerular filtration in adults with normal renal function is _____ mL/minute.

    A. 10
    B. 50
    C. 70
    D. 125
    E. 250

12. Which form of biotransformation is particularly prominent when intracellular oxygen tension is very low?

    A. Reduction
    B. Oxidation
    C. Hydrolysis
    D. Hydroxylation
    E. Dealkylation

13. Which of the following statements concerning hepatic clearance is FALSE?

    A. If the extraction ratio (and intrinsic clearance) is very high, then total hepatic clearance will be proportional to hepatic blood flow.
    B. Clearance of drugs with low extraction ratios is relatively independent of the amount of hepatic blood flow.
    C. Only a drug that is unbound upon entering the hepatic circulation will be cleared by the liver.
    D. Only unbound drug can enter hepatocytes.
    E. Clearance of lidocaine is reduced in patients with congestive cardiac failure in proportion to the decrease in hepatic blood flow.

14. Each of the following has a high hepatic extraction ratio EXCEPT:

    A. rocuronium
    B. lidocaine
    C. metoprolol
    D. propofol
    E. meperidine

15. Which of the following statements concerning renal clearance is FALSE?

    A. Normally, only unbound drugs can pass through the glomerular membrane into the renal tubule.
    B. Renal clearance of drugs that are secreted rapidly and not reabsorbed is proportional to renal blood flow.
    C. Highly lipophilic drugs, such as thiopental, undergo virtually no renal clearance of the parent molecule.
    D. Changes in renal drug clearance are proportional to changes in creatinine clearance, even for drugs eliminated primarily by tubular secretion.
    E. Lipid-soluble drugs are not filtered across the glomerular membrane.

16. By 80 years of age, creatinine clearance is decreased by ____%.

    A. 10
    B. 30
    C. 50
    D. 70
    E. 80

17. Which of the following statements about pharmacokinetics is FALSE?

    A. In first-order kinetics, when the concentration is high it will fall faster than when it is low.

B. The brain, heart, lungs, and muscle make up the vessel-rich group.

C. A first-order kinetic process is one in which a constant fraction of the drug is removed during a finite period of time.

D. Awakening after a single dose of thiopental is primarily the result of redistribution.

E. The disadvantage of perfusion-based pharmacokinetic models is their complexity.

18. Which of the following has the least binding to albumin?

A. Diazepam
B. Pancuronium
C. Propofol
D. Bupivacaine
E. Fentanyl

19. The free fraction of thiopental typically is _____ % in young adults and _____ % in geriatric patients.

A. 18, 22
B. 18, 90
C. 2, 22
D. 2, 40
E. 2, 90

20. What is the half-time of elimination for a drug that undergoes first-order elimination with a rate constant of 0.1 minute?

A. 10 minutes
B. 100 minutes
C. 0.1 minutes
D. 6.93 minutes
E. 693 minutes

21. How many minutes are required for approximately 97% elimination of a drug undergoing first-order elimination with a half-time of 10 minutes?

A. 10
B. 30

C. 50
D. 70
E. 100

For questions 22 to 24, choose A if 1, 2, and 3 are correct; B if 1 and 3; C if 2 and 4; D if 4; E if all.

22. Which of the following have pharmacologically active metabolites that are excreted by the kidneys?

1. Pancuronium
2. Lidocaine
3. Meperidine
4. Thiopental

23. TRUE statements about agonists and antagonists include:

1. Competitive antagonists bind irreversibly to receptors.
2. Competitive antagonists do not change the maximum possible effect that can be elicited by an agonist.
3. Noncompetitive antagonists bind reversibly to receptors.
4. Noncompetitive antagonists change the maximum effect elicited by an agonist.

24. TRUE statements regarding drug infusions of propofol include:

1. A multicompartment model must be used to predict propofol concentration during an infusion.
2. The concentration of infused propofol reaches 90% of the steady-state in 3.3 half-lives.
3. Propofol's elimination half-life is 6 hours.
4. It takes 6 hours from the start of a propofol infusion to reach 50% of its steady-state concentration.

ANSWERS

---

1. **B.** The large spaces between capillaries allow for passage of water-soluble drugs, except in the brain, where there are tight interendothelial cell junctions (the so-called blood-brain barrier). Transcellular penetration is much easier for lipid-soluble drugs, which can more readily cross lipid membranes. This accounts for the greater CNS penetrability of thiopental and for the reabsorption of drugs across the cells of the renal tubule and intestine. Distribution of highly polar drugs, such as neuromuscular blockers, essentially is limited to the extracellular fluid. (See page 250: Drug Distribution and page 248: Transfer of Drugs Across Membranes.)

2. **A.** The pKa is the pH at which a weak acid or base is 50% in its ionized form and 50% in its nonionized form. It is characteristic of a given drug, regardless of the surrounding pH. Equation 1 illustrates why, in an acidic environment, a weak acid (e.g., salicylic acid and barbiturates) tends to be nonionized; an acidic environment drives the equation to the left and causes acidic drugs to be more lipid soluble. Equation 2 illustrates why, in an alkaline environment, a weak base (e.g., opioids, local anesthetics) tends to be nonionized; the equation is driven to the left. (1) $HA = H^+ + A^-$, (2) $HB = OH^- + B^+$. (See page 248: Effects of Molecular Properties.)

3. **C.** Lipid-soluble drugs are more effective at penetrating the cellular membrane of the skin and mucosal surfaces. For example, sublingual administration is effective only for nonionized, highly lipid-soluble drugs such as nitroglycerin. In contrast, water-soluble drugs easily penetrate most blood vessels, as is the case after an intramuscular injection. Dissolving diazepam in propylene glycol, a nonaqueous solution, is associated with erratic absorption. Volatile anesthetics have low molecular weight and high lipid solubility. (See page 249: Drug Absorption: Route of Administration.)

4. **E.** Recovery from thiopental largely depends on redistribution from the brain to other tissues (e.g., muscle); the effects of elimination are not noted until later in the course of recovery and are relatively minor unless large doses are employed. The distribution of lipid-soluble drugs into the CNS is very rapid and thus is directly proportional to cerebral blood flow (i.e., to the amount of drug that is delivered to the brain). Polar compounds do not pass into the brain readily because brain capillaries do not have the large aqueous channels typical of capillaries in other tissues. For more polar compounds, the rate of entry into the brain is proportional to the lipid solubility of the nonionized drug. (See page 250: Drug Distribution.)

5. **A.** The brain concentration of thiopental peaks within 1 minute because of high blood flow to the brain and the high lipid solubility of thiopental. Thiopental quickly diffuses back into the blood, where it is redistributed to other tissues that are still taking up drug. Its duration of action is thus very short, unless high doses are used and termination of drug action becomes dependent on drug elimination. (See page 250: Drug Distribution: Redistribution.)

6. **E.** Most drugs cross the placenta by simple diffusion. The fetal total drug level of a weak base (e.g., opioids and local anesthetics) may be higher than the maternal total drug level because of "ion trapping." The lower pH on the fetal side of the placenta causes increased ionization of weak bases. This increases the overall amount of drug as well as the ionized fraction. However, at equilibrium, the concentration of free (nonionized) drug is the same on both sides of the placenta; it is this free drug that equilibrates. (See page 250: Placental Transfer.)

7. **D.** Elimination is an inclusive term referring to all the processes that remove drugs from the body. Elimination occurs either by excretion of unchanged drug or by metabolism (biotransformation) and subsequent excretion of metabolites. The liver and kidneys are the most important organs for drug elimination. The liver eliminates drugs primarily by metabolism to less active compounds and, to a lesser extent, by hepatobiliary excretion of drugs or their metabolites. The primary role of the kidneys is the excretion of water-soluble, polar compounds. (See page 250: Drug Elimination.)

8. **A.** Drug clearance has units of flow (e.g., mL/minute). It is the portion of the volume of distribution (the theoretical volume of a drug) from which the drug is completely removed in a given time interval. (See page 250: Drug Elimination.)

9. **B.** Extensive tissue uptake of a drug is reflected by a large volume of the peripheral compartment. If there is binding to the tissues, then the calculated volume of distribution can exceed the actual volume of the body. It may be as small as the plasma volume. The volume of distribution is equal to the total amount of drug divided by the concentration. The volume of distribution does not provide any information regarding the tissues into which the drug distributes or the concentrations in those tissues. (See page 259: Volumes of Distribution.)

10. **A.** The volume of distribution is 5 L. V_d = total amount of drug/concentration. (See page 260: Volumes of Distribution: One-Compartment Model.)

11. **D.** In adults, renal blood flow is approximately 1200 mL/minute, renal plasma flow is 700 mL/minute, and glomerular filtration rate is 125 mL/minute. (See page 253: Renal Drug Clearance: Physiologic, Pharmacologic, and Pathologic Alterations in Renal Drug Clearance.)

12. **A.** Reductive biotransformation (i.e., where electrons are transferred to the drug molecule) is inhibited by oxygen. Thus, it is facilitated when intracellular oxygen tension is low. (See page 254: Phase I Reactions.)

13. **C.** A very high liver extraction ratio indicates that the liver is removing most of the drug that is passing through it. Until the liver's capacity is exceeded, drug removal increases as the blood flow increases. A decrease in liver perfusion, as may occur with congestive heart failure, will decrease the clearance of drugs that are highly extracted (e.g., lidocaine). Only free drug can enter the hepatocytes. However, if free drug is rapidly eliminated by the liver, bound drug is released and, likewise, is taken up by the liver; that is, the concentration of free drug may drop so quickly that a greater amount of drug dissociates from plasma binding sites during its passage through the liver. (See page 251: Hepatic Drug Clearance.)

14. **A.** The extraction ratios for lidocaine, meperidine, propofol, and metoprolol are very high; the extraction ratio for rocuronium is much lower. (See page 252: Hepatic Drug Clearance: Physiologic, Pathologic, and Pharmacologic Alterations in Hepatic Drug Clearance and Table 11.1, Classification of drugs encountered in anesthesiology according to hepatic extraction ratios.)

15. **E.**   All unbound drug is filtered by the glomerulus, with a glomerular filtration rate that is 20% of renal plasma flow. Lipid-soluble drugs undergo reuptake in the renal tubule. Renal clearance of drugs that are filtered, as well as those that are secreted by the renal tubules, is directly proportional to renal blood flow and, hence, creatinine clearance. Decreased glomerular function is associated with a proportional loss of tubular function. (See page 253: Renal Drug Clearance.)

16. **C.**   During adulthood, creatinine clearance progressively declines. By 80 years of age, it is approximately 50% of its maximum value. However, serum creatinine is not elevated in healthy elderly patients because muscle mass, the source of creatinine, also decreases with age. (See page 253: Renal Drug Clearance.)

17. **B.**   The term "pharmacokinetics" refers to the quantitative analysis of the relationship between the dose of a drug and the ensuing changes in drug concentration in the blood and other tissues. Physiologic pharmacokinetic models provide much insight into factors affecting drug action. In these models, body tissues are classified according to similarities in perfusion and affinity for drugs. Highly perfused tissues, including the brain, heart, lungs, liver, and kidneys, make up the vessel-rich group. Muscle and skin comprise the lean tissue group, and fat is considered a separate group. These models established that awakening after a single dose of thiopental was primarily the result of redistribution from the brain to muscle and skin. The disadvantage of perfusion-based models is their complexity. The disposition of most drugs follows first-order kinetics. A first-order kinetic process is one in which a constant fraction of the drug is removed during a finite period of time. Because a constant fraction is removed per unit of time in first-order kinetics, the absolute amount of drug removed is proportional to the concentration of the drug. When the concentration is high, it will fall faster than when it is low. (See page 259: Pharmacokinetic Concepts.)

18. **B.**   In general, more lipid-soluble drugs are more highly protein bound. Consistent with its polarity, <30% of pancuronium is bound to albumin. (See page 257: Factors Affecting Drug Binding.)

19. **A.**   The average free fraction of thiopental increases from about 18% in young adults to 22% in geriatric patients. (See page 258: Factors Affecting Drug Binding: Age and Sex)

20. **D.**   Half-life (minutes) = natural log of 2 ÷ rate constant of elimination = $0.693 \div 0.1$ minute = 6.93 minutes. Thus, it would take 6.93 minutes for the concentration to change by a factor of 2 for a drug with a rate constant of 0.1 minute. (See page 259: Rate Constants and Half-Lives.)

21. **C.**   When a drug is eliminated by first-order elimination, its concentration is generally reduced by 97% after five half-times of elimination. Conversely, if a drug is infused at a constant rate, the concentration approaches a steady state after approximately five half-lives. (See page 259: Rate Constants and Half-Lives.)

22. **A.**   Many drugs, including pancuronium, lidocaine, and meperidine, have pharmacologically active metabolites that are excreted by the kidneys. (See page 253: Physiologic, Pharmacologic, and Pathologic Alterations in Renal Drug Clearance.)

23. **D.**   Competitive antagonists bind reversibly to receptors, and their blocking effect can be overcome by high concentrations of an agonist. Therefore, competitive antagonists produce a parallel shift in the dose-response curve, but the maximum effect is not altered. Noncompetitive antagonists bind irreversibly to receptors. This has the same effect as reducing the number of receptors and shifts the dose-response curve downward and to the right, decreasing both the slope and the maximum effect. (See page 265: Drug–Receptor Interactions: Agonists, Partial Agonists and Antagonists.)

24. **B.**   In a one-compartment model, the rise of drug concentration during a constant infusion is the mirror image of its elimination profile. Using a single-compartment model, drug infusions will reach 90% of their steady-state in 3.3 half-lives. Propofol, however, partitions extensively to pharmacologically inert body tissues, so a multicompartment model must be used to predict its concentrations during infusions. The half-life of propofol is 6 hours, yet the multicompartment model of drug concentration predicts that it will reach 50% of steady state in less than 30 minutes from starting a constant infusion. (See page 267: Rise to Steady-State Concentration.)

CHAPTER 12 ■ AUTONOMIC NERVOUS SYSTEM: PHYSIOLOGY AND PHARMACOLOGY

1. Which of the following statements concerning the sympathetic nervous system (SNS) is TRUE?

   A. The preganglionic fibers originate in the gray column of the two lower cervical, 12 thoracic, and first lumbar segments of the spinal cord.
   B. There are 22 paired sympathetic ganglia.
   C. Preganglionic fibers only synapse with postganglionic fibers in ganglia at the level of exit.
   D. Preganglionic fibers also may synapse in a ganglion that can then traverse to the adrenal gland.
   E. All preganglionic fibers are unmyelinated fibers.

2. Which of the following statements concerning postganglionic fibers of the SNS is TRUE?

   A. Postganglionic nerve cell bodies are located only in the paired lateral ganglia.
   B. The celiac and inferior mesenteric ganglia are located along the spinal cord and are considered part of a sympathetic paired ganglion.
   C. All ganglia of the sympathetic chain are located closer to the spinal cord than the organs they innervate.
   D. Postganglionic myelinated fibers proceed from paired ganglia to the respective organs.
   E. Approximately 25% of the fibers in the average somatic nerve are sympathetic.

3. Which of the following statements concerning the SNS is TRUE?

   A. The first four to five thoracic spinal segments generate fibers that converge to form three special paired ganglia.
   B. The middle cervical ganglion also is known as the stellate ganglion.
   C. The stellate ganglion provides sympathetic innervation only to the head and neck.
   D. The response of the SNS is very discrete.
   E. One preganglionic fiber influences one postganglionic neuron.

4. Which of the following statements regarding the parasympathetic nervous system (PNS) is TRUE?

   A. The sacral fibers originate from the white matter of the second, third, and fourth sacral nerves.
   B. Preganglionic fibers are myelinated fibers analogous to those in the SNS and terminate in ganglia next to the spinal cord.
   C. The ratio of preganglionic to postganglionic fibers in the PNS is the same as in the SNS.
   D. Postganglionic neurons are located in or near the organ to be innervated.
   E. Cranial nerve X has the least innervation of all PNS nerves.

5. All of the following are functions of the autonomic innervation of the heart EXCEPT:

   A. The autonomic nervous system (ANS) changes the heart rate (chronotropism).
   B. The ANS changes the strength of contraction (inotropism).
   C. The ANS modulates coronary blood flow.
   D. There is parasympathetic innervation of the ventricles of the heart.
   E. The vagus affects the sinoatrial and atrioventricular nodes.

6. Which of the following statements regarding the ANS and peripheral circulation is TRUE?

   A. The SNS and PNS are equally distributed in the peripheral circulation.
   B. Distribution is equal among all tissues.
   C. SNS stimulation of the coronary arteries may produce vasoconstriction or vasodilation depending on the predominant receptor activity.
   D. Vascular tone is predominantly controlled by PNS activity.
   E. Local autoregulatory factors do not influence coronary vascular tone.

7. All of the following statements about neurotransmission in the ANS are true EXCEPT:

    A. The SNS and PNS commonly are designated as adrenergic and cholinergic, respectively.
    B. In the PNS, the postganglionic receptors secrete acetylcholine.
    C. Norepinephrine is the only neurotransmitter of the SNS at the postganglionic site.
    D. The preganglionic neurotransmitter is acetylcholine in both the PNS and the SNS.
    E. Terminations of postganglionic fibers are anatomically and physiologically similar in both the SNS and PNS.

8. Which of the following statements regarding the PNS is TRUE?

    A. In addition to acetylcholinesterase, pseudocholinesterase also plays a significant role in the termination of acetylcholine.
    B. Acetylcholine is stored in presynaptic vesicles and is released in small amounts called quanta.
    C. Once released, acetylcholine is taken up by the presynaptic membrane for release again.
    D. Drugs that alter calcium release do not affect the release of acetylcholine because its release is calcium independent.
    E. Acetylcholine is formed by acetylation of choline by the enzyme acetylcholinesterase.

9. All of the following statements regarding the SNS are true EXCEPT:

    A. Epinephrine and norepinephrine are mediators of the peripheral SNS.
    B. In the adrenal medulla, the preganglionic neurotransmitter is acetylcholine.
    C. Chromaffin cells in the adrenal medulla are responsible for release of epinephrine and norepinephrine.
    D. The massive release of norepinephrine and epinephrine is the "fight or flight" response and lasts approximately 10 times as long as local direct stimulation.
    E. Equal amounts of epinephrine and norepinephrine are released during stimulation of the adrenal medulla.

10. Which of the following statements about catecholamines is TRUE?

    A. Circulating catecholamines are responsible for stimulating receptors in the central nervous system (CNS) during the "fight or flight" response.
    B. The only brain catecholamine is dopamine.
    C. Endogenous catecholamines are dopamine, epinephrine, and norepinephrine.
    D. Catecholamines have only a direct effect on adrenergic receptors.
    E. Intermediate precursors of catecholamine synthesis have no effect on adrenergic receptors.

11. All of the following statements regarding autonomic receptors are true EXCEPT:

    A. Acetylcholine is the neurotransmitter in the PNS, at preganglionic receptors of the SNS, and at the neuromuscular junction.
    B. Muscarinic receptors in the myocardium are stimulated by acetylcholine and inhibit the release of norepinephrine.
    C. The two subdivisions of cholinergic receptors are muscarinic and nicotinic.
    D. Muscarinic stimulation causes tachycardia, inotropism, bronchodilation, and miosis.
    E. Nicotinic receptors are located in the SNS.

12. Which of the following statements regarding alpha receptors is TRUE?

    A. $Alpha_1$ receptors result in no positive inotropic effect on the myocardium.
    B. $Alpha_1$ receptors appear to be confined to the postsynaptic membrane, whereas $alpha_2$ receptors are located on presynaptic and postsynaptic membranes.
    C. Presynaptic $alpha_2$ receptors do not play a significant role in reducing sympathetic outflow.
    D. $Alpha_1$ agonists, such as phenylephrine, have an effect on coronary resistance by creating vasoconstriction and hence consistently contribute to coronary ischemia.
    E. Epinephrine is a more potent venoconstrictor than norepinephrine.

13. All of the following statements regarding beta-adrenergic receptors are true EXCEPT:

    A. Beta receptors are found in both presynaptic and postsynaptic membranes.
    B. Activation of the presynaptic β_2 receptor has the same physiologic response as antagonism of the presynaptic α_2 receptor.
    C. Postsynaptic $beta_2$ receptors are noninnervated and respond to circulating catecholamines.
    D. $Beta_2$ receptors are primarily located in myocardium, sinoatrial node, and ventricular conduction system.
    E. $Beta_1$ receptors are innervated receptors responding to neuronally released norepinephrine.

14. Which of the following statements regarding beta receptors in the heart and in peripheral vessels is FALSE?

    A. Both $beta_1$ and $beta_2$ receptors are coupled to adenylate cyclase.
    B. Increased catecholamine levels in heart failure leads to a larger downregulation of $beta_2$ receptors compared with $beta_1$ receptors.
    C. The inotropic effect of epinephrine is mediated via $beta_1$ and $beta_2$ receptors, whereas the inotropic effect of norepinephrine is mediated entirely through $beta_1$ receptors.

   D. Postsynaptic beta$_1$ receptors are predominantly
      found in the myocardium, sinoatrial node,
      and ventricular conduction system. The
      beta$_2$ receptors have the same distribution
      but are presynaptic.
   E. Beta$_2$ receptors approximate 20 to 30% of beta
      receptors in the myocardium.

15. Which of the following statements regarding
    dopamine receptors is TRUE?

    A. Dopamine-1 receptors are located postsynaptically.
    B. Dopamine-2 receptors are located only
       presynaptically.
    C. Dopamine receptors have been located in the
       myocardium and are responsible for increased
       inotropism.
    D. Dopamine receptors inhibit the release of prolactin
       in the hypothalamus.
    E. Dopamine-1 receptors are located on vascular
       smooth muscle of the kidneys and mesentery, and
       produce vasoconstriction.

16. Which of the following statements regarding the
    baroreceptors is true?

    A. Impulses from the carotid sinus and aortic
       arch reach the vasomotor center through
       the hypoglossal and the vagal nerve,
       respectively.
    B. Increased sensory traffic from the baroreceptors
       caused by decreased blood pressure inhibits SNS
       effector traffic.
    C. The Valsalva maneuver can be used to identify
       patients at risk for ANS instability.
    D. Dysfunction in the SNS is suspected if prolonged
       hypertension develops during the forced
       expiration phase of the Valsalva maneuver.
    E. The absence of "overshoot" in blood pressure at
       the end of the Valsalva maneuver indicates
       dysfunction of the PSN.

*For questions 17 to 23, choose A if 1, 2, and 3 are correct;
B if 1 and 3; C if 2 and 4; D if 4; E if all.*

17. Which of the following is/are interactions of the ANS
    with endocrine regulatory systems?

    1. Release of antidiuretic hormone secondary to
       changes in plasma osmolality
    2. Alpha- or beta-receptor stimulation in the pancreas
    3. Release of renin from the juxtaglomerular
       apparatus
    4. Adrenal cortical function

18. Which of the following is/are mechanisms by which
    drugs may act on prejunctional membranes?

    1. Interference with transmitter synthesis
    2. Interference with transmitter storage
    3. Interference with transmitter release

    4. Interference with the shape or composition of the
       receptor

19. Features of ganglionic drugs include:

    1. nonselective drugs that affect both the SNS and the
       PNS
    2. unpredictable side effects that limit their
       usefulness
    3. nicotine as the prototypical agonist
    4. histamine release at low doses

20. Which of the following is/are properties of
    trimethaphan?

    1. It is a drug equivalent to nitroprusside.
    2. It has a short duration of action because of
       hydrolysis by pseudocholinesterase.
    3. It causes pupillary constriction
    4. It affects the ability of acetylcholine to bind to
       receptor sites.

21. Which of the following statements regarding
    cholinomimetic drugs is/are TRUE?

    1. There are three groups of these agents: esters,
       alkaloids, and anticholinesterases.
    2. The choline esters (acetylcholine, methacholine,
       carbamylcholine, bethanechol) make up the group
       of indirect agents.
    3. Acetylcholine has no therapeutic application
       because of its diffuse action and rapid
       hydrolysis.
    4. Choline esters other than acetylcholine are
       metabolized at a faster rate.

22. Which of the following statements regarding
    anticholinesterases is/are TRUE?

    1. All anticholinesterases are tertiary amines
       and therefore readily cross the blood-brain
       barrier.
    2. There are two types of anticholinesterase drugs:
       reversible and nonreversible.
    3. Physostigmine is a quaternary ammonium
       compound and has no central muscarinic
       stimulation.
    4. The two types of anticholinesterase agents are
       categorized by their site of inhibition.

23. Which of the following statements regarding
    anticholinesterase is/are true?

    1. Most of the indirect-acting drugs inhibit both
       cholinesterase and pseudocholinesterase.
    2. Muscarinic activity is evoked at higher
       concentrations than are necessary to produce the
       desired nicotinic effect.
    3. Excess accumulation of acetylcholine at the motor
       end plate produces a depolarizing block similar to
       succinylcholine or high doses of nicotine.
    4. Edrophonium is an esteratic drug (works on the
       esteratic site of cholinesterase).

ANSWERS

1. **B.** The preganglionic fibers originate from T1–T12 and L1–L3 in the gray intermediolateral column. These fibers are myelinated nerve axons that leave the spinal cord with the motor fibers to form the white communicating rami. These fibers enter the 22 paired sympathetic ganglia. Once entering these ganglia, the fibers may take three possible courses: they may synapse with postganglionic fibers in the ganglion, they can move up and down the SNS to another ganglion, or they can track through the sympathetic chain and exit without synapsing to SNS collateral ganglia. The exception to this rule is the group of myelinated fibers that terminate in the adrenal medulla without first synapsing in a ganglion. Many of the postganglionic fibers pass from the lateral SNS chain back into the spinal nerves, to form the gray (unmyelinated) communicating rami at all levels of the spinal cord. They are distributed distally to sweat glands, pilomotor muscle, and blood vessels of the skin and muscle. (See page 278: Sympathetic Nervous System or Thoracolumbar Division.)

2. **C.** Postganglionic neuronal cell bodies of the SNS are located in the paired lateral ganglia or unpaired collateral ganglia. The celiac and inferior mesenteric ganglia are considered to be collateral ganglia. SNS ganglia are located primarily near the spinal cord, rather than near the organs they innervate. The postganglionic fibers are unmyelinated. The average somatic nerve has approximately 8% sympathetic fibers. (See page 278: Sympathetic Nervous System or Thoracolumbar Division.)

3. **A.** The first four to five thoracic segments' preganglionic fibers form three specialized paired ganglia. These are the superior cervical, middle cervical, and cervicothoracic ganglia. The latter is known as the stellate ganglion. It is a fusion of the inferior cervical and first thoracic SNS ganglia. This provides sympathetic innervation to the head, neck, upper extremity, heart, and lungs. The response from sympathetic system activation is diffuse. The preganglionic neurons are fewer than the postganglionic neurons. Hence, preganglionic fibers influence a number of postganglionic neurons. (See page 278: Sympathetic Nervous System or Thoracolumbar Division.)

4. **D.** The PNS consists of preganglionic and postganglionic neurons. The preganglionic nerve fibers originate in cranial nerves III (oculomotor), VII (facial), IX (glossopharyngeal), and X (vagus) nerves. In addition, fibers originate from the intermediolateral horn of second, third, and fourth sacral nerves. Preganglionic nerve fibers pass directly to the organ that is innervated. Postganglionic neurons are located in or near the organ to be innervated. Therefore, postganglionic innervation is limited, and responses are discrete. Cranial nerve X (vagus) accounts for 75% of the PNS activity. The ratio of postganglionic to preganglionic fibers in many organs appears to be 1:1 to 3:1, compared with the 20:1 found in the SNS system. (See page 280: Parasympathetic Nervous System or Craniosacral Division.)

5. **D.** The heart is well supplied by both the SNS and PNS. These fibers are responsible for changing rate of the heart (chronotropism), changing strength of contraction (inotropism), and modulating coronary blood flow. PNS innervation is to the sinoatrial and atrioventricular nodes. There is no PNS supply to the ventricles. (See page 280: Autonomic Innervation: Heart.)

6. **C.** The SNS is the predominant regulator of the peripheral circulation; PNS innervation is minimal. SNS can cause vasodilation or vasoconstriction, depending on receptor activity. Distribution of the SNS is not equal among all organs. Skin, kidney, spleen, and mesentery have extensive SNS distribution, as opposed to the heart, brain, and muscles, which have less. Vascular tone is highly influenced by local factors such as metabolites and hormones. Blood vessels have differing sensitivities to local or neurogenic tone. Local autoregulation is predominantly at precapillary and postcapillary sphincters. (See page 281: Peripheral Circulation.)

7. **C.** The SNS and PNS are designated as adrenergic and cholinergic, respectively. In the PNS, acetylcholine is secreted at the postganglionic receptor site. In the SNS, norepinephrine is the main neurotransmitter at postganglionic sites, with the exception of sweat glands. The preganglionic neurotransmitter for both PNS and SNS is acetylcholine. The postganglionic fibers of both the SNS and PNS are anatomically and physiologically alike. The terminals branch out into terminal effector plexuses. One terminal will branch to thousands of effector cells. The terminal ending is called a varicosity. Each varicosity contains vesicles within which the neurotransmitter is stored. (See page 281: Autonomic Nervous System: Neurotransmission; page 282: Parasympathetic Nervous System Neurotransmission; and page 282: Sympathetic Nervous System Neurotransmission.)

8. **B.** Acetylcholine was once thought to be the only neurotransmitter; however, it now is believed that vasoactive intestinal peptide may play a role as a secondary neurotransmitter. Acetylcholine is formed within the presynaptic membrane by acetylation of choline with acetylcoenzyme. This process is catalyzed

by choline acetyltransferase. The active product of this reaction, acetylcholine, is stored in presynaptic vesicles. The depolarization of the end plate results in mass quantum release of acetylcholine into the synaptic cleft. This release is dependent on calcium influx. Drugs that alter calcium influx may decrease the release of acetylcholine. Acetylcholine is removed by rapid hydrolysis by the enzyme acetylcholinesterase. This enzyme is found in neurons, at the neuromuscular junction, and in various other tissues of the body. A similar enzyme, pseudocholinesterase or plasma cholinesterase, is also found throughout the body but only to a limited extent in nervous tissue. It does not appear to be physiologically important in termination of the action of acetylcholine. Both acetylcholinesterase and pseudocholinesterase hydrolyze acetylcholine as well as other esters (such as the ester-type local anesthetics), but they may be distinguished by specific biochemical tests. (See page 282: Parasympathetic Nervous System Neurotransmission; and page 282: Metabolism.)

9. **E.** Epinephrine and norepinephrine are mediators of SNS peripheral activity. Adenosine triphosphate (ATP) may be an additional neurotransmitter. In the adrenal medulla, acetylcholine is the primary neurotransmitter at the preganglionic site. It causes release of norepinephrine and epinephrine from the chromaffin cells. These cells are considered the postganglionic neurons. Stimulation of the adrenal medulla results in massive release of epinephrine and norepinephrine, which lasts 10 times as long as local direct stimulation. Epinephrine release is greater in proportion to norepinephrine release. (See page 282: Sympathetic Nervous System Neurotransmission.)

10. **C.** A catecholamine is a compound consisting of a catechol nucleus and amine site chain. Endogenous catecholamines are dopamine, norepinephrine, and epinephrine. Epinephrine is the precursor of norepinephrine synthesis and has an effect on adrenergic receptor sites. Dopamine is the primary neurotransmitter of the brain. The brain contains both noradrenergic and dopaminergic receptors. Catecholamines may have a direct or indirect effect on receptors. The indirect effect is mediated through the release of stored neurotransmitter. Direct effects are independent of norepinephrine release. Some drugs may have a mixed mode of action. The brain contains both noradrenergic and dopaminergic receptors, but circulating catecholamines do not cross the blood-brain barrier. The catecholamines present in the brain are synthesized there. (See page 283: Catecholamines: The First Messenger.)

11. **D.** Acetylcholine is neurotransmitter at three classes of receptors. The first is in the PNS. The second and third are located in ganglia of SNS and in the neuromuscular junction of striated muscle. Cholinergic receptors are subdivided into muscarinic

and nicotinic receptors. Nicotinic receptors are located at the preganglionic receptors of the SNS. PNS muscarinic stimulation causes bradycardia, decreased inotropism, bronchoconstriction, miosis, salivation, gastrointestinal hypermotility, and increased gastric acid secretion. Muscarinic receptors are known to exist in sites other than PNS postganglionic junctions. They are found on the presynaptic membrane of sympathetic nerve terminals in the myocardium, coronary vessels, and peripheral vasculature. These are referred to as adrenergic muscarinic receptors because of their location; however, they are stimulated by acetylcholine. Stimulation of these receptors inhibits release of norepinephrine in a manner similar to alpha$_2$ receptor stimulation. (See page 285: Receptors.)

12. **B.** Alpha$_1$ Receptors are believed to have a positive inotropic effect on cardiac tissues in most mammals. Enhanced alpha$_1$ activity may play a role in malignant arrhythmia. Drugs such as prazosin may have antiarrhythmic properties. Alpha$_2$ receptors are located at both the presynaptic and postsynaptic membranes. The alpha$_1$ receptors are located postsynaptically. The ratio of postsynaptic alpha$_1$ to alpha$_2$ receptors is approximately 1:1. Alpha$_2$ presynaptic receptors play a significant role in reducing sympathetic outflow. This results in decreases in systemic vascular resistance, cardiac output, and heart rate. In the CNS, these receptors may contribute to analgesia and sedation. Alpha$_1$ receptors in the epicardial vessels only contribute 5% of the total resistance in the normal coronary circulation. Therefore, phenylephrine probably has minimal effect on coronary resistance. Norepinephrine is the most potent venoconstrictor. (See page 287: Alpha-Adrenergic Receptors.)

13. **D.** Beta$_1$ and beta$_2$ are the two subtypes of beta-adrenergic receptors. Beta$_1$ receptors are located in the myocardium, sinoatrial node, and ventricular conduction system. They are innervated and respond to neuronally released norepinephrine. Beta$_1$ receptors are located only postsynaptically. Beta presynaptic receptors are mostly of the beta$_2$ type. The effects of activation of presynaptic beta$_2$ receptors are diametrically opposed to alpha$_2$ presynaptic receptors. Beta$_2$ presynaptic receptors accelerate endogenous norepinephrine release. Antagonism of these receptors results in a physiologic response that is similar to activation of the beta$_2$ presynaptic receptor. (See page 291: Beta-Adrenergic Receptors.)

14. **B.** Both beta$_1$ and beta$_2$ receptors are functionally coupled to adenylate cyclase, a finding suggesting a similar involvement in the regulation of inotropism and chronotropism. Postsynaptic beta$_1$ receptors are distributed predominantly to the myocardium, the sinoatrial node, and the ventricular conduction system. The beta$_2$ receptors have the same distribution but are presynaptic. Activation of the

presynaptic beta$_2$ receptor accelerates the release of norepinephrine into the synaptic cleft. The beta$_2$ receptor approximates 20 to 30% of the beta receptors in the ventricular myocardium and up to 40% of the beta receptors in the atrium.

The effect of norepinephrine on inotropism in the normal heart is mediated entirely through the postsynaptic beta$_1$ receptor, whereas the inotropic effects of ephedrine are mediated through both the beta$_1$ and beta$_2$ myocardial receptors. (See page: 291: Beta Receptors in the Cardiovascular System.)

15. **A.**   Dopamine receptors are of two types, dopamine-1 and dopamine-2. Type 1 receptors are located postsynaptically; type 2 receptors are located both presynaptically and postsynaptically. Dopamine receptors have not been located in the myocardium. They are located in the hypothalamus where they enhance the release of prolactin. They also are located in the basal ganglia where they coordinate motor function. Dopamine receptors in the smooth muscle of the kidneys and mesentery produce vasodilation, resulting in increased blood flow to these organs. (See page 291: Dopaminergic Receptors.)

16. **C.**   Impulses from the carotid sinus and aortic arch reach the medullary vasomotor center by the glossopharyngeal and vagus nerves, respectively. Increased sensory traffic from the baroreceptors, caused by increased blood pressure, inhibits SNS effector traffic. The relative increase in vagal tone produces vasodilation, slowing of the heart rate, and a lowering of blood pressure. Real increases in vagal tone occur when blood pressure exceeds normal limits. The arterial baroreceptor reflex can best be demonstrated by the Valsalva maneuver. The arterial blood pressure rises momentarily as the intrathoracic blood is forced into the heart (preload). Sustained intrathoracic pressure diminishes venous return, reduces the cardiac output, and drops the blood pressure. Reflex vasoconstriction and tachycardia ensue. Blood pressure returns to normal with release of the forced expiration, but then briefly "overshoots" because of the vasoconstriction and increased venous return. A slowing of the heart rate accompanies the overshoot in pressure. The Valsalva maneuver has been used to identify patients at risk for ANS instability. Dysfunction of the SNS is implicated if exaggerated and prolonged hypotension develops during the forced expiration phase. In addition, the overshoot at the end of the Valsalva maneuver is absent. (See page 293: Baroreceptors.)

17. **E.**   The ANS is related to several endocrine systems that control blood pressure and homeostasis. Antidiuretic hormone is secreted by the hypothalamus in response to changes in plasma osmolality. However, many factors, such as stress, pain, hypoxia, anesthesia, and surgery, may stimulate release of antidiuretic hormone. Beta stimulation of the pancreas increases insulin release, whereas alpha stimulation decreases it.

The complex renin-angiotensin system modulates blood pressure and water and electrolyte homeostasis. Renin release from the juxtaglomerular complex acts on plasma angiotensinogen II, a potent vasoconstrictor. The ANS also is closely linked to adrenocortical function; glucocorticoids modulate epinephrine synthesis. (See page 295: Interaction With Other Regulatory Systems.)

18. **A.**   Drugs interact at the prejunctional membrane by a number of different mechanisms, which include interfering with transmitter synthesis, storage, release, or reuptake or modifying neurotransmitter metabolism. Drugs acting at postjunctional sites may directly stimulate postjunctional receptors and interfere with transmitter agonist at postjunctional receptors. (See page 296: Mode of Action.)

19. **A.**   Autonomic ganglia are similar in that acetylcholine is the primary neurotransmitter in both the PNS and the SNS. Most ganglionic drugs are nonselective. This property makes them undesirable and unpredictable and thus limits their clinical usefulness. Nicotine is the prototypical agonist. It stimulates autonomic ganglia and the neuromuscular junction at low concentrations. In high doses, it creates blockade. (See page 296: Ganglionic Drugs.)

20. **C.**   Trimethaphan is the only ganglionic blocker currently available in the United States. It affects the ability of acetylcholine to bind to receptor sites. Its side effects and short duration of action limit its usefulness, and tachyphylaxis develops quickly. Pupillary dilation limits its use in neurosurgical patients. It is not equivalent to nitroprusside. (See page 296: Antagonists.)

21. **B.**   Cholinomimetic drugs act where acetylcholine is a neurotransmitter. There are three groups of cholinergic drugs. The first two groups, which are direct muscarinic agents, are the choline esters (acetylcholine, methacholine, carbamylcholine, bethanechol) and the alkaloids (pilocarpine, muscarine, arecoline). The third group consists of the indirect-acting agents: the anticholinesterases (physostigmine, neostigmine, pyridostigmine, edrophonium, echothiophate). Acetylcholine has a diffuse action and is rapidly hydrolyzed; therefore, it has no therapeutic applications. Other choline esters are more resistant to inactivation and therefore are more clinically useful. (See page 297: Muscarinic Agonists.)

22. **C.**   Anticholinesterase drugs are classified as reversible and nonreversible. They are divided into two different types based on the site of inhibition on the cholinesterase enzyme. Agents that inhibit at the esteratic site are called acid transferring inhibitors. These drugs are long acting (physostigmine, neostigmine, pyridostigmine). Drugs acting at the

anionic site are called prosthetic, competitive inhibitors. These drugs tend to be short acting (edrophonium). Physostigmine is a tertiary amine and therefore crosses the blood-brain barrier. It is useful for reversing atropine poisoning, but it is not useful for reversing neuromuscular blockade. (See page 297: Indirect Cholinomimetics.)

23. **B.** The indirect-acting cholinomimetic drugs are of greater importance to the anesthesiologist than are the direct-acting drugs. These drugs produce cholinomimetic effects indirectly as a result of inhibition or inactivation of the enzyme acetylcholinesterase, which normally destroys acetylcholine by hydrolysis. They are referred to as cholinesterase inhibitors or anticholinesterases. Most of these drugs inhibit both acetylcholinesterase and pseudocholinesterase. The most prominent pharmacologic effects of the anticholinesterase drugs are muscarinic. Their most useful actions are their nicotinic effects. Muscarinic activity is evoked by lower concentrations of acetylcholine than are necessary to produce the desired nicotinic effect. For example, the anticholinesterase neostigmine reverses neuromuscular blockade by increasing acetylcholine concentration at the muscle end plate, a nicotinic receptor. Nicotinic reversal of neuromuscular blockade can usually be produced safely only when the patient has been protected by atropine or other muscarinic blockers. This prevents the untoward muscarinic effects of bradycardia, hypotension, bronchospasm, or intestinal spasm. Conversely, neuromuscular paralysis may be produced or increased if excessive anticholinesterase is used. Excess accumulation of acetylcholine at the motor end plates produces a depolarizing block similar to that produced by succinylcholine or nicotine. The differences in duration of various anticholinesterases apparently depend on whether they inhibit the anionic or esteratic site of acetylcholinesterase. Therefore, the anticholinesterase drugs have also been pharmacologically subdivided. Drugs that inhibit the anionic site are called competitive inhibitors. Their action is the result of competition between the anticholinesterase and acetylcholine for the anionic site. These drugs tend to be short acting. Edrophonium is an example of this type. (See page 297: Indirect Cholinomimetics.)

CHAPTER 13 ■ NONOPIOID INTRAVENOUS ANESTHESIA

1. The rapid onset of the central nervous system (CNS) effects of most intravenous anesthetics is best explained by their:

   A. low hepatic extraction ratio
   B. small volume of distribution
   C. high lipid solubility
   D. large ratio of ionized to unionized drug
   E. slow elimination half-life

2. Ketamine interacts with all of the following receptors EXCEPT:

   A. N-methyl-D-aspartate (NMDA)
   B. opioid
   C. gamma-aminobutyric acid (GABA)
   D. muscarinic
   E. monoaminergic

3. Which of the following intravenous anesthetic agents has the highest degree of plasma protein binding?

   A. Thiopental
   B. Propofol
   C. Ketamine
   D. Methohexital
   E. Etomidate

4. Which of the following has the lowest hepatic extraction ratio?

   A. Ketamine
   B. Propofol
   C. Thiopental
   D. Midazolam
   E. Etomidate

5. Recovery of cognitive function following general anesthesia is slowest when which of the following agents is used for induction?

   A. Thiopental
   B. Propofol
   C. Midazolam

D. Etomidate
E. Ketamine

6. Concerning the antiemetic effect of propofol, all of the following hypotheses have been postulated EXCEPT:

   A. It has antidopaminergic activity.
   B. It has a depressant effect on the chemoreceptor trigger zone.
   C. It increases the release of glutamate and aspartate in the olfactory cortex.
   D. It decreases the concentration of serotonin in the area postrema.
   E. It has a depressant effect on the vagal nucleus.

7. Context-sensitive half-time describes:

   A. the rate of fall of drug concentration at the effect site following discontinuation of continuous infusion
   B. the rate of fall of drug concentration in the bloodstream following discontinuation of continuous infusion
   C. the rate of fall of drug concentration in the body following discontinuation of continuous infusion
   D. the rate of fall of drug concentration in its volume of distribution following discontinuation of continuous infusion
   E. the rate of fall of drug concentration in the liver following discontinuation of continuous infusion

8. The involuntary myoclonus seen during induction with etomidate is:

   A. not associated with cortical seizure activity
   B. unaffected by prior administration of opioid analgesics
   C. unaffected by prior administration of benzodiazepines
   D. extremely uncommon
   E. best treated with intravenous phenytoin

9. Rank the following induction agents in order of their degree of cardiovascular depression.

   A. Propofol > etomidate > thiopental
   B. Thiopental > propofol > etomidate
   C. Propofol > thiopental > etomidate
   D. Etomidate > thiopental > propofol
   E. Thiopental > etomidate > propofol

10. Which of the following statements concerning the mechanisms of action of intravenous induction agents is NOT true?

    A. Barbiturates appear to increase the duration of GABA-activated opening of chloride ion channels.
    B. Benzodiazepines appear to increase the efficiency of coupling between GABA receptors and chloride ion channels.
    C. Ketamine produces dissociative amnesia through interaction with NMDA receptors.
    D. Thiopental appears to act as a competitive inhibitor at central nicotinic acetylcholine receptors.
    E. Propofol appears to have a mechanism of action similar to that of the benzodiazepines.

11. Which of the following is NOT a typical induction regimen for a healthy adult patient?

    A. Etomidate 0.3 to 0.6 mg/kg
    B. Ketamine 0.5 to 1.0 mg/kg
    C. Methohexital 3 to 5 mg/kg
    D. Midazolam 0.1 to 0.2 mg/kg
    E. Propofol 1.5 to 2.5 mg/kg

12. Ketamine is associated with all of the following physiologic effects EXCEPT:

    A. bronchodilation
    B. elevation of intracranial pressure
    C. decreased oral secretions
    D. sympathetic stimulation
    E. increased pulmonary artery pressure

13. Which of the following induction agents may facilitate the interpretation of somatosensory evoked potentials?

    A. Ketamine
    B. Propofol
    C. Methohexital
    D. Midazolam
    E. Etomidate

14. For which of the following patients would ketamine be LEAST appropriate as an induction agent?

    A. A 39-year-old woman with acute asthma exacerbation who is undergoing emergency appendectomy
    B. A 70-year-old woman with cardiac tamponade who is undergoing emergency thoracotomy
    C. A 50-year-old woman with glaucoma who is scheduled for elective cataract resection

    D. A 55-year-old man with mild renal insufficiency who is undergoing sigmoid resection for diverticulitis
    E. A 7-year-old child without intravenous access who is scheduled for elective tonsillectomy

For questions 15 to 24, choose A if 1, 2, and 3 are correct; B if 1 and 3; C if 2 and 4; D if 4; E if all.

15. TRUE statements about the use of propofol for sedation include:

    1. It produces more reliable amnesia than midazolam.
    2. It has little effect on hypoxic ventilatory response.
    3. It is the drug of choice for patients with hemodynamic instability.
    4. It allows for relatively rapid transitions from deeper to lighter levels of anesthesia.

16. Which of the following statements concerning the pharmacology of intravenous induction agents is/are TRUE?

    1. At typical clinical concentrations, the rate of drug elimination is described by zero-order kinetics.
    2. Termination of initial CNS effects is primarily the result of drug redistribution.
    3. At high steady-state plasma concentrations, the rate of drug elimination will decrease as the exponential function of the drug's plasma concentration.
    4. They typically undergo hepatic metabolism followed by renal excretion.

17. Which of the following statements concerning intravenous anesthetic agents in elderly patients compared with younger adults is/are TRUE?

    1. Redistribution from vessel-rich tissue compartments is slower.
    2. The steady-state volume of distribution is reduced.
    3. The rate of hepatic clearance is reduced.
    4. There is a decreased volume of the central compartment.

18. Which of the following statements concerning methohexital is/are TRUE?

    1. It is an oxybarbiturate.
    2. It is associated with a more profound degree of hypotension compared with thiopental.
    3. It can be used to evoke epileptic activity in patients with temporal lobe epilepsy.
    4. It is approximately one-third as potent at thiopental.

19. Accidental intra-arterial injection of barbiturates is commonly treated with:

    1. intra-arterial administration of papaverine
    2. intra-arterial administration of lidocaine
    3. heparinization
    4. tourniquet application to the affected limb

20. Concerning propofol, which of the following statements is/are TRUE?

    1. It is a reasonable induction agent for the malignant hyperthermia-susceptible patient.
    2. It can be used safely in a patient with a history of acute intermittent porphyria.
    3. It can be used to decrease the pruritus associated with administration of intrathecal opioids.
    4. Its effects are usually prolonged in patients with pre-existing hepatic disease.

21. Which of the following statements concerning etomidate is/are TRUE?

    1. It does not stimulate histamine release.
    2. It induces involuntary myoclonic movements, which can be attenuated by prior administration of opioid analgesics.
    3. It is associated with a high incidence of postoperative nausea and vomiting.
    4. A single induction dose does not cause any measurable adrenal suppression.

22. Which of the following statements concerning the cardiovascular effects of propofol is/are TRUE?

    1. It causes arterial dilation.
    2. It increases peripheral venous pooling.
    3. It impairs the baroreceptor reflex response.
    4. It is not a direct myocardial depressant.

23. Which of the following statements regarding the structure and metabolism of intravenous induction agents is/are correct?

    1. Pentobarbital is a potential metabolite of thiopental that can cause long-lasting CNS-depressant activity.
    2. Thiopental solution (2.5%) is highly acidic.
    3. The hydroxyl derivative of methohexital is inactive.
    4. The analgesic and anesthetic potency of the S(+) isomer of ketamine is less than that of the racemic mixture.

24. Which of the following intravenous agents has intrinsic analgesic properties?

    1. Ketamine
    2. Dexmedetomidine
    3. Clonidine
    4. Thiopental

ANSWERS

1. **C.** The rapid onset of intravenous anesthetics is primarily attributable to their high lipid solubility and the relatively high proportion of the cardiac output that perfuses the brain. Only the unionized fraction of a drug can cross the blood-brain barrier, hence onset is also affected by the pKa of the drug relative to the pH of body fluids; onset is also more rapid when the ratio of unionized to ionized drug is high. Although volume of distribution, elimination half-life, and hepatic extraction ratio contribute to drug pharmacokinetics, these factors are not primarily responsible for the rapid onset of anesthetic effects. (See page 335: General Pharmacology of Intravenous Hypnotics.)

2. **C.** Ketamine interacts with NMDA, opioid, muscarinic, and monoaminergic receptors, but it does not interact with GABA receptors. This is in contrast to most intravenous anesthetics, which exert their primary effect through GABA receptors. (See page 344: Ketamine.)

3. **B.** Approximately 98% of propofol is protein bound, whereas about 85% of the barbiturates methohexital and thiopental bind to protein, and 75% of etomidate is protein bound. In contrast, only about 12% of ketamine is protein bound. (See page 336: Pharmacokinetics and Metabolism.)

4. **C.** The hepatic extraction ratio is a measure of the rate at which anesthetics are cleared from the systemic circulation by the liver. The hepatic clearance of intravenous anesthetics may be categorized into three groups: high, intermediate, and low. Thiopental, diazepam, and lorazepam have low hepatic extraction ratios, whereas propofol, etomidate, and ketamine have high hepatic extraction ratios. Methohexital and midazolam have hepatic extraction ratios intermediate between these two groups. (See page 336: Pharmacokinetics and Metabolism.)

5. **C.** In general, benzodiazepines such as midazolam are associated with relatively prolonged time to recovery of cognitive function compared with other intravenous anesthetics. In contrast, recovery from propofol is usually quite rapid, making it an ideal induction agent for outpatient procedures. Recovery from ketamine, etomidate, and thiopental is somewhere intermediate between the benzodiazepines and propofol. (See page 346: Use of Intravenous Anesthetics as Induction Agents.)

6. **C.** Propofol has antidopaminergic activity and depresses the chemoreceptor trigger zone and vagal nucleus. It also decreases the release of glutamate and aspartate in the olfactory cortex and reduces

serotonin levels in the area postrema. All of these mechanisms are believed to contribute to propofol's antiemetic properties. (See page 341: Propofol.)

7. **A.** Context-sensitive half-time is defined as the time necessary for the effect-compartment concentration of drug to decrease by 50% following discontinuation of continuous infusion. (See page 336: Pharmacokinetics and Metabolism.)

8. **A.** A common reaction to induction with etomidate is involuntary myoclonic movements, which occur as a result of subcortical disinhibition. This response is not associated with cortical seizure activity and may be attenuated by prior administration of opioid analgesics or benzodiazepines. The use of antiseizure drugs such as phenytoin is not indicated. (See page 344: Etomidate.)

9. **C.** The cardiovascular effects of propofol are more profound than those of thiopental or etomidate. Etomidate is the induction agent considered to have the least impact on the cardiovascular system. (See page 340: Comparative Physio-chemical and Clinical Pharmacologic Properties.)

10. **E.** Propofol appears to increase the duration of GABA-mediating chloride channel opening. Therefore, its mechanism of action is most similar to that of the barbiturates, not the benzodiazepines. However, benzodiazepines also act via the GABA receptor, increasing the efficiency of coupling between the GABA receptor and chloride ion channels. Thiopental is believed to exert its effect via competitive inhibition of nicotinic acetylcholine receptors in the CNS, whereas ketamine acts via NMDA receptors. (See page 335: General Pharmacology of Intravenous Hypnotics.)

11. **C.** The typical induction dose of methohexital is 1 to 1.5 mg/kg IV. All of the other choices represent typical induction drug dosages. (See page 340: Comparative Physio-chemical and Clinical Pharmacologic Properties.)

12. **C.** Ketamine is a sympathetic stimulant that increases peripheral arteriolar resistance, arterial blood pressure, heart rate, and pulmonary artery pressure. It also possesses bronchodilatory activity. In contrast to the other commonly used intravenous induction agents, ketamine increases cerebral blood flow, cerebral metabolic oxygen demand, and intracranial and intraocular pressures. Ketamine also increases oral secretions. Therefore, pretreatment with an antisialogogue is sometimes useful. (See page 344: Ketamine.)

13. **E.** Etomidate increases the amplitude of somatosensory evoked potentials and can be useful in the interpretation of somatosensory evoked potentials when signal quality is poor. (See page 344: Etomidate.)

14. **C.** Ketamine raises intraocular pressure and would therefore not be an appropriate induction agent in a patient with glaucoma. Ketamine is a sympathetic stimulant and has bronchodilatory effects. These properties make it a useful agent in a carefully defined subset of patients, such as those with acute bronchospasm, hypovolemic shock, right-to-left intracardiac shunts, and cardiac tamponade. Ketamine may be delivered intramuscularly in patients without intravenous access. (See page 344: Ketamine.)

15. **D.** Propofol is associated with relatively rapid recovery, facilitating transitions from deeper to lighter levels of anesthesia. In the intensive care unit setting, when compared with midazolam, propofol sedation has been associated with more rapid weaning from artificial ventilation. However, propofol produces less reliable amnesia and more pain on injection than midazolam. In addition, even at low concentrations, propofol depresses the normal hypoxic ventilatory response, and therefore supplemental oxygen should always be used in conjunction with propofol sedation. (See page 341: Propofol.)

16. **C.** Termination of the central effects of intravenous anesthetics is primarily related to redistribution from the brain, rather than elimination from the body. Most intravenous agents undergo hepatic metabolism into water-soluble compounds that are then excreted by the kidneys. At typical clinical concentrations, the rate of drug elimination decreases as the exponential function of the drug's plasma concentration—so-called first-order kinetics. However, at high steady-state concentrations, the rate of drug elimination becomes independent of drug concentration resulting from saturation of enzymes responsible for their metabolism—zero-order kinetics. (See page 336: Pharmacokinetics and Metabolism.)

17. **E.** Elderly patients have an increase in the steady-state volume of distribution of most intravenous anesthetics. They also have decreased hepatic clearance, decreased volume of the central compartment, and slower redistribution from vessel-rich tissue to intermediate compartments. As a result, the dose of anesthetic required to elicit effect is lower and the time to recovery is longer in elderly patients compared with younger patients. (See page 336: Pharmacokinetics and Metabolism.)

18. **B.** Methohexital is an oxybarbiturate that is two to three times more potent than thiopental. Compared with thiopental, it produces a relatively more robust tachycardic response, leading to a lesser degree of hypotension. Methohexital can produce epileptiform electroencephalographic (EEG) activity and is used to activate cortical EEG seizure discharges in patients

with temporal lobe epilepsy. (See page 340: Barbiturates.)

19. **A.** Treatments for accidental intra-arterial injection of thiobarbiturates include intra-arterial administration of papaverine and/or lidocaine, heparinization, and/or regional anesthesia–induced sympathectomy. Isolation of regional blood flow via tourniquet application is not appropriate. (See page 340: Barbiturates.)

20. **A.** Propofol is a reasonable induction agent in the patient who is susceptible to malignant hyperthermia, and it can be used safely in patients with acute intermittent porphyria. Propofol also decreases the pruritus associated with intrathecal opioids as well as cholestatic liver disease. Even though propofol is metabolized by the liver, its effects are generally not prolonged in patients with pre-existing hepatic disease. (See page 341: Propofol.)

21. **A.** Etomidate sometimes induces nonepileptogenic involuntary myoclonus during induction that can be attenuated by the preinduction use of an opioid analgesic. In addition, it is associated with a high incidence of postoperative nausea and vomiting and has been shown to depress adrenocortical function for several hours following a single induction dose. Etomidate does not induce histamine release and can be safely used in patients with reactive airway disease. (See page 344: Etomidate.)

22. **A.** Propofol causes arterial and venous dilatation as well as impairment of the baroreceptor reflex, all of which contribute to a decrease in systemic arterial pressure. In addition, propofol has myocardial depressant effects. All of these factors contribute to the decrease in systemic arterial pressure commonly observed following propofol induction. These cardiovascular effects are more profound than those associated with thiopental or etomidate. (See page 341: Propofol.)

23. **B.** Thiopental is metabolized in the liver to hydroxythiopental and a carboxylic acid derivative. However, at high doses, thiopental undergoes a desulfuration reaction that leads to the production of pentobarbital, a compound associated with long-lasting CNS depression. Methohexital is metabolized in the liver to inactive hydroxyderivates. Thiopental is available in a 2.5% solution that is highly alkalotic (pH >9), and as such, inadvertent extravenous injection causes tissue irritation. The anesthetic and analgesic potency of the S(+) isomer of ketamine is greater than that of the racemic mixture. (See page 340: Comparative Physio-chemical and Clinical Pharmacologic Properties.)

24. **A.** Ketamine, dexmedetomidine, and the alpha$_2$ agonist clonidine appear to possess analgesic properties. In contrast, thiopental appears to have a mild antianalgesic effect. (See page 338: Pharmacodynamic Effects.)

CHAPTER 14 ■ OPIOIDS

1. All of the following statements regarding opioid-receptor interactions are true EXCEPT:

   A. The analgesic effects of opioids are thought to result primarily from the activation of μ receptors in the brain and spinal cord.
   B. Opioid-receptor activation in peripheral tissues may play a role in the modulation of painful stimuli.
   C. Naloxone is highly specific for the μ subtype of opioid receptors.
   D. Most opioids clinically used are highly selective for the μ subtype opioid receptor.
   E. Opioid receptors are coupled to G proteins that regulate the activity of adenylate cyclase.

2. Which of the following statements regarding opioid-induced muscle rigidity is/are TRUE?

   A. Muscle rigidity does not occur with morphine doses <0.2 mg/kg.
   B. The phenomenon is seen only on induction of anesthesia without the utilization of neuromuscular blocking agents.
   C. Muscle rigidity is reduced by the addition of nitrous oxide.
   D. The effects are eliminated by naloxone.
   E. Opioid-induced muscle rigidity is mediated by sigma receptors.

3. Which of the following routes of opioid administration reliably reduces the incidence of opioid-induced nausea?

   A. Intramuscular
   B. Intrathecal
   C. Subcutaneous
   D. Transdermal
   E. None of the above

4. A 46-year-old man with a history of multiple uneventful general anesthetics is undergoing a spinal fusion procedure during which morphine 1 mg/kg is administered over 15 minutes. Shortly thereafter, the patient exhibits modest hypotension with a concomitant decrease in systemic vascular resistance, as well as an increase in pulmonary vascular resistance as measured by a pulmonary artery catheter. These findings are unaffected by the administration of naloxone 0.2 mg. The most likely cause of this clinical constellation is:

   A. morphine-induced histamine release
   B. previously undiagnosed anaphylaxis
   C. an opioid-mediated increase in vascular permeability
   D. central vagotonic effects of morphine
   E. direct myocardial depression by morphine

5. The occurrence of myoclonic activity and seizures observed after repeated or prolonged administration of meperidine is most likely the result of:

   A. direct central nervous system (CNS) effects resulting from the inherent local anesthetic actions of meperidine
   B. direct CNS excitation by meperidine
   C. neurotoxic effects of normeperidine, an active metabolite of meperidine
   D. insidious hypoxemia as a consequence of the prolonged clinical half-life of meperidine
   E. selective activation of spinal kappa receptors with increasing serum levels of meperidine

6. Which physical characteristic of fentanyl best accounts for its rapid onset of clinical effect as well as its brief duration of action?

   A. High lipid solubility
   B. High degree of ionization
   C. Relatively small molecular weight
   D. Negligible protein binding
   E. Low hepatic clearance

7. All of the following statements regarding clinical characteristics of alfentanil are true EXCEPT:

   A. On a milligram basis, the clinical potency of alfentanil is roughly 10 times that of morphine and one-tenth that of fentanyl.
   B. Alfentanil displays a significantly faster onset of action when compared with fentanyl or sufentanil.
   C. Alfentanil has a longer terminal half-life than fentanyl or sufentanil.
   D. The incidence of nausea and vomiting associated with alfentanil is no higher than that with either fentanyl or sufentanil.
   E. Like fentanyl and sufentanil, alfentanil may produce profound muscle rigidity when it is given in high doses.

8. Remifentanil exhibits a markedly shorter clinical duration of action when compared with other commonly used opioids because of:

   A. rapid redistribution resulting from high lipid solubility
   B. a lesser degree of opioid receptor affinity
   C. a high protein-bound (alpha$_1$-acid glycoprotein) fraction
   D. a relatively high volume of distribution
   E. metabolism of an ester side chain by blood and tissue esterases

9. All of the following statements regarding nalbuphine are true EXCEPT:

   A. The analgesic properties of nalbuphine exhibit a ceiling effect.
   B. Nalbuphine can be as effective as full mu agonists in providing postoperative analgesia in some instances.
   C. Significant respiratory depression is not seen with nalbuphine.
   D. Nalbuphine may be used to antagonize the respiratory depressant effects of another opioid while still providing analgesia.
   E. Nalbuphine may precipitate withdrawal symptoms in patients who are physically dependent on opioids.

10. Which of the following characteristics of remifentanil is FALSE?

    A. Remifentanil is about 40 times more potent than alfentanil.
    B. Remifentanil is devoid of muscle rigidity side effects because of its rapid metabolism.
    C. Remifentanil has less depressant effect on motor evoked potentials compared with other opioids.
    D. Remifentanil is associated with poor postoperative pain control if it is used intraoperatively because of its rapid metabolism.
    E. Shivering is more common with remifentanil compared with alfentanil.

11. Which of the following statements regarding opioid-induced nausea and vomiting is TRUE?

    A. Equipotent doses of opioids cause an equal incidence of nausea and vomiting.
    B. Morphine has no direct effect on the chemotactic trigger zone.
    C. Subcutaneous administration of opioid is associated with a lower incidence of nausea and vomiting compared with intravenous administration.
    D. Vestibular stimulation such as ambulation attenuates the nausea caused by morphine.
    E. All of the above

For questions 12 to 16, choose A if 1, 2, and 3 are correct; B if 1 and 3; C if 2 and 4; D if 4; E if all.

12. Which of the following statements regarding morphine-induced pupillary constriction (miosis) in humans is/are TRUE?

    1. The presence of miosis correlates with opioid-induced respiratory depression.
    2. The effect is thought to be mediated via the nucleus tractus solitarius of the oculomotor nerve.
    3. A near-maximal degree of miosis is seen with as little as 0.5 mg/kg of morphine.
    4. The absence of miosis virtually eliminates opioids as a cause of respiratory depression.

13. The clinical effects of meperidine that differ from those observed with other commonly used opioids include:

    1. absence of histamine release from tissue mast cells
    2. decrease in cardiac contractility after high doses
    3. less nausea and vomiting at equianalgesic doses
    4. direct local anesthetic effects

14. Common potential disadvantages of a high-dose opioid anesthetic technique using fentanyl as the sole agent for anesthesia include:

    1. hemodynamic instability and cardiac depression
    2. impaired ventilation resulting from intense chest wall muscle rigidity
    3. prolonged anterograde amnesia
    4. the need for protracted postoperative ventilatory support

15. Potential disadvantages to use remifentanil as a component to a balanced anesthetic technique include:

    1. prolonged respiratory depression with infusion techniques, resulting from accumulation of active metabolites
    2. ultrashort duration of analgesic effect
    3. that a single dose of 20 μg/kg reliably produces unconsciousness when used for induction
    4. intraoperative muscle rigidity

16. Potential hazards in the use of naloxone to reverse opioid-induced respiratory depression include:

 1. sudden severe pain in postoperative patients
 2. precipitation of withdrawal syndromes in patients who are physically dependent on opioids

 3. late respiratory depression
 4. acute pulmonary edema

ANSWERS

1. **C.**   Most observed opioid effects involve interactions with receptor systems at spinal and supraspinal sites, although clinical studies suggest that morphine can produce analgesia by peripheral mechanisms, especially when inflammation is present. Intrinsic activity, or efficacy, of an opioid is described by the dose-response curve resulting from drug-receptor interaction, whereas affinity describes the ability of a drug to bind a receptor to produce a stable complex. Most opioids used in current clinical practice are highly selective for μ receptors, whereas naloxone, the most commonly used opioid antagonist, is not selective for opioid receptor type. For this reason, identification of an opioid receptor-mediated drug effect requires demonstration of naloxone reversibility. (See page 354: Endogenous Opioids and Opioid Receptors.)

2. **D.**   Large doses of opioids can produce profound muscle rigidity, an effect that appears to be mediated by μ receptors at supraspinal sites, most notably the nucleus raphe pontis and sites lateral to it in the hindbrain. Such muscle rigidity most often is witnessed on induction with large doses of opioids, although postoperative occurrences have been observed, as have feelings of muscle tension after small doses (10–15 mg) of morphine. Opioid-induced muscle rigidity is drastically increased by the addition of 70% nitrous oxide, but it is reduced or eliminated by naloxone, drugs that facilitate gamma-aminobutyric acid (GABA) agonist activity, and muscle relaxants. (See page 358: Muscle Rigidity.)

3. **E.**   Opioid-induced nausea is thought to be a result of input to the vomiting center from stimulation of the chemotactic trigger zone (CTZ) in the area postrema of the medulla, which is rich in opioid receptors. Not only does the incidence of opioid-induced nausea appear to be irrespective of the route of administration, but also clinical studies reveal no differences among opioid species, including morphine, meperidine, fentanyl, sufentanil, and alfentanil. (See page 358: Nausea and Vomiting.)

4. **A.**   Opioids stimulate the release of histamine from mast cells and basophils in a dose-dependent manner, an effect seen commonly after high doses of morphine. Decreases in peripheral vascular resistance and corresponding increases in pulmonary vascular resistance after morphine administration have been shown to correlate well with elevated plasma histamine concentrations. Opioid-induced histamine release is not prevented by pretreatment with naloxone, a finding suggesting a mechanism independent of opioid receptor activation. In clinically relevant doses, morphine does not depress myocardial contractibility. It does, however, produce dose-dependent bradycardia, probably by both sympatholytic and parasympathomimetic mechanisms. (See page 359: Histamine Release.)

5. **C.**   Meperidine is metabolized primarily in the liver by N-methylation to form normeperidine, an active metabolite, and by hydrolysis, to a lesser extent, to form meperidinic acid. In humans, CNS effects such as restlessness and agitation have been associated with increased serum levels of normeperidine, as have tremors, myoclonus, and seizures. Normeperidine, which has a considerably longer elimination half-life than its parent compound, is more apt to accumulate with repeated or prolonged administration of meperidine or in patients with renal dysfunction. (See page 360: Active Metabolites.)

6. **A.**   Fentanyl's high degree of lipid solubility enables it to cross biologic membranes very rapidly and to permeate highly perfused tissue groups, such as the brain, heart, and lung. This same characteristic accounts for the relatively brief clinical duration of effect seen with fentanyl, because redistribution of the drug to other tissues, including muscle and fat, also results from high lipid solubility. Similarly, accumulation of fentanyl in such tissue compartments can be extensive with prolonged administration, thus creating "reservoirs" of drug. (See page 360: Disposition Kinetics.)

7. **C.**   Alfentanil is a synthetic tetrazole derivative of fentanyl, with a clinical potency nearly 10 times that of morphine and from one-fourth to one-tenth that of fentanyl. Alfentanil is a weaker base than other opioids, with a pKa of 6.8. As such, nearly 90% of unbound plasma alfentanil is nonionized at physiologic pH. This property, in addition to its moderately high lipid solubility, allows alfentanil to cross the blood-brain barrier rapidly and accounts for

its rapid onset of action. Alfentanil has a terminal elimination half-life of 84 to 90 minutes, considerably shorter than that of fentanyl or sufentanil, mainly because of its relatively small volume of distribution. The incidences of clinical side effects with alfentanil have been shown to be similar to those with fentanyl and sufentanil when compared at equianalgesic doses. Early reports of a higher incidence of nausea and vomiting with alfentanil have not been substantiated. (See page 368: Alfentanil.)

8. **E.** Remifentanil is a recently synthesized 4-anilidopiperidine opioid with a methyl ester side chain susceptible to metabolism by blood and tissue esterases. A unique property of remifentanil as compared with other clinically useful opioids is its lack of accumulation with repeated dosing or prolonged infusion. This is because its ultrashort duration of action is the result of metabolism to a substantially less active compound, rather than simply redistribution of an unchanged opioid. (See page 371: Remifentanil.)

9. **C.** Nalbuphine is a partial opioid agonist at both κ and μ receptors. Administered alone, partial agonists exhibit a more shallow dose-response curve and lower maximal effects than a full agonist. The respiratory depression produced by nalbuphine has a ceiling effect equivalent to that produced by 30 mg/70 kg morphine. Because of this, nalbuphine has been used to antagonize the adverse effects of other opioids while still providing analgesic effects. Indeed, nalbuphine has been shown to be as effective as full μ agonists in providing postoperative analgesia in some instances. As an opioid agonist-antagonist, nalbuphine may precipitate withdrawal symptoms in those patients who are dependent on opioids. (See page 376: Nalbuphine.)

10. **B.** Remifentanil is about 40 times as potent as alfentanil. A high incidence of muscle rigidity and purposeless movement was seen with remifentanil. Although all opioids and propofol depress motor evoked potentials in a dose-dependent fashion, remifentanil exerts less suppression than other opioids and propofol. One drawback of remifentanil use for general anesthesia is that patients require analgesics soon after an infusion is stopped. Shivering was less common with alfentanil than with remifentanil. (See page 371: Remifentanil.)

11. **A.** The incidence of opioid-induced nausea appears to be similar irrespective of the route of administration (including oral, intravenous, intramuscular, subcutaneous, transmucosal, transdermal, intrathecal, and epidural). Laboratory and clinical studies comparing the incidence and severity of nausea and vomiting have found no differences among opioids (including morphine, hydromorphone, meperidine, fentanyl, sufentanil, alfentanil, and remifentanil) in

equianalgesic doses. The CTZ is rich in opioid, dopamine (D2), serotonin (5-HT$_3$), histamine, and (muscarinic) acetylcholine receptors, and it also receives input from the vestibular portion of the eighth cranial nerve. Morphine and related opioids induce nausea by direct stimulation of the CTZ and can also produce increased vestibular sensitivity. Therefore, vestibular stimulation such as ambulation markedly increases the emetic effects of morphine. This can be especially problematic in outpatient surgery, when early ambulation is a clinical priority. (See page 358: Morphine: Nausea and Vomiting.)

12. **B.** Morphine produces dose-dependent miosis in humans, an effect that is believed to be mediated by the Edinger-Westphal nucleus of the third cranial nerve. Although significant differences exist between opioid species and their effects on pupillary size, morphine produces a near-maximal degree of constriction with 0.5 mg/kg. In the absence of other drugs, the resultant miosis appears to correlate with opioid-induced respiratory depression, although severe hypoxemia may result in pupillary dilation. (See page 372: Other Central Nervous System Effects.)

13. **C.** Meperidine is a synthetic opioid with an analgesic potency about one-tenth that of morphine. Although the analgesic effects are primarily mediated via mu receptor activation, meperidine has demonstrated local anesthetic properties, which has led to its increasing popularity for epidural and subarachnoid administration. This local anesthetic effect is thought to be responsible for decreases in cardiac contractility observed with high plasma concentrations of meperidine, a finding not consistent with other clinically used opioids. Meperidine administration does result in histamine release, an effect that may contribute to the hemodynamic instability often encountered when high doses are used in the clinical setting. At equianalgesic doses, the respiratory depression caused by meperidine is no different from that induced by morphine, hydromorphone, meperidine, fentanyl, sufentanil, alfentanil, or remifentanil. (See page 361: Side Effects.)

14. **C.** High-dose opioid-based anesthetic techniques, particularly those using synthetic opioids (such as fentanyl), initially gained popularity because of the reliable hemodynamic stability that is achieved with minimal cardiovascular depression. In addition, hormonal responses to surgical stimuli are significantly blunted with such a regimen. Notable disadvantages include prolonged respiratory depression, a high incidence of clinically significant muscle rigidity on induction, and frequent reports of intraoperative awareness and recall when opioids are used as the sole anesthetic agent. (See page 372: Effect on Minimum Alveolar Concentration of Volatile Anesthetics and Use in Anesthesia.)

15. C. Remifentanil is rapidly metabolized by blood and tissue esterases to a substantially less active compound. The duration of the respiratory depression seen with remifentanil has been shown to parallel the duration of its analgesic effects. Side effects of remifentanil, including a high incidence of muscle rigidity with high doses, are similar to those of other commonly used opioids at equianalgesic doses. Although an ultrashort duration of action makes remifentanil an appealing agent for opioid infusion techniques and ease of titration, this characteristic poses a potential disadvantage in that patients may require additional analgesics very soon after remifentanil is discontinued. Loss of consciousness is not reliably achieved with remifentanil alone. (See page 371: Remifentanil.)

16. E. Naloxone is a pure opioid antagonist at μ, κ, and δ opioid receptors, used most often in clinical practice to antagonize opioid-induced respiratory depression and sedation. Because naloxone antagonizes all opioid-receptor interactions, it interrupts μ- and/or κ-receptor–mediated analgesia and may lead to severe pain. In some instances, acute, and sometimes fatal, pulmonary edema may ensue, an effect that is believed to result from a centrally mediated catecholamine release causing acute pulmonary hypertension. Because the duration of clinical effect seen with naloxone ranges from 1 to 4 hours, it is possible for renarcotization to occur when pre-existing opioids reactivate receptors after the effects of naloxone have subsided. (See page 377: Opioid Antagonists (Naloxone and Naltrexone).)

CHAPTER 15 ■ INHALATION ANESTHESIA

For questions 1 to 11, choose the best answer.

1. Which of the following statements regarding minimum alveolar concentration (MAC) is FALSE?

   A. Pregnancy decreases MAC.
   B. MAC of inhaled drugs is additive.
   C. MAC is lowered in preterm neonates compared with term neonates.
   D. Acute ethanol administration increases MAC.
   E. MAC in an 80-year-old patient is only three-fourths that in a young adult.

2. Which of the following statements about MAC is FALSE?

   A. MAC-awake is the alveolar concentration at which 50% of patients respond to the command "open your eyes."
   B. Standard MAC values are roughly additive.
   C. MAC-block adrenergic response (BAR) is the alveolar concentration that blocks the adrenergic response to noxious stimuli in 50% of patients.
   D. MAC-awake for halothane is approximately equivalent to standard MAC.
   E. MAC-BAR is 1.5 times the standard MAC value.

3. Which of the following best relates the relative degree to which inhalational anesthetics decrease cerebral metabolic rate?

   A. Sevoflurane = halothane < isoflurane
   B. Isoflurane < halothane < sevoflurane
   C. Sevoflurane < isoflurane < halothane
   D. Isoflurane = sevoflurane > halothane
   E. Halothane < isoflurane = sevoflurane

4. Which of the following statements regarding the central nervous system effects of inhalational agents is FALSE?

   A. All potent inhalational agents depress the cerebral metabolic rate (CMR).
   B. Desflurane and sevoflurane cause a similar decrease in CMR.
   C. Once an isoelectric electroencephalogram (EEG) is achieved, a further increase in isoflurane concentration will further decrease the CMR of O_2 ($CMRO_2$).
   D. Isoflurane abolishes EEG activity at clinically used doses that are usually hemodynamically tolerable.
   E. Desflurane's effects on the central nervous system are similar to isoflurane's during deliberate hypotension.

5. True statements regarding inhalational agents include all of the following EXCEPT:

   A. A second gas effect exists for nearly every combination of inhaled drugs.
   B. The two major components of the second gas effect are (1) the concentration effect and (2) decreased solubility.
   C. For the more soluble anesthetics, augmentation of anesthetic delivery by increasing minute ventilation also increases the rate of rise in F_A/F_I.
   D. During emergence, washout of high concentrations of nitrous oxide can lower alveolar concentrations of O_2 and CO_2.
   E. The rate of alveolar concentration approaching the inspired concentration is inversely related to the blood solubility of the agent.

6. True statements regarding the effects of anesthetics on the chemical control of breathing include all of the following EXCEPT:

   A. Subanesthetic concentrations of potent inhalational agents will depress the hypoxic response in humans.
   B. The ventilatory response to CO_2 is depressed by all inhalational agents.
   C. With a 2 MAC inhalational agent in a spontaneously breathing patient, the apneic

threshold is generally 15 mm Hg below the resting Pa_{CO_2}.

    D. Residual effects of inhalation agents may impair ventilatory drive of patients in the recovery room.

    E. Nitrous oxide decreases Pa_{CO_2} during spontaneous breathing.

7. True statements concerning the hemodynamic effects of inhalational agents include all of the following EXCEPT:

    A. All potent inhaled agents decrease arterial pressure.

    B. Heart rate changes least with halothane and sevoflurane.

    C. Volatile anesthetics cause dose-dependent myocardial depression.

    D. Isoflurane causes greater slowing in the His-Purkinje system than does halothane.

    E. All inhalational agents attenuate baroreflex control of heart rate.

8. Which of the following statements regarding metabolism of inhaled agents is FALSE?

    A. The production of compound A is enhanced during low-flow anesthesia.

    B. Baralyme produces more compound A than soda lime.

    C. Compound A production is decreased by warm or very dry CO_2 absorbents.

    D. The potential effect of compound A is renal toxicity.

    E. CO_2 absorbents degrade all modern-day potent inhalational anesthetics.

9. Which statement is FALSE regarding fluoride-induced nephrotoxicity?

    A. The metabolism of sevoflurane to fluoride in the kidney is significantly greater than that of methoxyflurane.

    B. Sevoflurane transiently increases serum fluoride concentration.

    C. Fluoride-induced nephrotoxicity presents as high-output renal insufficiency.

    D. Inorganic fluoride produces renal injury.

    E. Metabolism resulting in nephrotoxicity is an accepted fact for methoxyflurane.

10. True statements regarding inhalational agents include all of the following EXCEPT:

    A. Inhalational agents have muscle relaxant properties of their own.

    B. Situations that decrease hepatic blood flow make a patient vulnerable to halothane's effects on hepatic blood flow.

    C. Of the volatile anesthetics, halothane is the most potent trigger of caffeine-induced contractions.

    D. Volatile anesthetics cause a dose-dependent decrease in uterine smooth muscle contractility.

    E. No inhalational anesthetic has been shown to be teratogenic in animals.

11. The FALSE statement concerning the effect of inhalational agents on cerebrospinal fluid (CSF) is:

    A. Sevoflurane at 1 MAC decreases CSF production.

    B. 1 MAC desflurane leaves CSF production unchanged or slightly increased.

    C. Halothane decreases the rate of CSF production and increases resistance to reabsorption.

    D. Isoflurane significantly increases CSF production and decreases resistance to reabsorption.

    E. The net effect of halothane is an increase in CSF volume.

For questions 12 and 13, choose A if 1, 2, and 3 are correct; B if 1 and 3; C if 2 and 4; D if 4, and E if all.

12. TRUE statements regarding the effects of inhaled anesthetics on circulation include:

    1. Enflurane is associated with myocardial depression.
    2. Sevoflurane provides a stable heart rate.
    3. Desflurane maintains cardiac output.
    4. Isoflurane is associated with an increase in heart rate.

13. TRUE statements regarding inhaled anesthetics include:

    1. The partial pressure is the pressure a gas exerts proportional to its fractional mass.
    2. A low-solubility agent results in a fast rise in F_A/F_I.
    3. Depth of anesthesia can be adjusted quickly.
    4. Fat has a slow time for equilibration with blood.

ANSWERS

1. **D.** MAC is influenced by age; in humans, the MAC is lower in preterm neonates than it is at term. It is higher in term infants than at any other age. Anesthetic requirements decrease with age; an 80-year-old patient requires only three-fourths the alveolar concentration of anesthetic that is required for a young adult. Pregnancy decreases the MAC in sheep. Acute ethanol administration decreases MAC. (See page 397: Minimum Alveolar Concentration [MAC].)

2. **D.** MAC-awake is the dose at which 50% of patients respond to the command "open your eyes." The alveolar concentration at this point is approximately one-half of the standard MAC value for halothane. MAC-BAR is the alveolar concentration required to block the adrenergic response to noxious stimuli in 50% of patients; this value is approximately 1.5 times the standard MAC value. MAC values are roughly additive. (See page 397: Minimum Alveolar Concentration [MAC].)

3. **D.** Each of the potent inhaled anesthetics decreases $CMRO_2$, with the order of effect from greatest to least being isoflurane = sevoflurane > halothane. (See page 398: Cerebral Metabolic Rate and Electroencephalogram.)

4. **C.** It has been shown that, once an isoelectric EEG is achieved with isoflurane, further increases in isoflurane's concentration do not lead to further decreases in CMR. Isoflurane abolishes EEG activity at clinically used doses that are usually hemodynamically tolerated. Desflurane and sevoflurane cause similar decreases in CMR. Desflurane's effects are similar to those of isoflurane during deliberate hypotension. (See page 398: Cerebral Metabolic Rate and Electroencephalogram.)

5. **B.** The rate at which the alveolar concentration approaches the inspired concentration is inversely related to the blood solubility of the anesthetic. Administration of high concentrations of one gas (e.g., nitrous oxide) facilitates the rise in alveolar concentration of another gas (e.g., halothane); this phenomenon is called the second gas effect. The two components of the second gas effect (increased ventilation [increased tracheal inflow] and the concentrating effect) are operative at the alveolar level. Although a second gas effect exists for nearly all combinations of inhaled drugs given simultaneously, it is most pronounced when nitrous oxide is used with a more soluble drug, such as halothane (the second gas). For more soluble anesthetics, increasing the minute ventilation will increase rate of rise in F_A/F_I. Emergence from anesthesia is more rapid with low blood or tissue anesthetic solubility, increased ventilation, and replacement of nitrous oxide with nitrogen. During washout of high concentrations of nitrous oxide, alveolar concentrations of O_2 and CO_2 can be lowered. This phenomenon is called diffusion hypoxia. (See page 392: Second Gas Effect.)

6. **C.** The ventilatory response to CO_2 is depressed more or less proportionately by all anesthetic agents. Apnea results if the anesthetic dose is high enough. If apnea occurs, the apneic threshold is approximately 4 to 5 mm Hg below the $Paco_2$ maintained during spontaneous breathing, regardless of the type of anesthesia. It should be anticipated that the $Paco_2$ will be 50 to 55 mm Hg at surgical planes of anesthesia when potent inhaled anesthetics are used. Surgical stimuli will decrease this level by 4 to 5 mm Hg at an equivalent level of anesthesia. Nitrous oxide maintains (or may slightly increase) the $Paco_2$ during spontaneous breathing. Subanesthetic concentrations of halothane, enflurane, and isoflurane depress the hypoxic response in humans. Residual effects of inhalational agents may impair ventilatory drive of patients in the recovery room. (See page 407: Response to Carbon Dioxide and Hypoxemia.)

7. **D.** Volatile anesthetics cause dose-dependent myocardial depression. All the potent inhaled agents decrease arterial pressure in a dose-related manner. The mechanism of the decrease in blood pressure includes vasodilation, decreased cardiac output resulting from myocardial depression, and decreased sympathetic nervous system tone. The heart rate changes least with halothane and increases most with desflurane. Halothane causes a greater slowing of the His-Purkinje system than does isoflurane. (See page 401: The Circulatory System.)

8. **C.** Sevoflurane is degraded by CO_2 absorbents to produce compound A. Baralyme produces more compound A than does soda lime, and this can be attributed to slightly higher absorbent temperatures during CO_2 extraction. The risk from compound A is renal tubular necrosis. Sevoflurane metabolism to compound A is enhanced in low-flow or closed-circuit breathing systems and by warm or very dry CO_2 absorbents. All the potent inhaled agents (halothane, sevoflurane, enflurane, desflurane, and isoflurane) are degraded by CO_2 absorbents. (See page 411: Anesthetic Degradation by Carbon Dioxide Absorbers.)

9. **A.** The metabolism of methoxyflurane to fluoride in the kidney is significantly greater than that of sevoflurane and enflurane. Metabolism with resultant nephrotoxicity is an accepted fact for methoxyflurane. Sevoflurane undergoes 5% metabolism that transiently increases serum fluoride concentrations. The inorganic fluoride causes nephrotoxicity, which presents as high-output renal insufficiency. (See page 413: Fluoride-Induced Nephrotoxicity.)

10. **E.** The potent inhaled anesthetic agents not only potentiate the action of neuromuscular blocking drugs, but also have muscle relaxant properties of their own. Situations that decrease hepatic blood flow or increase hepatic oxygen consumption make patients more vulnerable to the unwanted effects of halothane on hepatic blood flow. Virtually every volatile anesthetic agent has been shown to be teratogenic in animal studies, but none has been shown to be teratogenic in humans. Halothane causes a stronger contraction to the caffeine-induced contracture test than isoflurane or enflurane. Volatile anesthetics produce a dose-dependent decrease in uterine smooth

muscle contractility. (See page 409: Hepatic Effects.)

11. **D.** 1 MAC halothane decreases CSF production but increases resistance to reabsorption, the net being an increase in CSF volume. Isoflurane does not appear to alter CSF production but may increase, decrease, or leave unchanged the resistance to reabsorption depending on dose. Sevoflurane at 1 MAC depresses CSF production up to 40%. 1 MAC desflurane leaves CSF production unchanged or increased. In general, anesthetic effects on intracranial pressure via changes in CSF dynamics are clinically far less important than their effects on CBF. (See page 400: Cerebrospinal Fluid Production and Reabsorption.)

12. **E.** Enflurane is associated with some myocardial depression, a decrease in cardiac output, and an increase in right atrial pressure. Sevoflurane provides a stable heart rate. Desflurane, sevoflurane, and isoflurane are known to maintain cardiac output. Enflurane and isoflurane are associated with an increase in heart rate of 10 to 20% at 1 MAC. (See page 401: The Circulatory System.)

13. **E.** The partial pressure is the pressure a gas exerts proportional to its fractional mass. The inhaled anesthetics with the lowest solubilities in the blood show the fastest rise in Fa/Fi. Fat has a slow time for equilibration with blood. (See page 386: Pharmacokinetic Principles.)

CHAPTER 16 ■ NEUROMUSCULAR BLOCKING AGENTS

For questions 1 through 10, choose the best answer.

1. All of the following statements regarding a peripheral nerve are true EXCEPT:

   A. It is made up of a large number of axons of different threshold potentials.
   B. Each axon responds in an all-or-none fashion to a given stimulus.
   C. When a stimulating current reaches a high enough level, all axons are activated, and the amplitude of the action potential reaches a maximum level.
   D. There is a linear relationship between the amplitude of the muscle contraction and the current applied.
   E. Sodium channels in the nerve axon are activated in response to electrical stimulation.

2. The duration of the current delivered by a nerve stimulator should be approximately:

   A. 0.2 second
   B. 0.02 second
   C. 0.2 millisecond
   D. 0.02 millisecond
   E. 2.0 millisecond

3. Which of the following statements regarding acetylcholine is FALSE?

   A. The amount of acetylcholine released with repetitive stimulation decreases.
   B. Calcium is required for vesicle binding to docking proteins and subsequent release of acetylcholine.
   C. The action of magnesium augments the release of acetylcholine from vesicle stores.
   D. Acetylcholine is released in quanta, each of which contains 5,000 to 10,000 molecules.
   E. In the absence of stimulation, a small amount of acetylcholine is released at random.

4. Which of the following statements regarding neuromuscular blocking drugs (NMBs) is FALSE?

A. The ED_{50} is the median dose corresponding to a 50% depression in twitch.
B. The ED_{95} corresponds to the dose required to achieve neuromuscular blockade in 95% of patients.
C. The ED_{95} of vecuronium is approximately 0.05 mg/kg.
D. The time to maximal neuromuscular blockade can be shortened if the dose of NMB is increased.
E. The duration of action of NMBs increases with increasing dose.

5. Which of the following statements regarding the depolarizing blockade produced by succinylcholine is FALSE?

   A. During phase I block, fade in response to train-of-four stimulus is not observed.
   B. Phase II block is not antagonized by cholinesterase inhibitors.
   C. After administration of a 7 to 10 mg/kg dose of succinylcholine, train-of-four and tetanic fade become apparent.
   D. The prevalence of fasciculations after injection of succinylcholine is greater than 50%.
   E. Sinus bradycardia in response to succinylcholine is more common in children than in adults.

6. Regarding the clinical use of succinylcholine, all of the following statements are true EXCEPT:

   A. Infants and children are relatively resistant to succinylcholine compared with adults.
   B. The duration of neuromuscular blockade produced by succinylcholine is significantly increased in patients homozygous for an atypical form of plasma cholinesterase.
   C. Increases in serum potassium levels following succinylcholine injection can be mitigated by precurarization.

D. Precurarization may be effective at blocking the increase in intragastric pressure observed following succinylcholine administration.

E. At a dose of 1 mg/kg, the duration of action of succinylcholine is approximately 5 to 6 minutes.

7. All of the following statements regarding the pharmacokinetics of nondepolarizing NMBs are true EXCEPT:

   A. Termination of the clinical effects of vecuronium depends primarily on redistribution rather than elimination.

   B. Termination of the clinical effects of cisatracurium depends primarily on elimination.

   C. The volume of distribution of most nondepolarizing NMBs is approximately equal to extracellular fluid volume.

   D. More potent drugs have a faster onset of action than less potent agents.

   E. Onset and duration of action are determined by the concentration of drug at its site of action.

8. Which of the following muscle groups demonstrates the earliest recovery from neuromuscular blockade following administration of an anticholinesterase agent?

   A. Adductor pollicis
   B. Diaphragm
   C. Geniohyoid
   D. Pharyngeal
   E. Flexor hallucis

9. Which of the following is an acetylcholinesterase inhibitor with an onset of action most similar to atropine?

   A. Glycopyrrolate
   B. Edrophonium
   C. Neostigmine
   D. Pyridostigmine
   E. Physostigmine

10. All of the following are side effects associated with anticholinesterase drugs EXCEPT?

    A. Increased salivation
    B. Increased peristalsis
    C. Bradycardia
    D. Bronchodilation
    E. Increased bladder motility

For questions 11 through 17, answer A if 1, 2, and 3 are correct; B if 1 and 3; C if 2 and 4; D if 4; and E if all.

11. Which of the following statements about the nondepolarizing NMBs is/are TRUE?

    1. Laudanosine is a metabolite of cisatracurium.
    2. Pancuronium is associated with histamine release.
    3. Mivacurium is metabolized by plasma cholinesterase.

    4. Hypotension following administration of *d*-tubocurarine is mainly the result of autonomic ganglionic blockade.

12. Which of the following agents augment(s) neuromuscular blockade?

    1. Isoflurane
    2. Erythromycin
    3. Lidocaine
    4. Metronidazole

13. Which of the following statements regarding patients with myasthenia gravis is/are TRUE?

    1. They often demonstrate resistance to depolarizing NMBs.
    2. They often demonstrate resistance to nondepolarizing NMBs.
    3. The number of acetylcholine quanta at the neuromuscular junction is generally normal or increased.
    4. They demonstrate a voltage increment in response to repeated stimulation at 2 to 5 Hz.

14. In which of the following patients is a greater than average increase in serum potassium in response to succinylcholine administration found compared with the general population?

    1. A 57-year-old woman who sustained extensive burns 1 week ago
    2. A 19-year-old patient with T12 paralysis following a motor vehicle collision 1 month ago
    3. A 69-year-old man following a major stroke
    4. A 40-year-old woman diagnosed with myasthenia gravis 1 month ago

15. Which of the following statements regarding train-of-four response monitoring of the degree of nondepolarizing neuromuscular blockade is/are TRUE?

    1. The second twitch reappears when approximately 80 to 90% of receptors remained blocked.
    2. The third twitch reappears when approximately 75% of receptors remained blocked.
    3. All four twitches are visible when 65 to 75% of receptors are blocked.
    4. The single-twitch height has recovered to about 100% when the train-of-four ratio is approximately 70%.

16. Regarding the differential impact of NMBs on specific muscle groups, which of the following statements is/are TRUE?

    1. The adductor pollicis is relatively resistant to nondepolarizing NMBs compared with the diaphragm.
    2. Facial nerve stimulation with monitoring of response in the eyebrow is reliably predictive of intubating conditions.

3. Time to maximal response occurs more quickly in the adductor pollicis than in the diaphragm.
4. The diaphragm and laryngeal muscles are relatively resistant to nondepolarizing agents.

17. Which of the following acetylcholinesterase inhibitors can cross the blood-brain barrier?

1. Edrophonium
2. Pyridostigmine
3. Neostigmine
4. Physostigmine

ANSWERS

1. **D.**   A peripheral nerve is made up of a large number of axons of different thresholds and sizes. Each axon responds in an all-or-none fashion, but not all axons may respond to a given stimulus. Thus, the relationship between the amplitude of the muscle contraction and the current applied is sigmoid, not linear. At low currents, an insufficient number of axons is depolarized. As current increases, more and more axons are depolarized to threshold, and the strength of the muscle contraction increases up to a maximum level. The mechanism of action of nerve cell activation is via the opening of sodium channels. (See page 423: Physiology and Pharmacology: Structure.)

2. **C.**   The duration of the current delivered by a nerve stimulator should be 0.1 to 0.2 millisecond. (See page 424: Physiology and Pharmacology: Nerve Stimulation.)

3. **C.**   Acetylcholine is packaged into 45-nm vesicles, each of which contains 5,000 to 10,000 molecules of acetylcholine. A few vesicles are available for immediate release, but a much larger pool can be recruited with time. With repetitive stimulation, the amount of acetylcholine released decreases rapidly because of the limited availability of immediately releasable acetylcholine. Even in the absence of nerve stimulation, acetylcholine is released in small quantities called quanta, producing so-called miniature end-plate potentials. When an action potential reaches the nerve terminal, 200 to 400 quanta are released simultaneously, causing a rapid increase in the concentration of acetylcholine at the motor end plate. Calcium enters the nerve terminals through channels that open in response to depolarization and is responsible for release of acetylcholine from vesicles. Magnesium antagonizes the action of calcium and causes inhibition of acetylcholine release. (See page 424: Physiology and Pharmacology: Release of Acetylcholine.)

4. **B.** ED_{50} and ED_{95} are two measures of NMB potency. The ED_{50} is the median dose corresponding to a 50% depression in twitch. The ED_{95}, a more clinically relevant measure of potency, is defined as the amount of drug necessary to produce a 95% block in twitch response in half of patients. For example, the ED_{95} of vecuronium is approximately 0.05 mg/kg. The time needed to reach maximal neuromuscular blockade and duration of block are both affected by amount of drug given. Response time can be shortened and duration increased when an increased amount of drug is administered. (See page 426: Neuromuscular Blocking Agents: Pharmacological Characteristics of Neuromuscular Blocking Agents.)

5. **B.**   Administration of a usual intubating dose of succinylcholine produces a phase I block, marked by a decrease in single-twitch height, but sustained response to high-frequency stimulation and minimal if any train-of-four or tetanic fade. Phase I blockade is potentiated by inhibitors of acetylcholinesterase. After administration of larger doses of succinylcholine (7 mg/kg) or within 30 to 60 minutes after initiating infusion, train-of-four and tetanic fade become apparent. This is referred to as phase II blockade. In contrast to phase I block, phase II block can be antagonized by aceytlcholinesterase inhibitors. Succinylcholine produces a number of characteristic side effects. Fasciculations in response to succinylcholine injection occur in 60 to 90% of patients and can often be reduced with the prior administration of a small dose of nondepolarizing NMB such as rocuronium. Sinus bradycardia with nodal or ventricular escape beats is a relatively common cardiovascular side effect, more so in children than adults. (See page 427: Depolarizing Drugs: Characteristics of Depolarizing Blockade.)

6. **C.**   Succinylcholine is the only depolarizing NMB regularly used in clinical practice. It has an onset of action of approximately 30 to 60 seconds and a duration of action of 5 to 6 minutes, thus making it a useful agent for rapid sequence intubations and for patients in whom prolonged muscle relaxation is not desired. Side effects commonly observed following succinylcholine administration include muscle fasciculations and an elevation of intragastric and intraocular pressures. Both of these reactions can be blocked (but not with 100% consistency) by the prior administration of a small dose of nondepolarizing

NMB (precurarization). Succinylcholine also increases serum potassium levels by approximately 0.5 to 1 mEq/L. This effect is not prevented by precurarization. Therefore, succinylcholine should be used with caution in patients at risk of developing clinically significant hyperkalemia. Succinylcholine is metabolized by plasma cholinesterase. Patients with atypical versions of this enzyme experience prolongation of neuromuscular blockade caused by succinylcholine. However, this prolongation is only significant in patients homozygous for atypical cholinesterase. (See page 426: Depolarizing Drugs: Succinylcholine.)

7. **D.**   Duration of action of NMBs is a function of either their elimination from the body or redistribution away from the site of effect. Cisatracurium is an intermediate-duration drug whose effects are terminated as a result of elimination. By contrast, vecuronium has a long elimination half-life but an intermediate effect duration as a result of redistribution away from the motor end plate. The volume of distribution of nondepolarizing NMBs is about equal to the volume of the extracellular fluid compartment. The onset and duration of action of most NMBs are determined by the time required for drug concentrations to reach a critical level at their site of action. Drug concentration at the effect site approximately parallels plasma concentration, but drug onset lags behind peak plasma concentration slightly. More potent drugs actually have a slower onset of action than less potent ones because there are fewer molecules of the more potent agent than of an equivalent dose of a less potent agent. (See page 429: Nondepolarizing Drugs: Pharmacokinetics; page 431: Onset and Duration of Action.)

8. **B.**   The diaphragm exhibits the most rapid recovery from neuromuscular blockade. Recovery of upper airway and pharyngeal muscles (e.g., geniohyoid) and flexor hallucis muscle generally parallels that of the adductor pollicis. (See page 442: Monitoring Neuromuscular Blockade: Choice of Muscle.)

9. **B.**   Anticholinergic agents such as atropine or glycopyrrolate are frequently administered with neuromuscular reversal agents to blunt the cardiovascular effects of vagal stimulation produced by reversal agents. To achieve best effect, agents with similar pharmacokinetics should be paired. The onset of action of atropine is rapid (~1 minute) and closely parallels that of edrophonium. The onset of action of neostigmine is about 7 to 11 minutes, and that of pyridostigime is 15 to 20 minutes. Physostigmine has an onset of about 5 minutes. It is not used as a neuromuscular reversal agent because of its central side effects. The pharmacokinetic profile of glycopyrrolate (onset 2–3 minutes) is most similar to that of neostigmine. (See page 446: Antagonism of Neuromuscular Block: Reversal Agents.)

10. **D.**   Anticholinesterase agents produce vagal stimulation, leading to bradycardia and bradyarrythmias. Other cholinergic effects observed with anticholinesterase drugs include increased salivation, as well as increased bladder and bowel motility. Anticholinesterases may also be associated with bronchoconstriction, not bronchodilation. (See page 448: Antagonism of Neuromuscular Block: Anticholinesterases: Other Effects.)

11. **B.**   Laudanosine is a compound produced by the ester hydrolysis of atracurium and cisatracurium. Like succinylcholine, mivacurium is metabolized by plasma cholinesterase. Several of the nondepolarizing NMBs are associated with histamine release, which can cause transient hypotension following administration. This is the primary reason for the hypotension observed following administration of *d*-tubocurarine; it also causes ganglionic block. Pancuronium does not release histamine. However, it does appear to cause a transient increase in catecholamine release, leading to a temporary increase in heart rate, blood pressure, and cardiac output. (See page 432: Nondepolarizing Drugs: Individual Nondepolarizing Agents.)

12. **B.**   Several agents potentiate the effect of NMBs. These include the halogenated inhalational agents such as isoflurane and local anesthetics such as lidocaine. Aminoglycosides such as neomycin and streptomycin also potentiate neuromuscular blockade. Erythromycin, penicillins, and metronidazole, however, do not produce this effect. (See page 437: Drug Interactions.)

13. **B.**   Myasthenia gravis is an autoimmune disorder characterized by the production of antibodies to postsynaptic acetylcholine receptors. The number of acetylcholine quanta at the neuromuscular junction is normal or increased. However, muscle contraction in response to acetylcholine is blunted by a functional decline in acetylcholine receptors. The characteristic electromyographic finding in patients with myasthenia gravis is a voltage decrement in response to repeated stimulation at the 2- to 5-Hz level. Patients with myasthenia gravis have unpredictable responses to NMBs. They are often resistant to succinylcholine, in part because of the presence of higher concentrations of acetylcholine at the motor end plate. In contrast, sensitivity and prolonged duration of action are usually observed in response to nondepolarizing NMBs, as a result of the decreased number of functional acetylcholine receptors present on postsynaptic membranes. (See page 438: Altered Responses to Neuromuscular Blocking Agents.)

14. **A.**   An exaggerated increase in serum potassium concentration following succinylcholine administration is relatively more common in children with muscular dystrophies (e.g., Duchenne). It is also

observed as early as 24 to 48 hours following extensive burn injuries; this response usually resolves with healing. In addition, patients with upper motor neuron lesions are more susceptible to hyperkalemia induced by succinylcholine. This response is most prominent when the drug is given 1 week to 6 months following the injury, although it may occur at any time. Hyperkalemia following succinylcholine is not frequently associated with myasthenia gravis. (See page 428: Depolarizing Drugs: Side Effects.)

15. **E.** Train-of-four response monitoring to nondepolarizing neuromuscular blockade involves the application of four stimuli at 0.5-second intervals (2 Hz). Recovery from neuromuscular block is measured by the return of response to these stimuli. In general, the second twitch appears when 80 to 90% of receptors remain blocked, and the third appears when 75% are blocked. All four responses are usually visible and single-twitch height has recovered to 100% when blockade is about 65 to 75%. (See page 440: Monitoring Neuromuscular Block: Monitoring Modalities.)

16. **C.** Muscle groups demonstrate a differential response to NMBs. The adductor pollicis is relatively sensitive to nondepolarizing NMBs, whereas the diaphragm and laryngeal muscles are relatively resistant. The time to maximal blockade occurs somewhat later in the adductor pollicis compared with the more centrally located muscles. Facial nerve stimulation with response monitored in the eyebrow is thought to be indicative of the action of the corrugator supercilii muscle. The impact of nondepolarizing NMBs on this muscle approximates that of the laryngeal adductors, and therefore response monitoring to eyebrow movement may be a reliable predictor of adequate intubating conditions. (See page 442: Monitoring Neuromuscular Block: Choice of Muscle.)

17. **D.** Neostigmine, edrophonium, and pyridostigmine are all charged quaternary ammonium compounds that do not cross the blood-brain barrier. Physostigmine is an uncharged molecule that can cross the blood-brain barrier. (See page 446: Antagonism of Neuromuscular Block: Reversal Agents.)

CHAPTER 17 ■ LOCAL ANESTHETICS

1. Pick the FALSE statement regarding myelinated nerves.

   A. They have a diameter of >1 μm.
   B. They are surrounded by Schwann cells, which account for more than half of the nerve's thickness.
   C. They conduct impulses more slowly than similar-sized unmyelinated nerves.
   D. They have both afferent and efferent functions.
   E. The nodes of Ranvier are covered by negatively charged glycoproteins.

2. Pick the FALSE statement regarding neuronal conduction.

   A. The resting membrane potential is predominantly maintained by a potassium gradient with a 10 times greater concentration of potassium within the cell.
   B. Generation of action potentials is primarily the result of activation of voltage-gated sodium channels.
   C. Impulse generation is an all-or-nothing phenomenon.
   D. A three-state kinetic scheme conceptualizes the change in sodium channel conformation and accounts for changes in sodium conductance during depolarization and repolarization.
   E. The resting membrane potential of neural membranes averages −30 to −40 mV.

3. The rate of absorption from injection of local anesthetic to various sites generally increases in the following order:

   A. Intercostal, caudal, epidural, brachial plexus, sciatic/femoral
   B. Caudal, intercostal, epidural, brachial plexus, sciatic/femoral
   C. Intercostal, epidural, caudal, brachial plexus, sciatic/femoral

   D. Sciatic/femoral, brachial plexus, epidural, caudal, intercostal
   E. Intercostal, brachial plexus, epidural, caudal, sciatic/femoral

4. Which of the following descriptions of local anesthetics is FALSE?

   A. They are weak bases.
   B. The charged form of local anesthetics is lipid soluble.
   C. They have substituted benzene rings.
   D. They contain either an ester or amide linkage.
   E. They exert their effects on the intracellular side of the sodium channel.

5. Pick the FALSE statement concerning pKa.

   A. The pKa is the dissociation constant.
   B. When the pH equals the pKa of a compound, 50% of it is neutral and 50% of it is charged.
   C. Increasing the pKa of a local anesthetic increases the lipid-soluble form.
   D. Onset of action is slowed by increasing the pKa.
   E. Knowing the pKa of a local anesthetic lets one predict the relative speed of its onset of action.

6. Pick the FALSE answer concerning tachyphylaxis.

   A. It is a clinical phenomenon whereby repeat injection of the same dose of local anesthetic leads to decreased efficacy.
   B. A clinical feature of tachyphylaxis to local anesthetics is dependence on dosing interval.
   C. Pain is not important for the development of local anesthetic tachyphylaxis.
   D. Spinal cord sensitization is one theory of tachyphylaxis development.
   E. Prolonged exposure of peripheral nerves to local anesthetics does not affect the development of tachyphylaxis.

7. Pick the FALSE statement concerning clearance and elimination of local anesthetics.

    A. Ester local anesthetics are primarily cleared by plasma cholinesterases.
    B. Local anesthetics with higher rates of clearance will have a greater margin of safety.
    C. Renal disease is important in altering the pharmacokinetic parameters of local anesthetics.
    D. Protein binding of aminoamide local anesthetics is important in determining the rate of clearance.
    E. Correlation of resultant systemic blood levels between dose of local anesthetic and patient weight often is inconsistent.

8. Pick the FALSE answer concerning treatment of systemic toxicity from local anesthetics.

    A. Signs of central nervous system (CNS) toxicity typically occur before cardiovascular events.
    B. Propofol can terminate seizures from systemic local anesthetic toxicity.
    C. Succinylcholine can terminate seizure activity.
    D. Ventricular dysrhythmias may be difficult to treat.
    E. Amiodarone is indicated in the treatment of bupivacaine toxicity.

9. Pick the FALSE statement concerning transient neurologic symptoms (TNS) after spinal anesthesia.

    A. Increased risk of TNS is associated with lidocaine.
    B. The baricity of the local anesthetic is an important factor in the development of TNS.
    C. The dose of local anesthetic is not an important factor in the development of TNS.
    D. TNS may be a manifestation of subclinical neurotoxicity.
    E. The incidence varies with patient position.

10. Which of the following statements is FALSE?

    A. Bupivacaine 0.75% is not an acceptable concentration for obstetric use.
    B. CNS toxicity is more common with epidural local anesthetic injection than with peripheral nerve blocks.
    C. Levobupivacaine is approximately equipotent to racemic bupivacaine.
    D. Both ropivacaine and levobupivacaine appear to have approximately 30 to 40% less systemic toxicity than bupivacaine on a milligram-to-milligram basis.
    E. Levobupivacaine is an isomer of bupivacaine.

11. All of the following local anesthetics are racemic mixtures EXCEPT:

    A. lidocaine
    B. bupivacaine
    C. mepivacaine
    D. tetracaine
    E. chloroprocaine

For questions 12 to 18, choose A if 1, 2, and 3 are correct; B if 1 and 3; C if 2 and 4; D if 4; E if all.

12. Which of the following statements concerning spinal administration of opioids is/are TRUE?

    1. It is not dependent on supraspinal mechanisms.
    2. Combining a local anesthetic with opioids results in synergistic analgesia.
    3. 2-Chloroprocaine appears to decrease the effectiveness of epidural opioids.
    4. Spinal administration of opioids provides analgesia primarily by attenuating the Adelta fiber nociception.

13. Which of the following statements concerning peripheral opioid receptors is/are TRUE?

    1. Peripheral opioid receptors are found primarily at the end terminals of efferent fibers.
    2. Local tissue inflammation is important for analgesic effectiveness of peripheral opioid agonists.
    3. Intra-articular and peri-incisional opioids have not been found to provide postoperative analgesia.
    4. Combining local anesthetics with opioids for peripheral nerve blocks appears to be ineffective.

14. Which of the following statements concerning local anesthetics is/are TRUE?

    1. pKa determines onset of action.
    2. Lipophilicity influences potency.
    3. Protein binding influences duration of action.
    4. Clinically used local anesthetics cannot be alkalinized beyond a pH of 9 before precipitation occurs.

15. Systemic absorption and peak blood levels of local anesthetics are:

    1. linearly related to the total dose of local anesthetic injected
    2. reduced with the addition of epinephrine, especially for the less lipid-soluble, less potent, shorter-acting agents
    3. diminished with the more potent agents with greater lipid solubility and protein binding
    4. independent of anesthetic concentration

16. Which of the following statements concerning the CNS toxicity of local anesthetics is/are FALSE?

    1. CNS depression is a sign of high-dose local anesthetic toxicity.
    2. CNS excitation is a sign of low-dose local anesthetic toxicity.
    3. In general, decreased local anesthetic protein binding will decrease potential CNS toxicity.
    4. Seizure threshold is increased by administration of benzodiazepines.

17. Which of the following statements regarding the cardiovascular toxicity of local anesthetics is/are TRUE?

   1. In general, much greater doses of local anesthetics are required to produce cardiovascular toxicity than neurotoxicity.
   2. Bupivacaine cardiovascular toxicity is resistant to resuscitation.
   3. The central and peripheral nervous systems may be involved in the increased cardiotoxicity seen with bupivacaine
   4. Generally, the more potent, more water-soluble agents have increased cardiotoxicity.

18. Which of the following statements concerning allergic reactions to local anesthetics is/are TRUE?

   1. True allergic reactions to local anesthetics are rare.
   2. Allergic reactions to local anesthetics usually involve a type I reaction.
   3. The allergenic potential from esters may result from hydrolytic metabolism to *para*-aminobenzoic acid.
   4. Reactions are more common with amide than with ester anesthetics.

ANSWERS

---

1. **C.**   Myelinated nerves generally conduct impulses faster than unmyelinated nerves. The presence of myelin accelerates conduction velocity by increased electrical isolation of nerve fibers and by saltatory conduction. Increased nerve diameter accelerates conduction velocity both by increased myelination and by improved electrical cable conduction properties of the nerve. Myelinated and unmyelinated nerves carry both afferent and efferent functions. All nerves with a diameter >1 mm are myelinated. Myelinated nerve fibers are segmentally enclosed by Schwann cells forming a bilipid membrane that is wrapped several hundred times around each axon. Thus, myelin accounts for over half the thickness of large nerve fibers. The nodes of Ranvier are separated by the myelinated regions. The nodes are covered by interdigitations from nonmyelinated Schwann cells and by negatively charged glycoproteins. (See page 453: Anatomy of Nerves.)

2. **E.**   The resting potential of neural membranes averages −60 to −70 mV, with the interior being negative compared with the exterior. This resting potential is predominately maintained by a potassium gradient with 10 times greater concentration of potassium within the cell. An active protein pump transports potassium into the cell and sodium out of the cell through voltage-gated potassium channels. Generation of an action potential is primarily the result of voltage-gated sodium channels. Following activation (opening) of the sodium channel, it will spontaneously close into an inactive state and then revert to a resting confirmation. Thus, a three-state kinetic scheme conceptualizes the changes in the sodium channel confirmation that account for shifts in sodium conductance during depolarization and repolarization. An action potential is generated when the depolarization threshold of an axon is reached. This threshold is not an absolute voltage but depends on the dynamics of the sodium and potassium channels. Once an action potential is generated, propagation of the potential along nerve fibers is required for information to be transmitted. Both impulse generation and propagation are "all-or-nothing" phenomena. Nonmyelinated fibers require achievement of threshold potential at the immediately adjacent membrane, whereas myelinated fibers require generation of threshold potential at a subsequent node of Ranvier. (See page 454: Electrophysiology of Neural Conduction.)

3. **D.**   In general, local anesthetics with decreased systemic absorption will have a greater margin of safety in clinical use. The rate and extent of absorption will depend on numerous factors, of which the most important are the site of injection, the dose of local anesthetic, the physicochemical properties of the local anesthetic, and the addition of epinephrine. The relative amount of fat and vasculature surrounding the site of injection will interact with the physicochemical properties of the local anesthetic and will affect the rate of systemic uptake. In general, areas with greater vascularity will have more rapid and complete uptake as compared with those with more fat, regardless of type of local anesthetic. Hence, multiple injections near intercostal vascular bundles have a faster uptake than injections in the buttocks and groin. The greater the total dose of local anesthetic injected, the greater the systemic absorption and peak blood levels. (See page 457: Chemical Properties and Relationship to Activity and Potency.)

4. **B.**   The clinically used local anesthetics consist of a lipid-soluble substituted benzene ring linked to an amine group (tertiary or quaternary, depending on pKa and pH) via an alkyl chain containing either an amide or ester linkage. The type of linkage separates the local anesthetics into either aminoamides, which are metabolized in the liver, or aminoesters, which are metabolized by plasma cholinesterases. Several chemical properties of local anesthetics will affect their efficacy and potency. All clinically used local

anesthetics are weak bases that can exist as either the lipid-soluble (neutral) form or as the hydrophilic (charged) form. The primary site of action of local anesthetics appears to exist on the intracellular side of the sodium channel, and the charged form appears to be the predominately active form. Penetration of the lipid-soluble (neutral) form through the lipid neural membrane appears to be the primary form of access of local anesthetic molecules. Lipid solubility usually slows the rate of onset of action, increases duration of action, and increases potency. The degree of protein binding also affects activity of local anesthetics, because only the unbound form is free for pharmacologic activity. In general, increased protein binding is associated with increased duration of action. (See page 457: Chemical Properties in Relationship to Activity and Potency.)

5. **C.** The combination of pH of the environment and pKa, or dissociation constant, of a local anesthetic determines how much of the compound exists in each form. Decreasing pKa for a given environmental pH will increase the percentage of the lipid-soluble form and will hasten penetration of neural membranes and hence onset of action. (See page 457: Chemical Properties in Relationship to Activity and Potency.)

6. **C.** Tachyphylaxis to local anesthetics is a clinical phenomenon whereby repeated injection of the same dose of local anesthetic leads to decreasing efficacy. Tachyphylaxis has been described after central neuraxial blocks, after peripheral nerve blocks, and for different local anesthetics. An interesting clinical feature of local anesthetic tachyphylaxis is its dependence on dosing interval. If dosing intervals are short enough (such that pain does not occur), tachyphylaxis does not develop. Conversely, longer periods of patient discomfort before redosing hastens development of tachyphylaxis. Studies investigating the etiology of tachyphylaxis have found few pharmacokinetic or pharmacodynamic changes after repeated dose of local anesthetic. Prolonged exposure of peripheral nerve and neural cells to local anesthetic does not affect either flux through sodium channels or propagation of the action potential over time. Pain has been shown to be important for the development of tachyphylaxis; this has led to speculation of a central spinal mechanism via spinal cord sensitization. (See page 458: Tachyphylaxis to Local Anesthetic.)

7. **C.** Clearance of ester local anesthetics is primarily dependent on plasma clearance by cholinesterase, whereas amide local anesthetic clearance is dependent on hepatic metabolism. Thus, hepatic extraction, hepatic perfusion, hepatic metabolism, and protein binding will primarily determine the rate of clearance of amide local anesthetics. In general, local anesthetics with higher rates of clearance will have a greater margin of safety. Renal disease has little effect on pharmacokinetic parameters of local anesthetics. Correlation of resulting systemic blood levels between

dose of local anesthetic and patient weight often is inconsistent. (See page 462: Clinical Pharmacokinetics and Elimination.)

8. **C.** Treatment of systemic toxicity is primarily supportive. Injection of the local anesthetic should be stopped. Oxygenation and ventilation should be maintained, because systemic toxicity of local anesthetics is enhanced by hypoxemia, hypercarbia, and acidosis. If needed, the patient's trachea should be intubated and positive pressure ventilation instituted. Signs of CNS toxicity occur before cardiovascular events. Seizures can increase body metabolism and cause hypoxemia, hypercarbia, and acidosis. Intravenous administration of thiopental, midazolam, and propofol can all terminate seizures from systemic local anesthetic toxicity. Succinylcholine can terminate muscular activity from seizures and can facilitate ventilation and oxygenation; however, succinylcholine will not terminate seizure activity in the CNS, and increased cerebral metabolic demands will continue unabated. Potent local anesthetics (e.g., bupivacaine) can produce profound cardiovascular depression and malignant dysrhythmias that should be treated promptly. Oxygenation and ventilation must be immediately instituted, with cardiopulmonary resuscitation if needed. Ventricular dysrhythmias may be difficult to treat and may need large and multiple doses of electrical cardioversion, epinephrine, vasopressin, and amiodarone. (See page 466: Treatment of Systemic Toxicity from Local Anesthetics.)

9. **B.** There is a 4 to 40% incidence of TNS after lidocaine spinal anesthesia. These symptoms have been reported with other local anesthetics as well. The incidence of TNS varies with the type of surgical procedure and positioning. The incidence apparently is unaffected by baricity or dose. Reports of cauda equina syndrome after spinal anesthesia have led several authors to label TNS as a manifestation of subclinical neural toxicity. Other potential causes of TNS include patient positioning, early mobilization, needle trauma, neural ischemia, pooling of local anesthetics, and the addition of glucose. Clearly, the etiology of TNS remains undetermined, and further studies are needed to elucidate the underlying mechanism. Local anesthetics all have the potential to be neurotoxic, particularly in higher concentrations. (See page 467: Transient Neurologic Symptoms after Spinal Anesthesia.)

10. **B.** Enhanced awareness of potential cardiovascular toxicity with long-acting local anesthetics led to withdrawal of Food and Drug Administration approval for high concentrations of bupivacaine (0.75%) for obstetric use in the United States. The incidence of CNS toxicity with epidural injection is approximately three in 10,000, and with peripheral nerve blocks is 11 in 10,000. Levobupivacaine, an isomer of bupivacaine, appears to be approximately

equally potent to racemic bupivacaine for epidural anesthesia. Both ropivacaine and levobupivacaine appear to have approximately 30 to 40% less toxicity than bupivacaine on a milligram-to-milligram basis in both animal and human volunteer studies. This is likely the result of reduced affinity in brain and myocardial tissue. (See page 463: Systemic Toxicity of Local Anesthetics.)

11. A.   All currently available local anesthetics are racemic mixtures with the exception of lidocaine (achiral), ropivacaine (*S*), and *levo*-bupivacaine (*l* = *S*). Stereoisomers of local anesthetics appear to have potentially different effects on anesthetic potency, pharmacokinetics, and systemic toxicity. For example, *R* isomers appear to have greater in vitro potency for block of both neural and cardiac sodium channels and may thus have greater therapeutic efficacy and potential systemic toxicity. (See page 457: Pharmacology and Pharmacodynamics.)

12. A.   Opioids have multiple central neuraxial mechanisms of analgesic action. Supraspinal administration of opioids results in analgesia via opiate receptors in multiple sites (including activation of descending spinal pathways). Spinal administration of opioids provides the analgesia primarily by attenuating C-fiber nociception and is independent of supraspinal mechanisms. Coadministration of opioids with most local anesthetics results in synergistic analgesia. An exception to this analgesic synergy is 2-chloroprocaine, which appears to decrease the effectiveness of epidural opioids when used for epidural anesthesia. The mechanism for this action is unclear but does not appear to involve direct anatomization of opioid receptors. (See page 460: Opioids.)

13. C.   The recent discovery of peripheral opioid receptors offers yet another circumstance in which the coadministration of local anesthetics and opioids may be useful. The most promising clinical results have been from intra-articular and peri-incisional administration of local anesthetic and opioids for postoperative analgesia, whereas combining opioids and local anesthetics for nerve blocks appears to be ineffective. There are several reasons for a predicted lack of effective coadministration of local anesthetics and opioids for peripheral nerve blocks. Anatomically, peripheral opioid receptors are found primarily at the end terminals of afferent fibers. However, peripheral nerves are commonly blocked by deposition of anesthetic proximal to the end terminals of nerve fibers. In addition, common sites for peripheral nerve blocks are encased in multiple layers of connective tissue, which the anesthetic must traverse before accessing peripheral opioid receptors. Finally, previous studies have demonstrated the importance of concomitant local tissue inflammation for analgesic effectiveness of peripheral opioid receptor agonists. (See page 460: Opioids.)

14. E.   Physicochemical properties of local anesthetics will affect systemic absorption. In general, the more potent agents with greater lipid solubility and protein binding will result in lower systemic absorption and lower peak blood levels. Increased binding to neural and nonneural tissue probably explains this observation. (See page 457: Chemical Properties and Relationship to Activity and Potency.) pH of commercial preparations of local anesthetics ranges from 3.9 to 6.47 and is especially acidic if prepackaged with epinephrine. Because the pKa of commonly used local anesthetics ranges from 7.6 to 8.9, less than 3% of the commercially prepared local anesthetic exists as the lipid-soluble neutral form. However, clinically used local anesthetics cannot be alkalinized beyond a pH of 6.05 to 8 before precipitation occurs, and such a pH will increase the neutral form only to about 10%. (See page 459: Alkalinization of Local Anesthetic Solution.)

15. E.   Epinephrine can counteract the inherent vasodilating characteristics of most local anesthetics. The reduction in blood concentration with epinephrine is most effective for the less lipid-soluble, less potent, shorter-acting agents. The greater the total dose of local anesthetic injected, the greater the systemic absorption and peak blood levels will be. This relationship is nearly linear and is relatively unaffected by anesthetic concentration and speed of injection. (See page 460: Systemic Absorption.)

16. A.   Decreases in local anesthetic protein binding and clearance will increase potential CNS toxicity. Local anesthetics readily cross the blood-brain barrier, and generalized CNS toxicity may occur from systemic absorption or direct vascular injection. Signs of generalized CNS toxicity from local anesthetics are dose dependent. Low doses produce CNS depression, and higher doses result in CNS excitation and seizures. The rate of intravenous administration of local anesthetic will affect signs of CNS toxicity, because higher rates of infusion will lessen the appearance of CNS depression while leaving excitation intact. This dichotomous reaction to local anesthetics may be caused by a greater sensitivity of cortical inhibitory neurons to the impulse-blocking effects of local anesthetics. External factors, such as acidosis and increased P_{CO_2}, can increase CNS toxicity. Seizure thresholds of local anesthetics are increased by administration of barbiturates and benzodiazepines. (See page 463: Toxicity of Local Anesthetics: Central Nervous System Toxicity.)

17. A.   In general, much greater doses of local anesthetics are required to produce cardiovascular toxicity than CNS toxicity. Similar to CNS toxicity, potency for cardiovascular toxicity reflects the anesthetic potency of the agent. Recent attention has focused on the apparently exceptional cardiotoxicity of the more potent, more lipid-soluble agents (bupivacaine, etidocaine). These agents appear to have

a different sequence of cardiovascular toxicity than less potent agents. For example, increasing doses of lidocaine lead to hypotension, bradycardia, and hypoxia, whereas bupivacaine often results in sudden cardiovascular collapse from ventricular dysrhythmias that are resistant to resuscitation. (See page 464: Cardiovascular Toxicity of Local Anesthetics.)

18. **A.** True allergic reactions to local anesthetics are rare and usually involve type I (immunoglobulin E) or type IV (cellular immunity) reactions. Type I reactions are worrisome, because anaphylaxis may occur. They are more common with ester than with amide local anesthetics. True allergy to amide agents is extremely rare. Increased allergenic potential with esters may result from hydrolytic metabolism to *para*-aminobenzoic acid (a documented allergen). Added preservatives, such as methylparaben and metabisulfite, also can provoke an allergic response. (See page 469: Allergic Reactions to Local Anesthetics.)

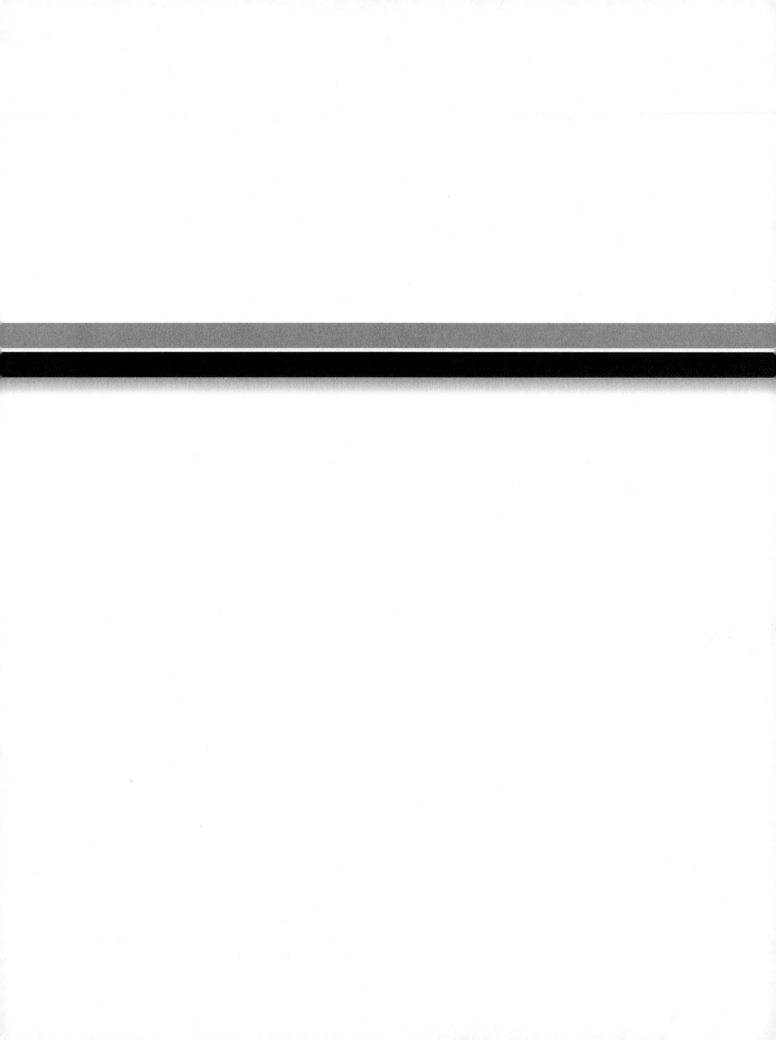

SECTION IV ■ PREPARING FOR ANESTHESIA

CHAPTER 18 ■ PREOPERATIVE EVALUATION AND MANAGEMENT

For *questions 1 to 6, choose the best answer.*

1. All of the following are important predictors of cardiac postoperative complications EXCEPT:

   A. preoperative serum creatinine of 1.0 mg/dL
   B. history of cerebrovascular accident
   C. preoperative treatment with insulin
   D. history of congestive heart failure
   E. major vascular surgery

2. After an episode of asthma, airway hyperreactivity may persist up to:

   A. 24 hours
   B. 48 hours
   C. 72 hours
   D. 4 days
   E. several weeks

3. The current recommendation of the National Blood Resource Education Committee is that a hemoglobin of _____ is acceptable in patients without systemic disease.

   A. 9 g/dL
   B. 6 g/dL
   C. 7 g/dL
   D. 10 g/dL
   E. 8 g/dL

4. Which of the following tests, if done preoperatively in a patient without risk factors, can lead to more harm than benefit?

   A. Electrocardiogram (ECG)
   B. Blood urea nitrogen (BUN)/creatinine
   C. Chest radiograph (CXR)
   D. Urinalysis (U/A)
   E. None of the above

5. Postoperatively, functional residual capacity may take up to _____ to return to baseline.

A. 24 hours
B. 48 hours
C. 3 days
D. 7 days
E. 14 days

6. As a general rule, oral medications should be given to the patient _____ before arrival in the operating room.

   A. 60 to 90 minutes
   B. 30 to 60 minutes
   C. 20 minutes
   D. 10 minutes
   E. 5 minutes

For *questions 7 to 12, choose A if 1, 2, and 3 are correct; B if 1 and 3; C if 2 and 4; D if 4; and E if all are correct.*

7. Which of the following place(s) a patient at risk for increased perioperative cardiovascular morbidity and should be considered in a preoperative evaluation?

   1. Peripheral arterial disease
   2. Diabetes mellitus
   3. Hypertension with left ventricular hypertrophy (LVH)
   4. At least one coronary artery with critical stenosis

8. The hallmark features of Cushing syndrome include:

   1. easy bruisability
   2. truncal "thinning"
   3. moon facies
   4. hypotension

9. Which of the following should be included in the preoperative history to rule out a bleeding abnormality?

   1. Easy bruising
   2. Unusual bleeding after a tooth extraction

3. Liver disease
4. Use of chemotherapeutic agents

10. A preoperative ECG should be ordered and evaluated in which of the following patient populations?

1. Patient with a prior myocardial infarction
2. Patient with a history of hypertension, diabetes mellitus, or peripheral vascular disease
3. Men >60 years of age
4. Women >70 years of age

11. TRUE statements about cessation of smoking include:

1. Stopping for 48 hours reduces the amount of carboxyhemoglobin.

2. Cessation between 48 hours and 6 weeks is associated with increased mucociliary clearance.
3. Cessation for 48 hours abolishes the effects of nicotine.
4. Stopping for 1 week is sufficient to eliminate the increased incidence of postoperative pulmonary complications.

12. A resting echocardiogram provides information about:

1. ventricular function
2. regional wall motion
3. ventricular wall thickness
4. valvular function

ANSWERS

---

1. **A.** The Revised Cardiac Risk Index identified six independent predictors of complications: high-risk type of surgery, history of ischemic heart disease, history of congestive heart failure, history of cerebrovascular disease, preoperative treatment with insulin, and preoperative serum creatinine >2.0 mg/dL. (See page 478: Evaluation of the Patient with Known Cardiac Disease.)

2. **E.** After an episode of asthma, airway hyperreactivity may persist for several weeks. (See page 484: Asthma.)

3. **C.** The current recommendation of the National Blood Resource Education Committee is that a hemoglobin of 7 g/dL is acceptable in patients without systemic disease. (See page 487: Complete Blood Count and Hemoglobin Concentration.)

4. **C.** A preoperative CXR can identify abnormalities that may lead to either delay or cancellation of the planned surgical procedure or modification of perioperative care. However, routine testing in the population without risk factors can lead to more harm than benefit. The American College of Physicians suggests that a CXR is indicated in the presence of active chest disease or before an intrathoracic procedure, but not solely on the basis of advanced age. (See page 488: Chest X-Rays.)

5. **E.** Functional residual capacity may take up to 2 weeks to return to baseline. (See page 483: Pulmonary Disease.)

6. **A.** As a general rule, oral medications should be given to the patient 60 to 90 minutes before arrival in the operating room. It is acceptable to administer oral drugs with up to 150 mL of water. Intravenous agents produce effects after a few circulation times, whereas for full effect, intramuscular medications should be given at least 20 minutes and preferably 30 to 60 minutes before the patient's arrival in the operating room. (See page 489: Pharmacologic Preparation.)

7. **E.** Peripheral arterial disease has been shown to be associated with coronary artery disease in multiple studies; at least 60% of the patients scheduled for major vascular surgery exhibit at least one coronary vessel with critical stenosis. Diabetes mellitus is common in the elderly, represents a disease that affects multiple organ systems, is associated with coronary artery disease, and increases the chance of silent myocardial ischemia and infarction. Hypertension also can be associated with an increased risk of silent myocardial ischemia and infarction, especially if the hypertension is associated with LVH with a strain pattern on ECG. A strain pattern usually suggests a chronic ischemic state. (See page 478: Cardiac Disease.)

8. **B.** The prolonged use of glucocorticoids can lead to Cushing syndrome. Truncal obesity, moon facies, skin striations, easy bruisability, and hypertension are hallmark signs of Cushing syndrome. Preoperative preparations include correction of fluid and electrolyte abnormalities (e.g., hypokalemia, hyperglycemia). In patients with long-term corticosteroid use, perioperative steroid supplementation is indicated to cover the stress of anesthesia and surgery. (See page 484: Endocrine Disease.)

9. **E.** Coagulation disorders can have significant impact on the surgical procedure and perioperative management. However, abnormal laboratory studies in the absence of clinical abnormalities will rarely lead to perioperative problems. It is important to identify

such disorders from a prior history of bleeding problems. Prothrombin time/partial thromboplastin time analysis is indicated in the presence of previous bleeding disorders (e.g., following injuries and after tooth extraction or surgical procedures), in patients with known or suspected liver disease, in patients with malabsorption or malnutrition, and in patients taking certain medications (e.g., chemotherapeutic agents). (See page 488: Coagulation Studies.)

10. E.   The preoperative 12-lead ECG can provide important information on the status of the patient's myocardium and coronary circulation. Abnormal Q waves in high-risk patients are highly suggestive of a past myocardial infarction. Patients with Q-wave infarctions are known to be at increased risk of a perioperative cardiac event and have a worse long-term prognosis. Patients who exhibit LVH or ST segment changes on a preoperative ECG also are at an increased risk of a perioperative cardiac event. Reasonable recommendations for a preoperative ECG include patients with systemic cardiovascular disease, diabetes mellitus, men >60 years, and women >70 years. (See page 481: Cardiovascular Tests.)

11. B.   Cessation of smoking for 2 days can decrease carboxyhemoglobin levels, abolish the nicotine effects, and improve mucous clearance. Between 2 days and 6 weeks, there is no real improvement because mucociliary clearance does not improve during this time. A prospective study showed that smoking cessation for at least 8 weeks was necessary to reduce the rate of postoperative pulmonary complications. (See page 484: Tobacco.)

12. E.   A resting echocardiogram can determine the presence of ventricular dysfunction, regional wall abnormalities, ventricular wall thickness, and valvular function. Pulsed-wave Doppler can be used to obtain the velocity time integral. Ejection fraction then can be calculated by determining the cross-sectional area of the ventricle. (See page 482: Assessment of Ventricular and Valvular Function.)

CHAPTER 19 ■ ANESTHESIA FOR PATIENTS WITH RARE AND COEXISTING DISEASES

1. Which of the following statements about Duchenne muscular dystrophy is TRUE?

   A. The underlying defect is the lack of the muscle protein dystrophin, a major component of the muscle membrane.
   B. Cardiac muscle is spared from the disease process.
   C. Painful degeneration of skeletal muscle is a hallmark of the disease.
   D. It is a genetic dominant trait.
   E. Death rarely occurs.

2. Anesthetic management of muscular dystrophy involves attention to all of the following EXCEPT:

   A. myocardial depressant sensitivity to inhalational agents
   B. avoidance of succinylcholine
   C. malignant hyperthermia precautions
   D. use of high doses of nondepolarizing agents, because of resistance to these drugs
   E. use of drugs for aspiration precautions

3. All of the following statements about myotonia are true EXCEPT:

   A. Myotonia results in delayed muscle relaxation, which is not reliably treatable by regional anesthesia, muscle relaxants, or deep anesthesia.
   B. Myotonia diseases are similar to muscular dystrophy in that the underlying defect is a membrane-stabilizing protein.
   C. Reversal with neostigmine may provoke a myotonic contracture.
   D. Quinine, tocainide, and mexiletene have all been used to relax myotonic contractures.
   E. Myotonic dystrophy (Steinert disease) is the most common of the dystrophies.

4. What is an important consideration in the anesthetic management of a patient with familial periodic paralysis?

   A. Maintenance of hypokalemia in both forms of periodic paralysis
   B. Use of succinylcholine is acceptable in the presence of normokalemia
   C. Maintaining mild hypothermia
   D. No change in dosing of nondepolarizing muscle relaxants (NDMRs)
   E. Avoidance of large carbohydrate loads

5. All of the following facts about myasthenia gravis are true EXCEPT:

   A. It is a disease of the neuromuscular junction involving the muscarinic acetylcholine receptors.
   B. It is an autoimmune disorder.
   C. The mainstay of medical therapy involves medical therapy with the cholinesterase inhibitor pyridostigmine.
   D. Coexisting diseases associated with myasthenia are systemic lupus erythematosus, rheumatoid arthritis, pernicious anemia, and thyroiditis.
   E. The process most likely originates in the thymus gland.

6. Intraoperative management of myasthenia gravis would include all of the following EXCEPT:

   A. consideration of increased sensitivity to NDMRs
   B. use of a defasiculating dose of NDMR to facilitate intubation
   C. use of a short-acting NDMR with neuromuscular monitoring
   D. consideration of resistance to succinylcholine
   E. use of an anesthetic technique that avoids the use of muscle relaxants

7. All of the following statements about Lambert-Eaton syndrome are true EXCEPT:

   A. It is a disorder of neuromuscular transmission associated with carcinomas.
   B. Antibodies against the acetylcholine receptor are produced.
   C. Treatment involves treating the underlying malignancy.
   D. 3,4-Diaminopyridine may be used in the treatment to increase release of acetylcholine.
   E. Patients with this syndrome are sensitive to the effects of both depolarizing muscle relaxants and NDMRs.

8. Which of the following statements about Guillain-Barré syndrome (polyradiculoneuritis) is TRUE?

   A. It is an autoimmune disorder triggered by a bacterial or viral infection.
   B. The autoimmune response is against myocytes of skeletal muscle.
   C. Ventilatory support is rarely needed.
   D. Eighty-five percent of patients do not recover.
   E. Administration of succinylcholine is not associated with hyperkalemia.

9. Multiple sclerosis may have all of the following anesthetic considerations EXCEPT:

   A. The effect of anesthesia and surgery on the disease process is controversial.
   B. A patient may have a relapse of symptoms after spinal anesthesia.
   C. A thorough neurologic examination before surgery/anesthesia is helpful.
   D. Autonomic dysfunction is not a concern in patients with multiple sclerosis.
   E. Multiple sites of demyelination of the brain and spinal cord are the hallmarks of the disease.

10. All of the following statements concerning epilepsy are true EXCEPT:

    A. Many different types of central nervous system (CNS) disorders may manifest with seizures.
    B. Grand mal seizures are characterized by tonic-clonic motor activity with respiratory arrest and hypoxemia.
    C. Status epilepticus is associated with a high mortality if not effectively treated.
    D. Use of muscle relaxants are an adequate method of treatment.
    E. Maintenance of chronic antiseizure medication is critical throughout the perioperative period.

For questions 11 to 20, choose A if 1, 2, and 3 are correct; B if 1 and 3; C if 2 and 4; D if 4; E if all are correct.

11. Anesthetic management of patients with a medically treated seizure disorder involves which of the following considerations?

    1. Consideration of significant drug interactions between the antiseizure medication and anesthetic agents is indicated.
    2. Propofol may raise seizure threshold in patients undergoing electroconvulsive therapy.
    3. Potent opioids may produce myoclonic activity or chest wall rigidity, which can be confused with seizure activity.
    4. Use of ketamine for induction is indicated.

12. Which of the following statements regarding Parkinson disease is/are TRUE?

    1. It is a disease of the CNS primarily affecting those >65 years of age.
    2. It is characterized by excessive dopaminergic fiber activity in the basal ganglia of the brain.
    3. Gamma-Aminobutyric acid (GABA) levels increase with resultant suppression of cortical motor function.
    4. Decreasing dopamine levels in the brainstem results in resolution of the symptoms.

13. Management of anesthesia in a patient with Parkinson disease will include which of the following?

    1. Use of phenothiazines and butyrophenones is contraindicated.
    2. Gastrointestinal dysfunction is manifested by salivation, dysphagia, and esophageal dysfunction.
    3. Autonomic dysfunction is a common manifestation.
    4. Drug therapy should be discontinued before anesthesia.

14. Which of the following statements regarding Huntington chorea is/are TRUE?

    1. Disordered movement and dementia are clinical hallmarks of the disease.
    2. Mental depression and suicide are common.
    3. Specific therapy is directed at control of the movement disorder.
    4. Duration of disease averages <20 years from the time of diagnosis to death.

15. Amyotrophic lateral sclerosis is manifested by which of the following?

    1. It is a degenerative disease involving anterior horn cells of the spinal cord.
    2. Although the etiology is unknown, glutamate excitotoxicity and impaired neural protein repair are among the theories that have been proposed.
    3. There is an increased sensitivity to NDMRs.
    4. There is sparing of pulmonary function.

16. Which of the following facts should be considered when anesthetizing a patient with anemia?

    1. Healthy individuals do not develop symptoms until hemoglobin (Hgb) levels fall to <7 g/dL.
    2. Physiologic compensation includes increased plasma volume, increased cardiac output, and increased 2,3-diphosphoglycerate (2,3-DPG) levels.
    3. Symptoms are highly variable and depend upon concurrent disease processes and the speed of developing anemia.
    4. There is no accepted Hgb level at which transfusion should be administered.

17. Which of the following facts is/are TRUE regarding nutritional deficiency anemias?

    1. All deficiency anemias result in microcytic hypochromic red blood cells (RBCs).
    2. Ferritin levels and Hgb measurements are good markers to detect iron deficiency anemia.
    3. The use of nitrous oxide (N_2O) is contraindicated in patients with iron deficiency anemia.
    4. Causes of folic acid deficiency include alcoholism, pregnancy, and malabsorption syndromes.

18. Which of the following statements regarding hemolytic anemias is/are TRUE?

    1. Spherocytosis is a disorder of all proteins of the RBC membrane.

    2. Glucose-6-phosphate dehydrogenase (G6PD) deficiency results in the inability to reduce methemoglobin, and therefore sodium nitroprusside is contraindicated.
    3. The life span of an RBC in a patient with hereditary spherocytosis is 120 days.
    4. Splenectomy may be indicated in patients with hereditary spherocytosis.

19. Anesthetic management of a patient with sickle cell disease involves which of the following:

    1. Adequate systemic oxygenation and hydration
    2. Avoiding barbiturates because they cause sickling
    3. Maintenance of normothermia for all types of surgery
    4. Always avoiding tourniquets

20. Which of the following statements concerning rheumatoid arthritis is/are TRUE?

    1. It is characterized by chronic inflammation of multiple organ systems.
    2. Polyarthropathy is the hallmark of the disease.
    3. Pericarditis and pulmonary nodules are manifestations of the disease.
    4. Rheumatoid arthritis may be associated with Felty syndrome.

ANSWERS

---

1. **A.**   Duchenne muscular dystrophy is a sex-linked recessive disorder that is evident in boys and young men. In Duchenne muscular dystrophy, the underlying defect is a lack of the muscle protein dystrophin. Progressive painless muscle degeneration with atrophy of skeletal muscle occurs. Cardiac muscle and smooth muscle are not spared. Pneumonia and congestive heart failure are common causes of death, which may occur between the ages of 15 and 25 years. (See page 503: Duchenne Muscular Dystrophy.)

2. **D.**   Patients with muscular dystrophy have increased susceptibility to the myocardial depressant effects of inhalation anesthetics. Use of NDMRs should be modified because of increased sensitivity to these drugs from pre-existing muscle weakness. Use of succinylcholine may result in increased potassium, secondary to membrane instability. Some patients with muscular dystrophy may be susceptible to malignant hyperthermia, but this is unpredictable. (See page 505: Muscular Dystrophy: Management of Anesthesia.)

3. **B.**   The myotonias are a group of illnesses characterized by delayed relaxation of skeletal muscle. Quinine, tocainide, mexiletene, and local anesthetic injected directly into the muscle will result in

relaxation of the muscle. Myotonic dystrophy is the most common form. The underlying defect is secondary to defects in sodium channels that alter ion channel function. Reversal with neostigmine may provoke a myotonic contracture. Steinert disease is the most common of the dystrophies. (See page 505: Myotonias.)

4. **E.**   Familial periodic paralysis is an autosomal dominant inherited disease. There are two forms: hyperkalemic and hypokalemic. Each is characterized by intermittent periodic muscle weakness. Both have different cellular mechanisms. Anesthetic management consists of maintenance of a normal potassium level and avoiding precipitating weakness. During weakness episodes, patients will be more sensitive to NDMRs. Succinylcholine should be avoided to prevent changes in serum potassium levels. Serial potassium measurements during the perioperative period are recommended. Avoidance of hypothermia and of large carbohydrate loads also is recommended. (See page 506: Familial Periodic Paralysis.)

5. **A.**   Myasthenia gravis is a disease of the neuromuscular junction where antibodies are formed against the nicotinic acetylcholine receptors; T-helper

cells assist in this antibody production. Systemic lupus erythematosus, pernicious anemia, and thyroiditis are associated with myasthenia. The disease probably originates in the thymus gland; 90% of patients have histologic abnormalities such as thymoma, thymic hyperplasia, or thymic atrophy. Thymectomy may help in controlling the symptoms. Mainstay therapy is medical treatment with the cholinesterase inhibitor pyridostigmine. Other treatment modalities may include corticosteroids, immunosuppressants, plasmapharesis, and thymectomy. (See page 507: Myasthenia Gravis.)

6. **B.**   Patients with myasthenia gravis are exquisitely sensitive to NDMRs; therefore, a defasiculating dose of an NDMR may result in excessive muscle relaxation. Use of a short-acting NDMR is recommended to avoid prolonged postoperative paralysis. Response to succinylcholine includes greater resistance and prolonged duration of action (which may partially be attributable to use of pyridostigmine in the treatment of the disease). Use of regional anesthesia may avoid respiratory depression associated with opioids. Use of an anesthetic technique that avoids use of muscle relaxants may be useful. (See page 508: Myasthenia Gravis: Management of Anesthesia.)

7. **B.**   Lambert-Eaton syndrome is a disorder of neuromuscular transmission associated with carcinomas, especially small cell carcinoma of the lung. Onset may precede carcinoma by years. Treatment of the underlying neoplasm may improve the neurologic condition. Immunoglobulin G antibodies are produced against presynaptic calcium channels; this inhibits the proper release of acetylcholine. Autonomic dysfunction also may occur. Patients are sensitive to both depolarizing muscle relaxants and NDMRs. Pyridostigmine may be used to treat symptoms of weakness. Treatments include immunoglobulin, plasmapharesis, and treating the underlying malignancy. 3,4-Diaminopyridine improves synaptic transmission by opening voltage-gated potassium channels and increasing release of acetylcholine. It is the most effective treatment. (See page 509: Myasthenic Syndrome [Lambert-Eaton Syndrome].)

8. **A.**   Guillain-Barré syndrome is an autoimmune disorder triggered by bacterial or viral infections. Antibodies are produced by the body against myelin, which results in demyelination of nerve tissue. Symptoms include subacute or acute skeletal muscle weakness, which may result in respiratory weakness. Prognosis is good, with 85% of patients achieving full recovery. Treatment consists of plasmapharesis or high-dose immunoglobulin. Patients are exquisitely sensitive to succinylcholine, and therefore this drug should be avoided. This response may persist after symptoms have resolved. (See page 510: Guillain-Barré Syndrome.)

9. **D.**   Multiple sclerosis is an acquired disease of the CNS that results in demyelination of the brain and spinal cord. The cause is multifactorial, and the disease occurs in genetically susceptible individuals. A viral etiology has been suspected but not proven. Symptoms of multiple sclerosis are related to the site of demyelination. The course of the disease process is characterized by waxing and waning of symptoms. Corticosteroids are used to control acute exacerbations of symptoms but have no influence on long-term outcome. The effect of anesthesia and surgery on the disease process is highly controversial. Patients with multiple sclerosis may experience worsening of symptoms with spinal anesthesia. Hyperthermia and metabolic and hormonal changes induced by surgery or anesthesia may exacerbate symptoms. Autonomic dysfunction caused by multiple sclerosis may exaggerate the hypotensive effects of volatile anesthetics. (See page 510: Multiple Sclerosis.)

10. **D.**   Seizures may be the manifestation of many disorders of the CNS. Seizures result from excessive discharge of neurons that synchronously depolarize. Symptoms are related to the area of neuronal activity. There are >40 different types of epilepsy based on clinical features. Grand mal seizures are characterized by tonic-clonic motor activity that results in respiratory arrest and arterial hypoxemia. Patients with status epilepticus have recurrent grand mal seizures with loss of consciousness lasting >30 minutes; mortality is high unless the condition is treated effectively. Lack of muscular activity may confuse and prevent proper diagnosis as a seizure progresses. During the perioperative period, antiseizure medication should be continued. In the event of seizure activity, benzodiazepines are the drug of choice for treatment. Use of muscle relaxants will abolish muscular activity; however, CNS neuronal activity will continue. (See page 511: Epilepsy.)

11. **A.**   Antiseizure medication may induce hepatic enzymes; therefore, fentanyl requirements may be greater with patients receiving anticonvulsant therapy. There is a potential for significant drug interaction for the same reason. Potent opioids may produce myoclonic activity or chest wall rigidity, which may be confused with seizure activity. Use of ketamine also may produce seizure-like activity and is relatively contraindicated in these patients because better alternative medicines exist. Propofol may raise seizure threshold in patients undergoing electroconvulsive therapy. (See page 512: Epilepsy: Management of Anesthesia.)

12. **B.**   Parkinson disease is a disabling neurologic disease, primarily affecting adults >65 years of age. It is a result of loss of dopaminergic fibers in the basal ganglia of the brain. Deficiency of dopamine results in increases in activity of GABA. This acid results in inhibition of brainstem nuclei, which suppress cortical motor function. This causes the characteristic features

of the disease, such as resting tremor, akinesia, and postural abnormalities. Treatment of the disease is directed at increasing dopamine levels in the brain with minimal peripheral side effects. (See page 513: Parkinson Disease.)

13. **A.** In Parkinson disease, use of butyrophenones (droperidol) and of phenothiazines is contraindicated because of their effect on dopamine levels in the CNS. Autonomic dysfunction is common; symptoms include orthostatic hypotension, gastrointestinal dysfunction, and an exaggerated response to inhalational agents. Drug therapy should not be discontinued because muscular rigidity can interfere with the ability to extubate a patient. Gastrointestinal manifestations include dysphagia, esophageal dysfunction, and salivation. Patients with Parkinson disease should be considered at risk of aspiration pneumonitis. (See page 513: Parkinson Disease.)

14. **E.** Huntington disease is a neurodegenerative disease of the corpus striatum and cerebral cortex. It is an inherited disorder that is autosomal dominant. Clinical symptoms include disordered movement, dementia, clinical depression, athetosis, and dystonia. Mental depression and suicide are common. Duration of the disease averages approximately 17 years from diagnosis to death. There is no specific therapy; treatment is directed at both depression and control of movement disorders. (See page 514: Huntington Disease.)

15. **A.** Amyotrophic lateral sclerosis is a degenerative disease of the anterior horn cell (motor cells) throughout the CNS. It is believed to be viral in origin and bears similarity to poliomyelitis. Glutamate excitotoxicity, free radical stress, impaired neural protein repair, viral or prion infection, heavy metal exposure, or an autoimmune response have all been proposed as etiologies. It is a rapidly progressive disorder in which death results within 3 to 5 years of diagnosis. Pulmonary function is severely affected, with all patients eventually requiring mechanical ventilation. Neuromuscular transmission is altered, and patients have increased sensitivity to NDMRs. These patients can also exhibit a hyperkalemic response to succinylcholine (because of the emergence of extrajunctional acetylcholine receptors). (See page 515: Amyotrophic Lateral Sclerosis.)

16. **E.** There are numerous causes of anemia. Compensations include an increase in plasma volume, cardiac output, and 2,3-DPG levels. Symptoms depend upon concurrent disease processes, and most healthy individuals can asymptomatically tolerate an Hgb level of 7 g/dL. No specific Hgb level exists below which a transfusion should be administered. Concurrent disease and the need for increased oxygen-carrying capacity should dictate the need for transfusion. (See page 516: Anemias.)

17. **C.** Nutritional deficiency anemias are categorized as iron, vitamin B_{12}, and folic acid deficiency. Only iron deficiency anemia produces RBCs that are microcytic and hypochromic. This anemia may be from poor iron intake or from rapid turnover of RBCs. Hgb levels and ferritin levels are good clinical tests for iron deficiency. N_2O is not contraindicated in iron deficiency anemia. In vitamin B_{12} and folate deficiency, the RBCs are enlarged. The clinical significance of an N_2O effect on vitamin B_{12} metabolism is controversial. Causes of folic acid deficiency include alcoholism, pregnancy, and malabsorption syndromes. (See page 516: Nutritional Deficiency Anemia.)

18. **C.** Hereditary spherocytosis is a disorder of the protein spectrin that renders the RBC membrane unstable. Chronic hemolysis occurs. G6PD deficiency is a hemolytic disorder in which NADPH is not produced. This results in an increased sensitivity to oxidation. G6PD deficiency also results in a reduced level of glutathione. The cells become rigid, which accelerates clearance by the spleen. Numerous drugs induce hemolysis. Patients with G6PD deficiency are unable to reduce methemoglobin. Therefore, nitroprusside and prilocaine should not be administered. Splenectomy is rarely indicated before age 6 because of the high incidence of pneumococcal infection. The life span of a normal RBC is 120 days. Because the RBC membrane in hereditary spherocytosis is altered, the life span of the RBC is shortened. (See page 517: Hemolytic Anemias.)

19. **B.** Sickle cell disease is a hereditary disorder associated with the formation of abnormal Hgb. This Hgb has the tendency to sickle under specific environmental conditions (e.g., hypoxia, hypothermia, and acidosis). Individuals who are homozygous have a greater tendency to develop sickling because of the greater proportion of abnormal Hgb. Arterial tourniquets have been used safely in patients with sickle cell disease; however, these devices should be used only when they are critical to the surgical procedure because of the possibility of local hypoxia and acidosis. Most commonly used anesthetic medications do not have an effect on the sickling process. (See page 518: Sickle Cell Disease.)

20. **E.** Rheumatoid arthritis is a chronic inflammatory disease with symmetric polyarthropathy and involvement of other systemic organs. Polyarthropathy initially occurs with the hands and wrists but may involve lower extremity joints, atlantoaxial joints, temporomandibular joint, cervical spine, and joints of the larynx. Other systemic manifestations include pericarditis, aortitis, pulmonary nodules, interstitial lung disease, renal failure, and anemia. Felty syndrome is the clinical triad of rheumatoid arthritis, leukopenia, and hepatosplenomegaly. (See page 521: Rheumatoid Arthritis.)

CHAPTER 20 ■ MALIGNANT HYPERTHERMIA AND OTHER PHARMACOGENETIC DISORDERS

For questions 1 and 2, choose the best answer.

1. What is the earliest sign of malignant hyperthermia (MH) in an intubated, paralyzed patient?

   A. Ventricular arrhythmia
   B. Tachycardia
   C. Tachypnea
   D. Fever
   E. Increased end-tidal CO_2

2. What percentage of patients with masseter muscle rigidity (MMR) is at risk for developing MH?

   A. 10
   B. 20
   C. 30
   D. 40
   E. 50

For questions 3 to 13, choose A if 1, 2, and 3 are correct; B if 1 and 3; C if 2 and 4; D if 4; E if all.

3. Which of the following are signs and symptoms of neuroleptic malignant syndrome?

   1. Bradycardia
   2. Flaccid paralysis
   3. Hypotension
   4. Acidosis

4. Which of the following can occur during an MH episode?

   1. Hyperkalemia
   2. Myoglobinuria
   3. Lactic acidosis
   4. Hypocalcemia

5. Which of the following statements regarding MMR is/are TRUE?

   1. It most commonly is seen in children.

2. Peripheral nerve stimulation typically does not reveal muscle relaxation.
   3. Tachycardia is frequent.
   4. Repeat doses of succinylcholine will cause relaxation.

6. Which of the following should be considered as a possibility in the differential diagnosis of MMR?

   1. Myotonic syndrome
   2. Low dose of succinylcholine
   3. Insufficient time to intubation after succinylcholine administration
   4. Temporomandibular joint syndrome

7. Which of the following statements regarding neuroleptic malignant syndrome is/are TRUE?

   1. Symptoms usually occur after an acute exposure to a triggering agent.
   2. Haloperidol is a cause.
   3. Bromocriptine is a treatment.
   4. Sudden withdrawal of levodopa may cause onset of symptoms.

8. Which of the following can trigger MH?

   1. Ether
   2. Succinylcholine
   3. Methoxyflurane
   4. Decamethonium

9. Which of the following regarding treatment of MH is/are TRUE?

   1. A reasonable initial dose of dantrolene is 2 to 2.5 mg/kg.
   2. Calcium channel blockers are useful in acute-phase treatment.
   3. Lidocaine is effective in managing dysrhythmias.
   4. The recommended maximum dose of dantrolene is 7.5 mg/kg.

10. Which of the following statements regarding
    dantrolene is/are TRUE?

    1. It acts intracellularly.
    2. It inhibits excitation contraction coupling.
    3. It has little effect on myocardial contractility.
    4. It increases the reuptake of intracellular calcium.

11. Which of the following can result in successful
    litigation if an MH episode occurs?

    1. Failure to obtain complete history
    2. Not having a temperature monitor
    3. Having an inadequate supply of dantrolene
    4. Not investigating unexplained fever

12. Which of the following statements regarding
    porphyria is/are TRUE?

1. It is a defect in heme synthesis.
2. Inducible porphyria may cause a neurologic
   syndrome.
3. Conjugation of succinyl coenzyme A is the limiting
   step.
4. All barbiturates are contraindicated in porphyria.

13. Which of the following is/are characteristic of
    glucose-6-phosphate deficiency?

    1. Hyperglycemia
    2. Poor tolerance to fasting
    3. Alkalosis
    4. Prolonged bleeding time

ANSWERS

1. **E.** Elevation of end-tidal CO_2 is one of the earliest
signs of MH. Tachypnea does not occur in an
intubated, paralyzed patient. Tachycardia and
hypertension result from sympathetic nervous system
stimulation secondary to underlying hypermetabolism
and hypercarbia. Ventricular dysrhythmias can occur
and are induced by sympathetic nervous system
stimulation, hypercarbia, hyperkalemia, or
catecholamine release. (See page 530: Classic
Malignant Hyperthermia.)

2. **E.** Muscle biopsy with caffeine-halothane
contracture testing has shown that approximately
50% of patients who experience MMR also are
susceptible to MH; therefore, one may elect to
discontinue anesthesia and postpone surgery after an
episode of MMR. (See page 531: Masseter Muscle
Rigidity.)

3. **D.** The symptoms and signs of neuroleptic malignant
syndrome include fever, rhabdomyolysis, tachycardia,
hypertension, agitation, muscle rigidity, and acidosis.
The mortality rate is unknown but may be significant.
Dantrolene is an effective therapeutic modality in
many cases of neuroleptic malignant syndrome.
(See page 533: Neuroleptic Malignant Syndrome and
Other Drug-Induced Hyperthermia Reactions.)

4. **A.** Hyperkalemia, hypercalcemia, lactic acidosis,
and myoglobinuria are characteristic of an MH
episode. A mixed venous sample will show even more
dramatic evidence of increased CO_2 production and
metabolic acidosis. (See page 530: Classic Malignant
Hyperthermia.)

5. **B.** Although MMR probably occurs in patients of all
ages, it is distinctly most common in children and

young adults. Several studies have shown a peak age
incidence at 8 to 12 years. A peripheral nerve
stimulator usually reveals flaccid paralysis. However,
increased tone of other muscles also may be noted.
Repeat doses of succinylcholine do not relieve the
problem. Tachycardia and dysrhythmias are not
infrequent. (See page 531: Masseter Muscle
Rigidity.)

6. **E.** The differential diagnosis of MMR includes (1)
myotonic syndrome, (2) temporomandibular joint
dysfunction, (3) underdosing with succinylcholine, or
(4) not allowing sufficient time for succinylcholine to
act before intubation. (See page 531: Masseter Muscle
Rigidity.)

7. **C.** Although the resemblance of neuroleptic
malignant syndrome to MH is striking, there are
significant differences between the two. MH is acute,
whereas neuroleptic malignant syndrome often occurs
after long-term drug exposure. Phenothiazines and
haloperidol or other antipsychotic agents are the usual
triggering agents for neuroleptic malignant syndrome.
Sudden withdrawal of drugs used to treat Parkinson
disease also may trigger neuroleptic malignant
syndrome. Electroconvulsive therapy with
succinylcholine does not appear to trigger the
syndrome. (See page 533: Neuroleptic Malignant
Syndrome and Other Drug-Induced Hyperthermia
Reactions.)

8. **E.** It is clearly established that potent inhalational
agents, including sevoflurane, desflurane, isoflurane,
halothane, methoxyflurane, cyclopropane, and ether,
may trigger MH. Succinylcholine and decamethonium
also are triggers. (See page 533: Drugs That Trigger
Malignant Hyperthermia.)

9. **B.** Initial intravenous therapy should be started with a minimum dose of 2.5 mg/kg, with repeat doses as needed. Although it often is recommended that the maximum dose of dantrolene is 10 mg/kg, more should be given as dictated by clinical circumstances. Dysrhythmia control usually follows hyperventilation, dantrolene therapy, and correction of acidosis. Lidocaine can be safely used during an MH crisis. Calcium channel blockers should not be used in the acute treatment of MH. Several studies have shown that verapamil can interact with dantrolene to produce hyperkalemia and myocardial depression. (See page 538: The Treatment of Malignant Hyperthermia.)

10. **A.** Dantrolene acts within the muscle cell itself by reducing intracellular levels of calcium. Most likely this results from a reduction of calcium release by the sarcoplasmic reticulum. In usual clinical doses, dantrolene has little effect on myocardial contractility. (See page 538: Dantrolene.)

11. **E.** Most of the common themes underlying the basis of litigation in MH cases include failure to obtain a thorough personal history, failure to monitor temperature continuously, failure to have an adequate supply of dantrolene, and failure to investigate an unexplained increase in body temperature. (See page 539: Medicolegal Aspects.)

12. **E.** All the porphyrias result from a defect in heme synthesis. The very limiting step in heme synthesis is the conjugation of succinyl coenzyme A with glycine to form D-aminolevulinic acid. The inducible porphyrias are those in which the acute symptoms are precipitated during drug exposure. These porphyrias may cause an acute neurologic syndrome. Barbituates are contraindicated in porphyria. (See page 549: The Porphyrias.)

13. **C.** Glucose-6-phosphate deficiency is an autosomal recessive disorder. The prognosis is moderately good, with many patients surviving into adulthood. These patients tolerate fasting very poorly. Hypoglycemia, acidosis, and convulsions may be a problem. Prolonged bleeding time has been described. (See page 551: Defects in Glucose Metabolism.)

CHAPTER 21 ■ DELIVERY SYSTEMS FOR INHALED ANESTHETICS

1. To comply with the 2000 ASTM (American Society for Testing Materials) standards, newly manufactured anesthesia work stations must have all of the following EXCEPT:

    A. exhaled tidal volume monitors
    B. anesthetic vapor concentration monitors
    C. a prioritized alarm system
    D. a way to measure supplied O_2 pressure
    E. a low-pressure circuit leak alarm

2. Considering the O_2 cylinder supply source, which of the following statements is TRUE?

    A. Anesthesia machines hold reserve D cylinders.
    B. The hanger yoke assemblies that attach the cylinders to the anesthesia machine are equipped with a Pin Index Safety System to eliminate cylinder interchange.
    C. The cylinder supply source is the primary gas source for the anesthesia machine.
    D. A cylinder exchange cannot take place while gas is flowing from another cylinder into the machine.
    E. The cylinder should be left open when the machine is in use in case of a pipeline failure.

3. Flow meter assembly includes all of the following EXCEPT:

    A. the physically distinguishable O_2 flow control knob
    B. the high-flow alarm to prevent turbulent flow
    C. series arrangement when two flow tubes are present for a single gas
    D. float stops at the top and bottom of the flow tubes
    E. flow meter scales individually hand calibrated using a specific float

4. Considering the flush valve, which of the following statements is TRUE?

    A. Using it intraoperatively can lead to patient awareness.

    B. Using it intraoperatively can cause barotrauma if it is used during the expiratory phase of positive-pressure ventilation.
    C. It is never suitable as a high-pressure O_2 source for jet ventilation.
    D. Flow from the flush valve enters the low-pressure circuit upstream from the vaporizer.
    E. Using it never leads to retrograde flow.

5. Most modern vaporizers are classified as all of the following EXCEPT:

    A. out-of-circuit
    B. temperature compensated
    C. flow-over
    D. pressure compensated
    E. variable bypass

6. When considering flow rate and vaporizer output, which of the following statements is TRUE?

    A. The vaporizer output is most consistent at extremes of flow rates.
    B. The output of variable bypass vaporizers is less than the dial setting at high flow rates.
    C. At high flow rates, the vaporizer output can be higher than the dial setting secondary to increased resistance to bypass flow.
    D. Incomplete mixing leads to the output's being higher than the dial setting at extremely high flow rates.
    E. The low level of turbulence at low flow rates affects the number of molecules vaporized.

7. Considering desflurane and the Datex-Ohmeda Tec 6 vaporizer for desflurane, which of the following statements is FALSE?

    A. The vapor pressure of desflurane is six to seven times that of contemporary inhaled anesthetics.
    B. Desflurane has a low blood gas coefficient, making recovery from anesthesia more rapid.

C. Desflurane can boil at room temperature.

D. The Tec 6 is electrically heated and pressurized.

E. The Tec 6 output is affected by carrier gas composition.

8. Considering the Mapleson circuits and their relative efficiency with respect to prevention of rebreathing CO_2, which of the following statements regarding spontaneous ventilation is TRUE?

A. A > DFE > BC

B. DFE > A > BC

C. BC > DFE > A

D. DFE > BC > A

E. A > BC > DFE

9. Regarding the circle system, which statement is FALSE?

A. Circle systems prevent rebreathing of CO_2.

B. Circle systems prevent rebreathing of all exhaled gases.

C. A circle system can be semiopen.

D. Numerous variations of the circle arrangement are possible.

E. The semiclosed system is the most commonly used application of the circle system.

10. All of the following factors can lead to increased production of compound A from the interaction of sevoflurane and CO_2 absorbent EXCEPT:

A. low fresh gas flow

B. high absorbent temperature

C. barium hydroxide lime (Baralyme) versus soda lime

D. dehydration of the Baralyme absorbent

E. old absorbent

11. When considering breathing circuits, which of the following statements is TRUE?

A. Absorbent canister leaks are the leading cause of critical incidents in anesthesia.

B. The most common site of disconnection is the inspiratory limb.

C. Leaks in the disposable anesthesia circuit can be detected through the high-pressure system leak test.

D. The effectiveness of electronic pressure monitors in diagnosing a disconnection is independent of the threshold pressure alarm limit.

E. Pressure monitors are probably the best device for revealing patient disconnection.

12. Considering the scavenging interfaces:

A. Positive-pressure and negative-pressure reliefs are mandatory if an active system is used.

B. Neither positive-pressure nor negative-pressure relief is necessary if using an active system.

C. Negative-pressure but not positive-pressure relief is necessary when using an active system.

D. Positive-pressure but not negative-pressure relief is necessary when using an active system.

E. Positive-pressure and negative-pressure relief is mandatory for a passive system.

For questions 13 to 25, choose A if 1, 2, and 3 are correct; B if 1 and 3; C if 2 and 4; D if 4; E if all.

13. Considering the O_2 and nitrous oxide pipeline supply source, which of the following statements is/are TRUE?

1. The O_2 cylinder supply source should not be regulated from the cylinder pressure upon entering the machine.

2. The hospital piping system supplies gases to the anesthesia machine at 50 pounds per square inch gauge (psig).

3. The fail-safe valve links the O_2 and nitrous oxide flow control valves.

4. The second-stage O_2 regulator in the Ohmeda machine supplies a constant pressure to the O_2 flow control valve regardless of the fluctuating pipeline pressure.

14. Considering flow meter assembly, which of the following statements is/are TRUE?

1. The space between the float and the wall of the flow tube varies with different flow rates.

2. The flow meters are referred to as constant pressure because the pressure across the float does not change with changing flow rates.

3. They are made up of tapered tubes and a mobile indicator float.

4. Flow through the annular space can only be laminar.

15. Which of the following is/are the safest configuration(s) for the flow meter sequence?

1. Nitrous oxide → air → O_2 → outlet

2. O_2 → nitrous oxide → air → outlet

3. Air → nitrous oxide → O_2 → outlet

4. O_2 → air → nitrous oxide → outlet

16. A hypoxic mixture can be delivered even with a proportioning system if:

1. The wrong gas is in the O_2 pipeline.

2. There is a leak downstream from the flow valves.

3. There are defective pneumatics or mechanics in the system.

4. An inert gas (helium, CO_2) is being delivered.

17. Saturated vapor pressure:

1. is independent of temperature

2. is dependent on atmospheric pressure

3. is the same for all inhalation agents

4. is equal to atmospheric pressure at the boiling point of a liquid

18. The pumping effect is increased with which of the following?

    1. Low flow rates
    2. Rapid respiratory rates
    3. Low levels of liquid anesthetic in the vapor chamber
    4. High peak inspiratory pressure

19. Which of the following vaporizer hazards are correctly matched with their safety features?

    1. Misfilling-keyed filling devices
    2. Tipping-interlock system
    3. Overfilling-filler port location
    4. Simultaneous inhaled anesthetic administration–fail-safe system

20. Considering the Bain circuit, which of the following statements is/are TRUE?

    1. The fresh gas inflow rate necessary to prevent rebreathing is 2.5 times the minute ventilation.
    2. It is a modification of the Mapleson D circuit.
    3. The major hazard of the Bain circuit is kinking or disconnection of the inner fresh gas hose.
    4. Fresh gas enters the circuit near the reservoir bag.

21. When considering CO_2 absorption, which of the following statements is/are TRUE?

    1. The absorption of CO_2 by soda lime is a chemical process, not a physical one.
    2. The maximum amount of CO_2 that can be absorbed is 26 L of CO_2/100 g of absorbent.
    3. The size of the absorptive granules is very important and takes both resistance to airflow and absorptive efficiency into consideration.
    4. It is not necessary for all closed and semiclosed circle systems.

22. Problems associated with the bellows assembly include which of the following?

    1. A bellows leak can lead to a change in the delivered FiO_2.
    2. Hypoventilation may occur if the ventilator relief valve is incompetent.
    3. A bellows leak can cause barotrauma if ventilators use a high-pressure driving gas.
    4. Hypoventilation may occur if the ventilator relief valve is stuck in the closed position.

23. Which of the following anesthetic techniques is/are associated with increased operating room contamination?

    1. Failure to turn off gas flow at the end of an anesthetic
    2. Filling of vaporizers
    3. Use of uncuffed endotracheal tubes
    4. Jackson-Reese circuits

24. The low-pressure circuit test:

    1. can detect loose filler caps
    2. evaluates the portion of the machine that is downstream from all safety devices, except the O_2 analyzer
    3. evaluates the integrity of the machine from the flow control valves to the common gas outlet
    4. evaluates the portion of the machine with least possibility of leaks

25. Considering the new breathing system technology of fresh gas decoupling, which of the following statements is TRUE?

    1. Nitrous oxide and O_2 are decoupled at the fresh gas inflow site.
    2. The expiratory and inspiratory limbs of the breathing circuit are no longer connected at the Y-piece.
    3. The O_2 flush valve is eliminated.
    4. The fresh gas flow is no longer added to the volume of gas delivered to the patient during inspiration.

ANSWERS

1. **E.** To comply with the 2000 ASTM standards, newly manufactured workstations must have monitors that measure the following parameters: continuous breathing system pressure, exhaled tidal volume, ventilatory CO_2 concentration, anesthetic vapor concentration, inspired O_2 concentration, O_2 supply pressure, arterial hemoglobin oxygen saturation, arterial blood pressure, and continuous electrocardiogram. The anesthesia workstation must have a prioritized alarm system that groups alarms into three categories: high, medium, and low priority. (See page 559: Standards for Anesthesia Machines and Workstations.)

2. **B.** The anesthesia machines hold reserve E cylinders if a pipeline supply source is not available or if the pipeline fails. Each hanger yoke is equipped with the Pin Index Safety System. It is a safeguard to eliminate cylinder interchanging and the possibility of accidentally placing the incorrect gas on a yoke designed to accommodate another gas. A check valve is located downstream from each cylinder. It minimizes gas transfer from a cylinder at high pressure to one with low pressure. It also allows an empty cylinder to be exchanged for a full one while gas continues to flow from another cylinder. The cylinder should be turned off except during the preoperative

machine checking period or when a pipeline source is unavailable. (See page 563: Cylinder Supply Source.)

3. **B.** Contemporary flow control valve assemblies have numerous safety features. The O_2 flow control knob is physically distinguishable from other gas knobs. It is distinctively fluted, projects beyond the control knobs of the other gases, and is larger in diameter than all the other flow control knobs. If a single gas has two flow tubes, the tubes are arranged in series and are controlled by a single control valve. Flow tubes are equipped with float stops at the top and bottom of the tube. The upper stop prevents the float from ascending to the top of the tube and plugging the outlet. It also ensures that the float will be visible at maximum flows (instead of being hidden in the manifold). The bottom float provides a central foundation for the indicator when the flow control valve is turned off. Flow meter scales are individually hand calibrated using a specific float. There is no high-flow alarm to prevent turbulent flow. (See page 566: Components of Flow Meter Assembly.)

4. **A.** The O_2 flush valve is associated with several hazards. Improper use of a normally functional O_2 valve also can result in problems. Overzealous intraoperative O_2 flushing can dilute inhaled anesthetics and lead to patient awareness. O_2 flushing during the inspiratory phase of positive-pressure ventilation can cause barotrauma. Flow from the O_2 flush valve enters the low-pressure circuit downstream from the vaporizers and downstream from the Ohmeda machine check valve. Inappropriate preoperative use of the O_2 flush valve to evaluate the low-pressure circuit for leaks can be misleading, particularly on the Ohmeda machine, which has the check valve at the common outlet. Back-pressure from the breathing circuit closes the check valve airtight, and large low-pressure circuit leaks can go undetected. Some machines, including the Ohmeda Modulus 2+, do not have check valves; thus, O_2 can flow in retrograde fashion through an internal relief valve located upstream from the O_2 flush valve. The O_2 flush valve can provide a high-pressure O_2 source suitable for jet ventilation. (See page 569: Oxygen Flush Valve.)

5. **D.** Most modern vaporizers, including the Ohmeda Tec 4, the Ohmeda Tec 5, and the North American Drager Vapor 19.1, are classified as variable bypass, flow-over, temperature-compensated, agent-specific, out-of-circuit vaporizers. Variable bypass refers to the method of regulating output concentration. As gas enters the vaporizer's inlet, the setting of the concentration control valve determines the ratio of flow that goes through the bypass chamber and through the vaporizing chamber. The gas channel to the vaporizing chamber flows over the liquid anesthetic and becomes saturated with vapor. Thus, flow-over refers to the method of vaporization. These vaporizers are temperature compensated because they are equipped with an automatic temperature-compensating device that maintains a constant vapor output over a wide range of temperatures. These vaporizers are agent specific and out-of-circuit because they are designed to accommodate a single agent and to be located outside the breathing circuit. Most modern vaporizers are not pressure compensated. However, vaporizers for desflurane, including the Datex-Ohmeda Tec 6 vaporizer, do need to be pressure compensated, because desflurane has a vapor pressure three to four times that of other contemporary inhaled anesthetics. (See page 571: Variable Bypass Vaporizers.)

6. **E.** With a fixed dial setting, vaporizer output varies with the rate of gas flowing through the vaporizer. This variation is particularly notable at extremes of flow rates. The output of all variable bypass vaporizers is less than the dial setting at low flow rates (<250 mL/minute). This results from a relatively high density of volatile inhaled anesthetics. At low flows, insufficient turbulence is generated in the vaporizing chamber to upwardly advance the vapor molecules. At extremely high flow rates, such as 15 L/minute, the output of most variable bypass vaporizers is less than the dial setting. This discrepancy is attributed to incomplete mixing and saturation in the vaporizing chamber. The resistant characteristics of the bypass chamber and the vaporizing chamber can vary as flow increases. These changes can result in decreased output concentration. (See page 572: Variable Bypass Vaporizers, Flow Rate.)

7. **A.** Desflurane has unique physical properties compared with other inhalation anesthetics. It has a minimal alveolar concentration value of 6 to 7%. Desflurane is valuable because it has a low blood gas solubility coefficient of 0.45 at 37°C and thus promotes rapid recovery from anesthesia. The vapor pressure of desflurane is three to four times that of contemporary inhaled anesthetics. It boils at 22.8°C, which is near room temperature. To achieve controlled vaporization of desflurane, Ohmeda has introduced the Tec 6 vaporizer, which is electrically heated and pressurized. Vaporizer output approximates the dial setting when O_2 is the carrier gas because the Tec 6 vaporizer is calibrated using 100% O_2. At low flow rates when a carrier gas other than 100% O_2 is used, however, a clear trend toward reduction in vaporizer output emerges. This reduction parallels the proportional decrease in viscosity of the carrier gas. (See page 574: Datex Ohmeda Tec 6 Vaporizer for Desflurane.)

8. **A.** To summarize the relative efficiency of different Mapleson systems with respect to prevention of rebreathing, during spontaneous ventilation, A > DFE > BC. During controlled ventilation, DFE > BC > A. (See page 578: Mapleson Systems.)

9. **B.**   The circle system prevents rebreathing of CO_2 by use of CO_2 absorbents but allows partial rebreathing of other gases. A circle system can be semiopen, semiclosed or closed, depending on the amount of fresh gas inflow. A semiclosed system is associated with some rebreathing of exhaled gases and is the most commonly used application in the United States. Numerous variations of the circle arrangement are possible, depending on the relative positions of the components. (See page 579: Circle Breathing System.)

10. **E.**   Sevoflurane has been shown to produce degradation products upon interaction with CO_2 absorbents. The major degradation product produced is fluoromethyl-2, 2-difluoro-1(trifluoromethyl) vinyl ether, or compound A. During sevoflurane anesthesia, factors apparently leading to an increase in the concentration of compound A include (1) low-flow or closed-circuit anesthetic techniques, (2) use of Baralyme rather than soda lime, (3) higher concentrations of sevoflurane in the anesthetic circuit, (4) higher absorbent temperatures, and (5) fresh absorbent. Baralyme dehydration increases the concentration of compound A, and soda lime dehydration decreases the concentration of compound A. (See page 581: Interactions of Inhaled Anesthetics with Absorbents.)

11. **C.**   Breathing circuit disconnections are the leading cause of critical incidents in anesthesia. The most common disconnection site is the Y-piece. Disconnections can be complete or partial. The disposable anesthesia circuit must be fully expanded before the circuit is checked for leaks. This is done to detect leaks in the high-pressure system, not the low-pressure system. Pneumatic and electronic pressure monitors are helpful in diagnosing disconnections. Factors influencing monitor effectiveness include the disconnection site, pressure sensor location, threshold pressure alarm limit, inspiratory flow rate, and resistance of the disconnected breathing circuit. When an adjustable-threshold pressure alarm limit is available, the operator should set the alarm limit to within 5 cm H_2O of the peak inspiratory pressure. CO_2 monitors are probably the best devices for revealing patient disconnections. (See page 584: Traditional Circle System Problems.)

12. **A.**   Positive-pressure relief is mandatory in both active and passive systems to vent excess gas in case of occlusion downstream from the scavenging interface. If the system is active, negative-pressure relief also is necessary. It protects the breathing circuit or ventilator from excessive subatmospheric pressure. Passive systems need only a single positive-pressure relief valve. In this system, transfer of the waste gas from the interface to the basal system relies on pressure of the waste gas itself, because the vacuum is not used positively. The positive-pressure relief valve opens at a preset value, such as 5 cm H_2O, if an

obstruction between the interface and disposal system occurs. (See page 589: Scavenging Interface.)

13. **C.**   The hospital piping system provides gases to the machine at approximately 50 psig, which is the normal working pressure of most machines. The cylinder supplies are the source of backup if the pipeline fails. The O_2 cylinder source is regulated from 2,200 to approximately 45 psig, and the nitrous oxide cylinder source is regulated from 745 to approximately 45 psig. Most Ohmeda machines have a second-stage O_2 regulator located downstream from the O_2 supply source. This regulator supplies a constant pressure to the O_2 flow control valve regardless of fluctuating O_2 pipeline pressures. A safety device, traditionally referred to as the fail-safe valve, is located downstream from the nitrous oxide supply source. It serves as an interface between the O_2 and nitrous oxide supply source. This valve shuts off, or proportionally decreases, the supply of nitrous oxide and other gases if the O_2 supply pressure decreases. A *proportioning system* is a safety feature that links O_2 and nitrous oxide flow control valves either mechanically or pneumatically so the minimum O_2 concentration at the common outlet is 25%. (See page 562: Anesthesia Workstation Pneumatics.)

14. **A.**   The flowmeter assembly precisely controls measured gas flow to the common gas outlet. The flow control valve regulates the amount of gas that enters the tapered transparent tube known as the flow tube. A mobile indicator located inside the flow tube indicates the amount of gas passing through the flow control valve. The flow meters are commonly referred to as constant-pressure flow meters, because the pressure decrease across the float remains constant for all positions in the tube. The term "variable orifice" designates the type of unit, because the annular space between the float in the flow tube varies with the position of the float. Flow through the constriction created by the float can be laminar or turbulent, depending on the flow rate. (See page 565: Flowmeter Assembly and page 566: Operating Principles of the Flowmeters.)

15. **B.**   It has been demonstrated that, in the presence of a flow meter leak, a hypoxic mixture is less likely to occur if the O_2 flowmeter is located downstream from all other flowmeters. A potentially dangerous arrangement has the nitrous oxide flowmeter located in the downstream position. A hypoxic mixture can result, because a substantial portion of O_2 flow passes through the leak, and all the nitrous oxide is directed to the common outlet. A safer configuration has the O_2 flow meter located in the downstream position. A portion of the nitrous oxide flow escapes through the leak and the remainder goes toward the common outlet. A hypoxic mixture is less likely, because all of the O_2 flow is advanced by the nitrous oxide. A leak in the O_2 flow tube can produce a hypoxic mixture

even when O_2 is located in the downstream position. (See page 567: Problems With Flowmeters.)

16. **E.**   All of the conditions can lead to hypoxic mixture delivery even with a proportioning system. The proportioning system will be fooled if a gas other than O_2 is present in the O_2 pipeline. Normal operation of the proportioning system is contingent upon the pneumatic and mechanical integrity. A leak downstream from these devices, such as a broken O_2 flow tube, can cause delivery of a hypoxic mixture. In this case, the O_2 analyzer is the only machine safety device that can detect the problem. Also, administration of a third inert gas, such as helium, nitrogen, or CO_2, can cause a hypoxic mixture because contemporary proportioning systems link only nitrous oxide and O_2. (See page 568: Proportioning Systems.)

17. **D.**   Saturated vapor pressure is the pressure created by the molecules in the vapor phase of a volatile liquid. As more molecules enter the vapor phase from the volatile liquid, the vapor pressure increases. Vapor pressure is dependent on the temperature and physical characteristics of the liquid; it is independent of the atmospheric pressure. The boiling point of a liquid is that temperature at which the vapor pressure equals the atmospheric pressure. All inhalation agents have a unique saturated vapor pressure. (See page 570: Physics: Vapor Pressure.)

18. **E.**   Intermittent back-pressure associated with positive-pressure ventilation or O_2 flushing can cause higher vaporizer output concentration than the dial setting. This phenomenon, known as the pumping effect, is more pronounced at low flow rates, low dial settings, and low levels of liquid anesthetics in the vaporizing chamber. Additionally, the pumping effect is increased by rapid respiratory rates, high peak inspired pressures, and rapid drops in pressure during expiration. (See page 572: Intermittent Back Pressure.)

19. **B.**   Agent-specific, key filling devices help prevent filling a vaporizer with the wrong agent. Overfilling of these vaporizers is minimized because the filler port is located at the maximum safe liquid level. Today's vaporizers are firmly secured to the vaporizer manifold, and there is little need to move them. Thus, problems associated with tipping are minimized. Some vaporizers are equipped with extensive baffles to make them even more immune to the problems associated with tipping. Administration of more than one inhaled anesthetic at a time is prevented by an interlock system that will not allow more than one vaporizer at a time to be operational. (See page 576: Vaporizer Safety Feature.)

20. **A.**   The Bain circuit is a modification of the Mapleson D circuit. It is a coaxial circuit in which the fresh gas flows through a narrow tube within the outer corrugated tubing. The central tube originates near the reservoir bag, but the fresh gas actually enters the circuit at the patient end. Exhaled gases enter the corrugated tubing and are vented through the respiratory valve near the reservoir bag. The Bain circuit may be used for both spontaneous and controlled ventilation. The fresh gas inflow rate necessary to prevent rebreathing of CO_2 is 2.5 times the minute ventilation. The main hazard of the Bain circuit is unrecognized disconnection or kinking of the inner fresh gas hose. (See page 579: Bain Circuit.)

21. **A.**   The closed and semiclosed circle systems both require the CO_2 be absorbed from exhaled gases. Two formulations of CO_2 absorbents are commonly used today: soda lime and Baralyme. The size of the absorptive granules has been determined by trial and error, which represents a compromise between resistance to airflow and absorptive efficiency. The absorption of CO_2 by soda lime is a chemical process, not a physical process. The maximum amount of CO_2 that can be absorbed is 26 L of CO_2/100 g of absorbent. However, channeling of gas through the granules may substantially decrease efficiency and allow only 10 to 20 L of CO_2 actually to be absorbed. (See page 580: Carbon Dioxide Absorbents.)

22. **A.**   Many problems can occur with bellows assembly. Leaks can occur from improper seating of the plastic bellows resulting in inadequate ventilation, because a portion of the driving gas is vented to the atmosphere. A hole in the bellows can lead to alveolar hyperventilation and possibly barotrauma when high-pressure driving gas is used. The value of delivered O_2 may increase when the driving gas is 100% O_2, but it also may decrease if the driving gas is composed of an air-O_2 mixture. The ventilator relief valve can cause problems as well. Hypoventilation occurs if the valve is incompetent, because the anesthetic gas is delivered to the scavenging system during the inspiratory phase instead of to the patient. If the ventilator relief valve is stuck in the closed position, it can produce barotrauma. (See page 586: Bellows Assembly Problems.)

23. **E.**   The two major causes of waste gas contamination in the operating room are the anesthetic technique used and the equipment used. Regarding the anesthetic technique, the following factors cause operating room contamination: failure to turn off gas flow control valves at the end of an anesthetic, poorly fitting mask, flushing of the circuit, filling anesthetic vaporizers, use of uncuffed endotracheal tubes, and use of breathing circuits such as the Jackson-Reese circuit, which is difficult to scavenge. (See page 588: Scavenging Systems.)

24. **A.**   The low-pressure leak test checks the integrity of the machine from the flow control valves to the common outlet. It evaluates the portion of the machine that is downstream from all safety devices

except for the O$_2$ analyzer. The components located in this area are precisely the ones that may be subject to breakage and leaks. Leaks in the low-pressure system can cause hypoxia and patient awareness. The North American Drager uses a positive-pressure leak test, and the Ohmeda uses a negative-pressure leak test on the low-pressure circuit. (See page 560: Low-Pressure Circuit Leak Test.)

25. **D.** The technology of fresh gas decoupling refers to a new breathing system that does not allow the volume of gas that enters the circuit via the fresh gas inlet to be part of the volume of gas delivered to the patient during inspiration. (See page 569: Oxygen Flush Valve.)

CHAPTER 22 ■ AIRWAY MANAGEMENT

1. Which of the following statements regarding airway anatomy is FALSE?

   A. The right principal bronchus is larger in diameter than the left.
   B. Cartilaginous rings support only the first two generations of the bronchi.
   C. The larynx is innervated bilaterally by two branches of each vagus nerve.
   D. The laryngeal "skeleton" consists of nine cartilages.
   E. The trachea measures approximately 15 cm in adults.

2. The maximum recommended inflation pressure for a number 4 laryngeal mask airway (LMA) is:

   A. 20 cm H_2O
   B. 40 cm H_2O
   C. 60 cm H_2O
   D. 80 cm H_2O
   E. none; a volume of air (30 mL) is inserted regardless of pressure

3. All of the following statements regarding endotracheal intubation in children are true EXCEPT:

   A. Elevation of the head on a pillow is not usually necessary.
   B. Cricoid pressure may be needed to displace an anterior appearing larynx into view.
   C. A Macintosh blade is generally more useful because of a larger tongue-to-mouth ratio.
   D. The cricoid cartilage is the narrowest part of the child's airway.
   E. Hyperextension at the atlanto-occipital joint may cause airway obstruction.

4. Which of the following statements regarding innervation of the airway is TRUE?

   A. The oropharynx is innervated by branches of the facial, glossopharyngeal, and vagus nerves.
   B. The oropharynx is innervated by branches of the vagus, glossopharyngeal, and hypoglossal nerves.
   C. The hypoglossal nerve provides for sensation over the posterior third of the tongue, vallecula, and epiglottis.
   D. The internal branch of the superior laryngeal nerve provides all sensory innervation below the vocal cords.
   E. The external branch of the superior laryngeal nerve provides all sensory innervation above the vocal cords.

For questions 5 to 12, choose A if 1, 2, and 3 are correct; B if 1 and 3; C if 2 and 4; D if 4; E if all are correct.

5. Laryngospasm is commonly caused by:

   1. saliva
   2. hypercapnia
   3. light anesthesia
   4. hypoxemia

6. Which of the following statements regarding use of an LMA and gastroesophageal reflux is/are TRUE?

   1. The LMA fits in the esophageal inlet but does not reliably seal it.
   2. There is a high incidence of aspiration when an LMA is used in the presence of a "full stomach."
   3. Aspiration is more common when a bag-valve mask device is used for cardiopulmonary resuscitation than when an LMA is used.
   4. If regurgitation is noted when an LMA is in place, it should be removed immediately.

7. Which of the following statements regarding the LMA is/are TRUE?

   1. Positive-pressure ventilation is generally not useful.
   2. Gastric inflation is much more likely when positive-pressure ventilation (with pressures of

10 cm H_2O) is used with an LMA than with an endotracheal tube (ETT).

3. An LMA cannot be used in the lateral position.
4. Tidal volumes of up to 8 mL/kg and airway pressure <20 cm H_2O can be used in positive-pressure ventilation with an LMA.

8. Which of the following statements regarding the Sellick maneuver is/are TRUE?

   1. It can obliterate the esophageal lumen while maintaining the tracheal opening.
   2. It is contraindicated when there is active vomiting.
   3. It can be used in conjunction with gentle positive-pressure ventilation.
   4. It should be used for rapid sequence induction in patients with laryngeal fracture.

9. Which of the following statements regarding laryngospasm is/are TRUE?

   1. It may be triggered by abdominal visceral stimulation.
   2. It accounts for approximately 75% of all critical postoperative respiratory events in adults.
   3. It is a possible cause of pulmonary edema.
   4. It should always be treated with muscle relaxants.

10. Which of the following statements regarding the local anesthetic cocaine is/are TRUE?

    1. It may be especially useful in blunting the

exaggerated blood pressure response to intubation often seen in hypertensive patients.
    2. It is an excellent topical anesthetic as well as a potent vasodilator.
    3. It is poorly absorbed from tracheal mucosa and must be given in larger doses to be effective (10% solution).
    4. It is metabolized by pseudocholinesterase and should not be given to patients with this enzyme deficiency.

11. Which technique(s) is/are almost always useful for endotracheal intubation in the patient with gross blood in the airway?

    1. Retrograde wire intubation
    2. Intubating LMA
    3. Esophageal Combitube
    4. Fiber-optic bronchoscopy

12. Which of the following statements regarding airway management is/are TRUE?

    1. The BURP maneuver helps to expel air entrained in the stomach following bag mask ventilation.
    2. In general, the Miller blade provides a better laryngeal view in the patient with a smaller mandibular space.
    3. The best treatment for laryngospasm is the Sellick maneuver.
    4. Cricoid pressure (the Sellick maneuver) can be effectively used with an LMA in place.

ANSWERS

---

1. **B.** The laryngeal skeleton consists of nine cartilages (three paired and three unpaired); together, these house the vocal folds, which extend in an anterior-posterior plane from the thyroid cartilage to the arytenoid cartilages. The larynx is innervated bilaterally by two branches of each vagus nerve: the superior laryngeal nerve and the recurrent laryngeal nerve. The trachea measures approximately 15 cm in adults and is circumferentially supported by 17 to 18 C-shaped cartilages, with a posterior membranous aspect overlying the esophagus. The right principal bronchus is larger in diameter than the left and is deviated from the plane of the trachea at a less acute angle. Cartilaginous rings support the first seven generations of the bronchi. (See page 596: Review of Airway Anatomy.)

2. **C.** Before attachment of the anesthesia circuit, the LMA is inflated with the minimum amount of gas to form an effective seal. Although it is difficult to suggest a particular volume of gas to be used, the operator should be accustomed to the feel of the pilot

bulb when it is inflated to 60 cm H_2O pressure, the maximum suggested seal pressure. (See page 602: LMA Insertion.)

3. **C.** Because of the relatively larger size of the occiput in children, which produces an "anatomic sniffing position," elevation of the head (as done in the adult) is not needed. On occasion, one may need to elevate the thorax instead. The relatively short neck gives the impression of an anterior position of the larynx. Posterior cricoid pressure often is helpful to place the laryngeal inlet into view. A straight blade is more helpful than a curved blade in displacing the stiff, omega-shaped, high epiglottis. Because the cricoid cartilage is the narrowest aspect of the airway until the child is 6 to 8 years of age, one must be sensitive to resistance to advancement of the ETT that has easily passed the vocal folds. Hyperextension at the atlanto-occipital joint, as done in adults, may cause airway obstruction because of the relative pliability of the trachea. (See page 610: Tracheal Intubation: Use of the Laryngoscope Blade.)

4. **A.** The oropharynx is innervated by branches of the vagus, facial, and glossopharyngeal nerves. The glossopharyngeal nerve travels anteriorly along the lateral surface of the pharynx. Its three branches supply sensory innervation to the posterior third of the tongue, the vallecula, the anterior surface of the epiglottis (lingual branch), the walls of the pharynx (pharyngeal branch), and the tonsils (tonsillar branch). The internal branch of the superior laryngeal nerve, which is a branch of the vagus nerve, provides sensory innervation to base of the tongue, epiglottis, aryepiglottic folds, and arytenoids. The remaining portion of the superior laryngeal nerve, the external branch, supplies motor innervation to the cricothyroid muscle. (See page 621: Awake Airway Management.)

5. **B.** Obstruction to mask ventilation may be caused by laryngospasm, which is a reflex closure of the vocal folds. Laryngospasm may occur as a result of foreign body (oral or nasal airway), saliva, blood, or vomitus touching the glottis, or it can occur during a light plane of anesthesia. (See page 600: The Anesthesia Facemask.)

6. **B.** Although the distal tip of the LMA's mask sits in the esophageal inlet, it does not reliably seal it. A predominant clinical perception is that the LMA does not protect the trachea from regurgitated gastric contents. During cardiopulmonary resuscitation, the incidence of gastroesophageal regurgitation is four times greater with a bag-valve mask as compared with the LMA. If regurgitated gastric contents are noted in the LMA, maneuvers similar to those applied when using an ETT should be instituted: Trendelenburg position, 100% oxygen, and leaving the LMA in place and using a flexible suction device down the barrel. When populations of patients considered to have a "full stomach" are studied (in controlled trials, prospective series, or case reports), there is a very low incidence of aspiration noted with elective or emergency LMA use. (See page 604: The LMA and Gastroesophageal Reflux.)

7. **D.** Although first introduced for use with spontaneous ventilation, the LMA has shown to be useful when positive-pressure ventilation is either desired or preferred. There is no difference found in gastric inflation with positive pressure (<17 cm H_2O pressure) when comparing the LMA and the ETT. When using the LMA, one should limit tidal volumes to 8 mL/kg and airway pressure to 20 cm H_2O, because this is the sealing pressure of the device under normal circumstances. Patients' airways have been managed with the LMA in the supine, prone, lateral, oblique, Trendelenburg, and lithotomy positions. (See page 604: LMA and Positive-Pressure Ventilation.)

8. **A.** Cricoid pressure entails the downward displacement of the cricoid cartilage, against the vertebral bodies. In this manner, the lumen of the esophagus is ablated while the completely circular nature of the cricoid cartilage maintains the tracheal lumen. Early cadaveric studies showed that correctly applied cricoid pressure was effective in preventing gastric fluids, <100 cm H_2O pressure, from leaking into the pharynx. Cricoid pressure is contraindicated in patients with active vomiting (risk of esophageal rupture), cervical spine fracture, and laryngeal fracture. If there are difficulties in securing the airway during rapid sequence induction, gentle positive-pressure ventilation may be used while maintaining cricoid pressure. (See page 613: NPO Status and the Rapid Sequence Induction.)

9. **B.** As a cause of ventilatory compromise, laryngospasm deserves special attention because of its prevalence in children and because it accounts for 23% of all critical postoperative respiratory events.in adults. Laryngospasm may be triggered by respiratory secretions, vomitus, or blood in the airway, pain in any part of the body, and pelvic or abdominal visceral stimulation. The cause of airway obstruction during laryngospasm is contraction of the lateral cricoarytenoids, the thyroarytenoid, and the cricothyroid muscles. Management of laryngospasm consists of immediate removal of the offending stimulus (if identifiable), administration of oxygen with continuous positive airway pressure, and, if other maneuvers are unsuccessful, use of a small dose of short-acting muscle relaxants. Negative-pressure pulmonary edema may result from any airway obstruction in a patient who continues to have a voluntary respiratory effort. Negative intrathoracic pressure is transmitted to the alveoli, which are unable to expand as a result of the more proximal obstruction. (See page 617: Difficult Extubation.)

10. **D.** Among otolaryngologists, cocaine is a popular topical agent. Not only is it a highly effective local anesthetic, it is the only local anesthetic that is a potent vasoconstrictor. It is commonly available in a 4% solution. The total dose applied to the mucosa should not exceed 200 mg in the adult. Cocaine should not be used in patients with known cocaine hypersensitivity, hypertension, ischemic heart disease, or pre-eclampsia or in those taking monoamine oxidase inhibitors. Because cocaine is metabolized by pseudocholinesterase, it is contraindicated in patients deficient in this enzyme. (See page 621: Awake Airway Management.)

11. **A.** Retrograde wire intubation has been described in a number of clinical situations as a primary intubation technique (elective or urgent) and after failed attempts at direct laryngoscopy, fiber-optic-aided intubation, and LMA-guided intubation. The most common indications are inability to visualize the vocal folds because of blood, secretions, or anatomic variations, unstable cervical spine, upper airway malignancy, and mandibular fracture. Contraindications to fiber-optic bronchoscope–aided intubation are relative and revolve around the limitations of the device. Because

the optical elements are small, minute amounts of airway secretions, blood, or traumatic debris can hinder visualization. Advantages to the esophageal tracheal Combitube include rapid airway control, airway protection from regurgitation, ease of use by the inexperienced operator, lack of requirement to visualize the larynx, and ability to maintain the patient's neck in a neutral position. This device has been shown to be useful in the patient with massive upper gastrointestinal bleeding or vomiting. The LMA-fastrach is indicated for routine elective intubation and for anticipated and unanticipated difficult intubation. Because it was designed to facilitate blind tracheal intubation, the presence of airway secretions, blood, or edema does not interfere with its use. (See page 631: Use of Retrograde Wire Intubation in Airway Management; page 635: Use of the Esophageal Tracheal Combitube; page 613: The Intubating Laryngeal Mask Airway; and page 624: Use of the Fiberoptic Bronchoscope in Airway Management.)

12. C.   Treatment of laryngospasm includes removal of an offending stimulus (if it can be identified), continuous positive airway pressure, deepening of the anesthetic state, and use of a rapidly acting muscle relaxant. If, during the laryngoscopy, a satisfactory laryngeal view is not achieved, the backward-upward-rightward pressure (BURP) maneuver may aid in improving the view. In this maneuver, a second operator displaces the larynx backward (B) against the cervical vertebrae, as superiorly (U) as possible and slightly lateral to the right (R), using external pressure (P) over the cricoid cartilage. As a generalization, the Macintosh blade is regarded as better wherever there is little room to pass an ETT (e.g., small mouth), whereas the Miller blade is regarded better in the patient who has a small mandibular space, large incisor teeth, or a large epiglottis. The major disadvantage of the LMA in resuscitation is the lack of mechanical protection from regurgitation and aspiration. Lower rates of regurgitation during cardiopulmonary resuscitation (3.5%) than with bag-valve mask ventilation (12.4%) have been shown. Even in the presence of regurgitation, pulmonary aspiration is a rare event with the LMA. Unfortunately, use of the Sellick maneuver may prevent proper seating of the LMA in a minority of instances. This may require brief removal of cricoid pressure until the LMA has been properly seated. Cricoid pressure is effective with an LMA in place. (See page 608: Direct Laryngoscopy; page 600: The Anesthesia Facemask; page 610: Use of the Laryngoscope Blade; and page 608: Preparing for Laryngoscopy and the "Best Attempt.")

CHAPTER 23 ■ PATIENT POSITIONING

For questions 1 to 9, choose the best answer.

1. A 67-year-old woman is scheduled for exploratory laparotomy because of a large pelvic mass.
   Before induction, she suddenly develops hypotension and tachycardia. What is the most appropriate next step?

   A. Immediately administer 500 μg epinephrine.
   B. Put the patient in the Trendelenburg position.
   C. Rapidly infuse 1000 mL of intravenous saline.
   D. Place a wedge underneath the patient's right hip.
   E. Administer 100 μg of phenylephrine.

2. All of the following statements concerning lithotomy position are true EXCEPT:

   A. It provides easy access to the perineum.
   B. Hip flexion to more than 90 degrees may impinge on lateral femoral cutaneous nerves.
   C. The legs should be brought together at the knees and ankles in the sagittal plane and then lowered slowly together at the end of the case.
   D. A high lithotomy position can potentially create a significant uphill gradient for arterial perfusion into the feet.
   E. Knees can be safely flexed more than 90 degrees to ensure surgical exposure.

3. All of the following statements concerning upper extremity injuries are true EXCEPT:

   A. The long thoracic nerve arises from nerve roots C5 to C7.
   B. Winging of the scapula is commonly associated with injury of the long thoracic nerve.
   C. The long thoracic nerve is routinely involved in stretch injuries of the brachial plexus.
   D. Hyperabduction of the arm may push the humerus into the axillary neurovascular bundle.
   E. A dampened pulse oximetry tracing may be a sign of neurovascular compression.

4. All of the following statements concerning radial nerve injury are true EXCEPT:

   A. Repeated compression of the upper arm may lead to radial nerve injury.
   B. Radial nerve injury results in wrist drop and weakness of thumb abduction.
   C. The most common site is at the olecranon groove.
   D. The patient with a radial nerve injury cannot extend the distal phalanx of the thumb.
   E. The patient with a radial nerve injury has decreased sensation in the web space between the thumb and index finger.

5. Which of the following statements concerning ulnar nerve injury is TRUE?

   A. The nerve is most susceptible to injury when the arm is on an arm board with the hand supinated.
   B. Elbow flexion can cause ulnar nerve damage by compression by the aponeurosis of the flexor carpi ulnaris muscle.
   C. The nerve is susceptible to injury as it passes in the ulnar groove of the lateral epicondyle.
   D. Injury causes loss of sensation in the thumb.
   E. Women have a statistically greater chance of postoperative ulnar neuropathy.

6. In order to have the pelvis retained in place on a fracture table, a vertical pole at the perineum should be placed:

   A. between the genitalia and the uninjured limb
   B. between the genitalia and the injured limb
   C. between the limbs at the midthigh level
   D. against the surface of the sacral prominence
   E. none of the above

7. All of the following may result from a compartment syndrome EXCEPT:

   A. deep venous thrombosis
   B. rhabdomyolysis

C. hypoxic edema and ischemia
D. lasting nerve damage
E. renal damage

8. Causes of a compartment syndrome include all of the following EXCEPT:

A. systemic hypotension augmented by elevation of the extremities
B. intrapelvic retractors
C. excessive flexion of knees or hips
D. Compression from a tight "draw sheet"
E. sequential compression device of the legs in the supine position

9. All of the following accurately describe problems resulting from the lateral decubitus position EXCEPT:

A. Contusion of the ear may occur.
B. There is the potential for excessive ventilation of the upside lung.
C. Respiratory compromise may be lessened if the point of flexion is at the iliac crest as opposed to the costal margin or flank.
D. There is the potential for winging of the scapula.
E. The saphenous nerve of the downside leg is likely to be compressed.

For questions 10 to 13, choose A if 1, 2, and 3 are correct; B if 1 and 3; C if 2 and 4; D if 4; E if all are correct.

10. Which of the following statements regarding postoperative complications of positioning is/are TRUE?

1. Severe postoperative macroglossia can be caused by prolonged marked neck flexion.
2. Neuropathies that result in motor function loss are generally associated with more prolonged or

permanent nerve dysfunction compared with those with isolated sensory loss.
3. Midcervical tetraplegia can occur after hyperflexion of the neck with or without head rotation.
4. The loss of functional residual capacity is less in the prone position than in either the supine or lateral position.

11. Which of the following statements concerning pulmonary perfusion zones is/are TRUE?

1. West zone 2 is the ideal portion to match perfusion with ventilation.
2. West zone 1 can be produced by excessive positive-end expiratory pressure and pulmonary hypotension.
3. When the patient is tilted head down, zone 3 is in the dorsal portion of the lung.
4. In the supine position, dorsal portions of the lung will have increased compliance and less ventilation–perfusion (V/Q) mismatch.

12. Which of the following may result from the prone position?

1. Decreased pulmonary compliance
2. Breast injuries, especially if the breast is displaced laterally
3. Distention of paravertebral vessels
4. Blindness

13. Which is/are the complication(s) associated with the sitting position?

1. Paradoxical air embolus
2. Tension pneumocephalus
3. Peripheral nerve injury
4. Postural hypotension

ANSWERS

---

1. **D.** With a patient in the supine position, a mobile abdominal mass, such as a very large tumor or a pregnant uterus, can rest on the great vessels of the abdomen and compromise circulation. This is known as the aortocaval syndrome, or the supine hypotensive syndrome. A significant degree of perfusion can be restored if the compressive mass is rolled toward the left hemiabdomen by a mechanical device that produces leftward displacement (e.g., a wedge under the right hip). (See page 644: Variations of the Dorsal Decubitus Positions.)

2. **E.** Flexion of either knees or hips more than 90 degrees can threaten to angulate and compress the

major vessels at either joint. Stretching of the inguinal ligament may impinge upon the lateral femoral cutaneous nerves and cause ischemia. When taking a patient out of the lithotomy position, the legs should be brought together and then lowered slowly to minimize torsion stress on the lumbar spine. This also permits gradual accommodation to the increase in circulatory capacitance, thereby avoiding sudden hypotension. A high lithotomy position, where the legs are almost fully extended on the thighs, produces an uphill perfusion gradient to the feet. To prevent the development of compartment syndromes, systemic hypotension and compressive leg wrapping should be avoided in high lithotomy. (See page 646: Lithotomy.)

3. **C.**   The long thoracic nerve arises from nerve roots C5 to C7 and innervates the serratus anterior muscle. Dysfunction of this nerve causes winging of the scapula. The effect of patient position is speculative, because the nerve is not routinely involved in a stretch injury of the brachial plexus and because the plexus is not routinely involved when long thoracic nerve dysfunction occurs. Hyperabduction of an arm can force the head of the humerus into the axillary neurovascular bundle and may be associated with dampening of the distal pulse and the ipsilateral pulse oximeter waveform. (See page 649: Brachial Plexus and Upper Extremity Injuries.)

4. **C.**   The radial nerve may be injured by compression against the underlying bone as it wraps around the humerus approximately 3 cm above the lateral epicondyle. Excessive cycling of an automatic blood pressure cuff has been implicated in causing damage to the radial nerve. Radial nerve injury results in wrist drop, weakness of thumb abduction, inability to extend the metacarpophalangeal joints, and loss of sensation in the web space between the thumb and the index finger. (See page 649: Brachial Plexus and Upper Extremity Injuries.)

5. **B.**   The ulnar nerve passes though the groove between the medial epicondyle and the olecranon process of the humerus. The nerve can be compressed as the arm lies abducted on a normal arm board with the hand pronated. Injury should be suspected if a pinprick of the fifth finger is not felt. Elbow flexion can cause ulnar nerve damage by several mechanisms: compression by aponeurosis of flexor carpi ulnaris muscle and cubital tunnel retinaculum or anterior subluxation of the ulnar nerve over the medial epicondyle of the humerus. Men are statistically more likely to have postoperative ulnar neuropathy than are women. (See page 649: Brachial Plexus and Upper Extremity Injuries.)

6. **A.**   The vertical pole on a fracture table should be well padded and placed against the pelvis between the genitalia and the uninjured limb. Damage to the genitalia and pudendal nerve and complete loss of penile sensation have been reported after improper use of the fracture table. (See page 652: Perineal Crush Injury.)

7. **A.**   Ischemia, hypoxic edema, and elevated tissue pressure within a fascial compartment characterize a compartment syndrome. This causes extensive rhabdomyolysis and lasting damage to nerves and muscles, and it releases nephrotoxic products of myoglobin destruction. Circulating debris from infections is apt to be filtered by the pulmonary microvasculature with injurious consequences for the lungs. (See page 652: Compartment Syndrome.)

8. **E.**   Position-related causes of a compartment syndrome include extremity elevation in the presence of hypotension, vascular obstruction of major vessels by intrapelvic retractors, excessive knee or hip flexion, and external compression on an elevated extremity. Tight straps or "draw sheets" on the arms may compress the anterior interosseous neurovascular bundle and may cause neuropathy or a hand compartment syndrome. A sequential compression device is used to prevent development of deep venous thrombosis in a prolonged case; this is not associated with compartment syndrome. (See page 652: Compartment Syndrome.)

9. **E.**   The lateral decubitus position may compromise ventilation and lead to injuries of the shoulder, scapula, and extremities. Damage of the peroneal nerve of the downside leg is common as it courses laterally around the neck of the fibula. The saphenous nerve courses medially and is less likely to be compressed. (See page 655: Complications of the Lateral Decubitus Positions.)

10. **E.**   Postoperative macroglossia can result from marked neck flexion. The prone position results in less of a loss of functional residual capacity than does either the supine or the lateral position. A midcervical tetraplegia can occur after hyperflexion of the neck. Motor neuropathies are generally more prolonged than are sensory neuropathies. (See page 643: Keypoints; page 663: Complications of the Head Elevated Positions; page 657: Physiology; and page 657: Ventral Decubitus Positions.)

11. **A.**   In West zone 1, alveolar pressure exceeds both arterial and venous pressure and prevents perfusion of the lung unit. It can be produced by pulmonary hypotension, excessive positive end-expiratory pressure, or overdistention of alveolar units from large tidal volumes. In West zone 2, arterial pressure exceeds alveolar pressure, and alveolar pressure remains higher than venous pressure. Perfusion is the result of fluctuation between arterial and alveolar pressure. In supine positions (especially when the head is down), gravity-induced vascular congestion forces the dorsal portions of the lung to function as a zone 3. Consequently, the compliance of the area is reduced, and passive ventilation tends to distribute gas preferentially to more easily dispensable substernal areas. (See page 644: Circulatory and Respiratory Physiology of the Dorsal Decubitus Positions.)

12. **E.**   Compression of the abdominal viscera and restricted chest expansion in the prone position decrease pulmonary compliance. Conjunctival edema is common in the prone patient whose head is at or below the level of the heart. It is usually transient; permanent loss of vision can occur. When intra-abdominal pressure approaches or exceeds venous pressure, return of blood from the pelvis and lower extremities is reduced or obstructed, and there is distention of paravertebral vessels. Finally, medial and cephalad displacement of breasts is better

tolerated than forced lateral displacement. (See page 659: Complications of the Ventral Decubitus Positions.)

13. E.   Postural hypotension may occur in the sitting position as the normal protective reflexes are inhibited by drugs used during anesthesia. The sitting position predisposes patients to air embolization when venous pressure becomes subatmospheric. Pneumocephalus occurs if air from the dural incision site spreads over the surface of the brain. There is risk of peripheral nerve injury, especially of the sciatic nerve, as a result of marked hip flexion. If the neck is excessively extended, diminished cervical spinal cord perfusion pressure may cause quadriplegia. (See page 663: Complications of the Head-Elevated Positions.)

CHAPTER 24 ■ MONITORING THE ANESTHETIZED PATIENT

1. The O_2 sensor location is on which part of the anesthesia circuit?

   A. Expiratory limb
   B. Inspiratory limb
   C. Fail-safe valve
   D. Second-stage O_2 pressure regulator
   E. O_2 pipeline supply

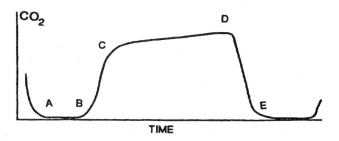

FIGURE 24.1. The normal capnogram. Point *D* delineates the end-tidal CO_2. End-tidal CO_2 (ETCO_2) is the best reflection of the alveolar CO_2 tension.

2. In the above capnograph, dead space ventilation occurs during which interval?

   A. A-B
   B. B-C
   C. C-D
   D. D-E
   E. C-E

3. In the above capnograph, the point defined as ETCO_2 occurs at:

   A. A
   B. B
   C. C
   D. D
   E. E

4. O_2 saturation determination by a pulse oximeter is based on what physical law?

   A. Charles' law
   B. Bohr law
   C. Beer-Lambert law
   D. Boyle law
   E. Bernoulli principle

5. The correct formula for determination of mean arterial pressure (MAP) based on systolic pressure (SP) and diastolic pressure (DP) is:

   A. DP + 1/3(SP − DP)
   B. SP − 1/3(SP − DP)
   C. DP − 1/2(SP − DP)
   D. (SP − DP) × 3
   E. (SP + DP)/3

6. Patients suffering from which condition are at increased risk of developing complete heart block during insertion of a pulmonary artery catheter (PAC)?

   A. Right bundle branch block
   B. Left bundle branch block
   C. Atrial fibrillation
   D. Anterior fascicular block
   E. Posterior fascicular block

7. Which of the following monitors is the most accurate indicator of ventricular preload?

   A. Central venous pressure (CVP) trends
   B. Pulmonary capillary wedge pressure (PCWP)
   C. Transesophageal echocardiogram (TEE)
   D. Mixed venous saturation
   E. Urine output

8. Which of the following is the most sensitive indicator of myocardial ischemia?

   A. CVP
   B. PAC

C. TEE
D. ST analysis of the electrocardiographic (ECG) tracing in leads II and V_5
E. Cardiac output

9. Which of the following is the correct ranking of evoked potentials according to their sensitivity to anesthetic depth from least affected to most affected?

A. Visual evoked potentials (VEP)/somatosensory evoked potentials (SSEP)/brainstem auditory evoked potentials (BAEP)
B. SSEP/VEP/BAEP
C. BAEP/VEP/SSEP
D. BAEP/SSEP/VEP
E. SSEP/BAEP/VEP

10. BAEPs are useful for monitoring neurologic function during which of the following surgical procedures?

A. Thoracic spine surgery
B. Frontal craniotomy
C. Cerebellar surgery
D. Middle cerebral artery clipping
E. Carpal tunnel surgery

11. Volatile general anesthetics produce what effects on the electroencephalogram (EEG)?

A. Increase amplitude and latency
B. Decrease amplitude and increase latency
C. Increase latency with no effect on amplitude
D. Decrease latency with no effect on amplitude
E. Decrease amplitude with no effect on latency

For questions 12 to 43, choose A if 1, 2, and 3 are correct; B if 1 and 3; C if 2 and 4; D if 4; E if all.

12. The use of monitoring devices on patients provides which of the following benefits?

1. Monitoring devices can allow for correction of derangements before irreversible injury occurs.
2. Monitoring devices are not subject to fatigue or distraction.
3. Monitoring devices make measurements at higher frequencies than is humanly possible.
4. Monitoring devices always enhance patient safety.

13. Methods of analyzing O_2 concentration include:

1. paramagnetic
2. galvanic cell
3. polarographic
4. photovoltaic

14. $ETCO_2$ values can be altered because of changes in which of the following?

1. Ventilation
2. Pulmonary blood flow
3. Metabolic activity
4. Cardiac output

15. Failure of the capnograph to return to baseline (zero) during inspiration can be caused by which of the following?

1. Failure of expiratory one-way valve
2. Cracked flow meter tubing
3. Exhaustion of CO_2 absorbent
4. Inadequate tidal volume

16. The assumption that $ETCO_2$ reflects $PaCO_2$ is dependent upon which of the following statements' being TRUE?

1. Ventilation and perfusion are appropriately matched.
2. No diffusion gradient exists for CO_2.
3. No sampling errors occur during measurement.
4. All alveoli empty at the same time.

17. Increasing dead space ventilation results in which change to $ETCO_2$?

1. Reduces the $ETCO_2$ value measured
2. Increases the baseline $ETCO_2$ value
3. Widens the $PaCO_2$-$ETCO_2$ gradient
4. Causes downsloping of the plateau phase of the capnogram

18. The presence of a stable (three breaths) CO_2 waveform via capnography can indicate which of the following?

1. Endotracheal tube (ETT) in the trachea
2. ETT in the pharynx
3. ETT in the right mainstream bronchus
4. ETT in the esophagus

19. Possible causes for a sudden loss of $ETCO_2$ include:

1. extubation
2. cardiac arrest
3. disrupted sample line
4. hyperventilation

20. Common clinical causes for a widened $PaCO_2$-$ETCO_2$ gradient include:

1. pulmonary embolism
2. hypoperfusion
3. chronic obstructive pulmonary disease
4. pulmonary shunt

21. The cause(s) of a sudden rise in nitrogen level in exhaled gases during O_2/N_2O anesthesia include(s):

1. failure of O_2 fail-safe alarm
2. leak in anesthesia circuit
3. failed inspiratory one-way valve
4. air embolism

22. During a laparoscopic cholecystectomy, an arterial blood gas sample is drawn because of difficulty maintaining O_2 saturation. When reviewed, the practitioner notes a large discrepancy between

$PaCO_2$ and $ETCO_2$. Possible causes for this include which of the following?

1. Air embolism
2. Hypoxic mixture
3. Baseline obstructive airway disease
4. Pre-existing restrictive airway disease

23. Which of the following statements regarding arterial pulse contour analysis is/are TRUE?

    1. It gives a beat-to-beat estimation of left ventricular output.
    2. It is not accurate in patients with septic shock.
    3. It requires calibration to a reference cardiac output determined by thermodilution or lithium dilution.
    4. Is not as precise or as accurate as cardiac outputs determined by thermodilution.

24. What alterations are seen in the arterial waveform measurement as one moves from the aorta to a distal artery?

    1. Later occurrence of the dicrotic notch
    2. Increase in DP
    3. Increase in SP
    4. Reduced slope of the initial systolic upstroke

25. Falsely high estimations of blood pressure determined by noninvasive cuff will occur in which of the following conditions?

    1. Cuff too small
    2. Loosely applied cuff
    3. Extremity below the heart
    4. Even compression applied to arm

26. The fidelity of fluid transducing systems (i.e., arterial lines) is constrained by which of the following properties?

    1. Damping
    2. Piezoelectric impedance
    3. Natural frequency
    4. Laminar flow

27. Which of the following can complicate placement of a radial arterial line?

    1. Median nerve injury
    2. Thrombosis of the artery
    3. Hematoma formation
    4. Ulnar nerve injury

28. Compared with the right internal jugular (IJ) vein, the left IJ vein is used less often for central venous access because of which of the following?

    1. Potential for damage to the thoracic duct
    2. Closer proximity to the carotid artery
    3. Difficulty passing through the jugular-subclavian junction
    4. Increased risk of injury to the phrenic nerve

29. Which of the following statements regarding the a wave seen in a CVP waveform are TRUE?

    1. Large a waves are seen in tricuspid stenosis.
    2. Cannon a waves are often seen in patients with atrial fibrillation.
    3. The a waves arise from atrial contractions.
    4. The a waves are preceded by the c wave.

30. Which of the following statements regarding CVP waveform monitoring are TRUE?

    1. CVP monitoring accurately estimates left ventricular (LV) filling pressures during ischemia.
    2. CVP and PCWP become similar during cardiac tamponade.
    3. CVP is more sensitive to thoracic pressure changes than is a PAC.
    4. Trends in CVP value reflect intravascular volume changes.

31. Determination of mixed venous O_2 saturation (SvO_2) allows one to assess which of the following?

    1. Adequacy of O_2 delivery
    2. Adequacy of cerebral perfusion
    3. Determination of intracardiac and pulmonary shunts
    4. Quantity of dead space within the lungs

32. Which of the following conditions can alter the PCWP-PAEDP relationship?

    1. Pulmonary embolism
    2. Alveolar hypoxia
    3. Acidosis
    4. Chronic pulmonary disease

33. Which of the following statements describes conditions in which a PAC is located in a West zone 3?

    1. PCWP > PAEDP
    2. Ability to aspirate blood from the distal port when the PAC is wedged
    3. Nonphasic PCWP tracing
    4. Chest radiograph showing the catheter tip above the level of the left atrium

34. PCWP is not a valid reflection of left ventricular end-diastolic pressure (LVEDP) in which of the following conditions?

    1. Ischemic left ventricle
    2. Aortic regurgitation
    3. Mitral valve stenosis
    4. Prolonged Q-T interval

35. Factors increasing risk of mortality following a PAC-induced pulmonary artery rupture include:

    1. coagulopathy
    2. pulmonary hypertension
    3. heparinization
    4. hypotension

36. A 67-year-old man is scheduled to have an infra-abdominal aortic aneurysm repaired. The surgeon desires a PAC to be placed in the patient, whereas the anesthesiologist wants to place a TEE probe. Which of the following statements regarding TEE are TRUE?

   1. TEE gives a more accurate estimation of LV preload than a PAC.
   2. Left arterial filling pressures can be calculated by measuring blood flow rates from the pulmonary veins into the left atrium.
   3. TEE can accurately identify myocardial ischemia.
   4. TEE is free from major complications.

37. Which of the following conditions produce a falsely elevated determination of cardiac output measured by thermodilution?

   1. Tricuspid regurgitation
   2. Intracardiac shunts
   3. Pulmonary regurgitation
   4. Aortic stenosis

38. Which of the following statements regarding the intracranial pressure (ICP) waveform is/are TRUE?

   1. The waveform is pulsatile.
   2. It varies with the respiratory cycle.
   3. The normal value is <15 mm Hg.
   4. A normal pressure indicates normal neurologic function.

39. Bispectral Index (BIS) monitoring of patients during anesthesia allows for which of the following:

   1. It improves speed of emergence and recovery from general anesthesia.
   2. It predicts movement in response to noxious stimulation.
   3. A BIS value <60 predicts lack of recall.
   4. It cannot be used if the patient is taking antiepileptic medications.

40. Which of the following statements regarding BIS monitoring is/are TRUE?

   1. BIS level reflects anesthetic depth.
   2. BIS value varies according to the type of anesthetic used.
   3. BIS integrates four different processed EEGs into a single numeric variable.
   4. BIS level >70 reflects loss of consciousness.

41. Loss of SSEPs during surgery could arise from which of the following?

   1. Increased depth of anesthesia
   2. Insufficient perfusion pressure at the dorsal horn of the spinal cord
   3. Sensory cortex stroke
   4. Insufficient perfusion pressure at the ventral horn of the spinal cord

42. When following SSEPs during thoracolumbar surgery, which of the following statements is/are TRUE?

   1. Monitoring both upper and lower limbs helps rule out physiologic causes of altered SSEP values.
   2. Monitoring SSEP makes the wake-up test redundant.
   3. A decrease in amplitude and increase in latency could indicate a deterioration in spinal cord function.
   4. Normal SSEP throughout surgery ensures normal motor function postoperatively.

43. Which of the following statements is/are TRUE?

   1. Convection is heat loss resulting from contact with surfaces.
   2. Radiation is heat loss resulting from infrared irradiation.
   3. Conduction is heat loss resulting from movement of air.
   4. Evaporation is heat loss resulting from energy required to vaporization of water.

ANSWERS

1. **B.** The O_2 monitor is located on the inspiratory limb of the anesthesia circuit. Beyond this point, the only alteration to the delivered anesthetic mixture would be the entrainment of room air, which would not produce a hypoxic mixture. The expiratory limb is downstream to the patient, thus providing no protection regarding what is delivered to the patient. The other possible answers are all upstream sites in the anesthesia circuit and, although they would ensure that the mixture was not hypoxic at that site, they could not ensure that downstream contamination will not occur. (See page 669: Inspiratory and Expired Gas Monitoring: Oxygen.)

2. **A.** During the initial phase of ventilation, the gases being expired are from the conducting airways, trachea, and anesthesia circuit. These areas are not involved in gas exchange and, thus, their composition will reflect the inspired mixture. Unless the inspired mixture contains CO_2, the initial phase of expiration will be a horizontal line at 0 mm Hg of CO_2. With further exhalation, alveolar gas reaches the sampling site and a rise in the capnograph will occur. (See page 670: Figure 24.1.

3. **D.** The end-tidal CO_2 value is recorded at the end of expiration, which on the capnograph occurs just

before the steep decline back to baseline. (See page 670: Figure 24.1.)

4. **C.** O_2 saturation detection via a pulse oximeter uses the physical principle described by the Beer-Lambert law. Beer law states that a parallel beam of light transmitted through a clear solution with a solute dissolved within it will fall exponentially as the solute level increases. Lambert law states that a parallel beam of light will have its intensity fall exponentially as the distance through which it must shine increases. (See page 672: Pulse Oximetry.)

5. **A.**   The formula for MAP is DP plus one-third the difference between the DP and SP. (See page 673: Indirect Measurement of Arterial Blood Pressure.)

6. **B.**   Individuals who have a left bundle branch block are relying on their right bundle branch to transmit the impulses from their atrioventricular node to the ventricular mass. In individuals with a left bundle branch block, passing a PAC through the right side of the heart could injure the right bundle and produce complete heart block. (See page 678: Complications of Pulmonary Catheter Monitoring.)

7. **C.**   The most accurate preload indicator for the left ventricle is the TEE probe, because it can assess actual intracardiac chamber size and thus preload. Urine output is also a very accurate method of detecting adequacy of LV preload; however, in healthy people with inadequate LV preload, urine output may be maintained. Conversely, in numerous conditions, urine output is inadequate despite adequate LV preload. CVP trends can be altered by abnormalities within the right ventricle, pulmonary circulation, and the left side of the heart. PCWP is accurate only if there are no complicating matters within the lungs (excessive positive end-expiratory pressure), left atrial abnormalities (mitral stenosis), and LV abnormalities (ischemia). Mixed venous O_2 saturation is an accurate indicator of total body O_2 balance but does not directly measure LV preload; it may be normal despite inadequate LV preload if the heart rate is increased to maintain cardiac output. (See page 681: Monitoring Applications.)

8. **C.**   Of all the answers, TEE and ST analysis of the ECG are the most accurate of the monitors for detecting myocardial ischemia. The most sensitive and specific of the two is TEE. The regional wall motion abnormalities that occur during ischemia are readily detected by TEE. Abnormal wall thickening and inward motion of the ischemic segment occur within seconds of the segment's becoming ischemic. However, not all wall motion abnormalities are caused by ischemia. Comparing TEE with ECG ST analysis, TEE picks up more ischemic episodes. ST analysis is very sensitive for ischemia. Increasing its sensitivity and specificity can be accomplished by placing the leads in the areas most likely to become ischemic. CVP, PAC readings, and cardiac output become abnormal with ischemia; however, they become abnormal late and are not very specific for ischemia. (See page 681: Monitoring Applications.)

9. **D.**   All evoked potentials are affected by anesthetics, but to varying degrees. BAEPs are least sensitive to anesthetic depth, followed by SSEPs; the most sensitive are VEPs. (See page 684: Evoked Potential Monitoring.)

10. **C.**   By keeping the anesthetic depth the same and keeping physiologic state near normal, evoked sensory potentials attempt to identify surgical effects on neural function. In order to detect changes secondary to the surgery, the evoked potential pathway must be within the surgical field. Thus, BAEPs are used during surgery on the base of the brain, SSEPs are used during extremity and spine surgery, and VEPs are used when surgery is located near the optical tracts. (See page 684: Evoked Potential Monitoring.)

11. **B.**   In general, volatile anesthetics produce a dose-dependent increase in latency and a decrease in amplitude. Isoflurane and desflurane can produce an isoelectric EEG. Enflurane is associated with an epileptic waveform at high levels. (See page 683: Electroencephalogram.)

12. **A.**   Because monitors are mechanical devices, they do not become distracted. They also can make repetitive measurements more often than humans because they do not fatigue. Monitoring the patient's vital sign allows one to detect derangements in the patient's early stages and make interventions to prevent irreversible injury. Monitors enhance patient safety only if an appropriate intervention is undertaken to correct the perturbation in the patient's physiology. (See page 668: Introduction.)

13. **A.**   The first three options are all methods used clinically to detect O_2 levels in the anesthetic mixture. Photovoltaics involve the generation of electrical current when certain metals are exposed to light. Examples of their use include the system that prevents elevator doors from closing on people within the threshold of the elevator. (See page 669: Paramagnetic Oxygen Analysis; page 669: Galvanic Cell Analyzers; and page 669: Polarographic Oxygen Analyzers.)

14. **E.**   The production of end-tidal CO_2 is dependent on its generation (i.e., metabolic rate), transportation from the cells to the lungs (i.e., cardiac output and pulmonary blood flow), and excretion from the lung (resulting from ventilation). (See page 670: Monitoring of Expired Gases.)

15. **B.**   Under normal conditions, the inspirate is free of CO_2. Hence, when it passes the sampling site, the capnograph registers zero. Failure to reach a zero

baseline value, when using a circle system, can occur as a result of any condition in which the one-way nature of the system is compromised. This will occur with damage to the inspiratory or expiratory one-way valves. Exhaustion of the CO_2 absorbent also will result in rebreathing of expired gases and a failure to reach a baseline of zero. Different anesthesia circuits, such as Bain circuit, can have rebreathing occur if their inspiratory fresh flow rates are insufficient to clear the expiratory limb of the circuit. Cracked flow tubes may cause altered inspirate composition or a hypoxic mixture, but this will not result in an altered inspiratory baseline of zero during capnographic measurement. Inadequate tidal volume will result in an elevation of $ETCO_2$ but will not alter the return to baseline during inspiration. (See page 670: Monitoring of Expired Gas: Carbon Dioxide.)

16. **A.**   Ventilation–perfusion ($\dot{V}/\dot{Q}$) mismatch results in an increase in dead space ventilation, which produces a situation in which alveolar gas is diluted by dead space gas (whose $PaCO_2$ value is zero). This will increase the $PaCO_2$-$ETCO_2$ gradient. Diffusion abnormalities, such as acute respiratory distress syndrome, will restrict the diffusion of CO_2 from the blood into the alveoli and thus widen the $PaCO_2$-$ETCO_2$ gradient. Sampling errors, such as excessive sampling rate in which fresh gas is entrained, or leaks in the system, will dilute the expired CO_2, resulting in a widened gradient. Alveolar emptying rate does not affect the gradient between $PaCO_2$ and $ETCO_2$, but it does produce the gentle upward trend of the plateau phase of the capnograph. (See page 670: Monitoring of Expired Gas: Carbon Dioxide.)

17. **B.**   Increasing dead space ventilation results in a larger reservoir or tidal volume, which is not involved in respiration. During exhalation, this reservoir of nonrespiratory gas mixes with alveolar gas and dilutes its concentration of CO_2. This results in a widening of the $PaCO_2$-$ETCO_2$ gradient. It will have no effect on the baseline value seen during inspiration. Downsloping of the capnograph plateau phase can be seen when the sampling rate exceeds exhaled volume. (See page 670: Monitoring of Expired Gas: Carbon Dioxide.)

18. **A.**   Three stable CO_2 waveforms on a capnograph indicate that the ETT is in such a position to be exposed to expired pulmonary gas. Thus, the ETT could be anywhere from the nose to the alveoli. Sampling gases from a ETT within the stomach may result in detection of CO_2; however, the quantity measured will fall rapidly with subsequent breaths. (See page 670: Monitoring of Expired Gas: Carbon Dioxide.)

19. **A.**   For $ETCO_2$ to be detected, there must be adequate pulmonary blood flow to deliver the CO_2 to the lungs for excretion, ventilation of the lungs, and an intact sampling system. Cardiac arrest will cease pulmonary

blood flow. Extubation in a mechanically ventilated patient would result in cessation of ventilation. A disrupted sampling line in a sidestream sampling system would result in a sudden loss of CO_2 waveform. Hyperventilation would result in a gradual lowering of $ETCO_2$, not a sudden decrease. (See page 670: Monitoring of Expired Gas: Carbon Dioxide.)

20. **E.**   Widening of the $ETCO_2$-$PaCO_2$ gradient can occur because of $\dot{V}/\dot{Q}$ mismatch, pulmonary shunt, diffusion abnormalities of CO_2, and sampling errors. (See page 670: Monitoring of Expired Gas: Carbon Dioxide.)

21. **C.**   During an O_2/N_2O anesthetic, there should be no nitrogen detected in the system. Any nitrogen in the circuit must be coming from the air surrounding the patient or the anesthesia circuit. Thus, the possible causes include venous air embolism and leaks in the anesthesia or sampling circuit. Failure of the O_2 fail-safe alarm will prevent one from detecting a loss in sufficient pipeline O_2 pressure. A failure in the inspiratory one-way valve will result in the patient's rebreathing expired gases that, if the system is closed, will not contain nitrogen. (See page 670: Monitoring of Expired Gases.)

22. **B.**   The gradient between $PaCO_2$ and $ETCO_2$ is dependent on the degree of dead space ventilation. The common clinical causes associated with a widened $PaCO_2$-$ETCO_2$ gradient include embolic phenomena (thrombus, fat, air, amniotic fluid), hypoperfusion states with reduced pulmonary blood flow, and chronic obstructive pulmonary disease. Hypoxic mixture and restrictive pulmonary disease do not affect $ETCO_2$-$PaCO_2$ gradient. (See page 670: Monitoring of Expired Gases: Carbon Dioxide.)

23. **B.**   Pulse contour analysis of arterial waveform allows one to estimate left ventricular output. It does require calibration using thermodilution or lithium dilution cardiac output determinations as a reference. Numerous clinical studies have demonstrated that the precision and accuracy of arterial pulse contour analysis are acceptable when compared with thermodilution cardiac output measurements obtained by PACs. (See page 681: Noninvasive Techniques for Cardiac Output: Arterial Pulse Contour Analysis.)

24. **B.**   As one moves from the large central arteries to the peripheral arteries, the arterial waveform changes. This occurs because of the narrowing of the vascular tree, which results in different impedance and harmonic resonances compared with the larger arteries. This results in the phenomenon called distal pulse amplification. This amplification manifests itself in higher systolic but lower diastolic blood pressure readings, widened pulse pressure, steeper systolic upstroke, and a later occurrence of the dicrotic notch. MAP is just slightly lower in a peripheral artery when

compared with the aorta. (See page 673: Figure 24.3.)

25. **A.** For a noninvasive blood pressure cuff to give accurate blood pressure readings, the cuff must be appropriately sized, with the width of the cuff bladder being 40% of the arm's circumference. Excessively large or small cuffs will result in falsely low and falsely high pressures, respectively. The cuff must be applied appropriately tight, because a loose cuff will result in an artificially high reading. Deflation of the cuff must be slow enough to detect the Korotkoff sounds and the resultant changes with deflation. Excessively quick deflation will result in falsely low pressure readings. (See page 673: Indirect Measurement of Arterial Blood Pressure.)

26. **B.** Natural frequency and damping are the two primary conditions that influence reproduction of the arterial wave measured by a fluid-filled transducer system. The natural frequency of the monitoring systems must be higher than the frequency within the arterial waveform. If the frequency within the arterial pulse wave approaches the natural frequency of the fluid-filled transducer, resonance will occur. This will be seen as overshoot or ringing. This produces amplification of the original signal by the monitoring device. SP will be overestimated in such situations. Damping within the system impedes the transducer from detecting the changes of the pressure within the arterial waveform. This impedance results in a loss of the fine details contained within the arterial waveform. An overdampened arterial waveform will result in blunting of the pulse pressure, little change in MAP, and loss of the dicrotic notch. Underdampened systems will produce an overshoot of the SP and the development of artifacts produced not by the waveform but rather secondary to the monitoring system. (See page 675: Figure 24.4.)

27. **A.** The radial artery can be damaged during placement of a catheter. Hematoma formation and thrombosis of the artery can occur during placement, while in situ, or during removal. The median nerve lies approximately 1 cm medially from the radial artery but is sufficiently close as to risk possible injury. The ulnar nerve lies on the opposite side of the wrist along with the ulnar artery. (See page 674: Complications of Invasive Arterial Monitoring.)

28. **B.** The right IJ vein is the jugular vein of choice for a number of reasons. It tends to be larger than the left IJ vein, and it travels in a more direct line path into the superior vena cava. The left IJ vein's more tortuous route and the presence of the thoracic duct at the left IJ vein-subclavian junction (which can lead to thoracic duct injury) make it a less desirable site. Both the right and left IJ veins are in similarly close approximation with the carotid artery and the phrenic nerve. (See page 676: Central Venous and Pulmonary Artery Monitoring.)

29. **B.** The CVP waveform measures pressures on the right side of the heart. The pattern seen with the CVP includes a, c, and v waves and both x and y descents. The a wave arises during atrial contraction, the c wave arises during ventricular isovolumic contraction (which results in the tricuspid valve moving toward the right atrium), and the v wave arises secondary to systolic filling of the atrium (when the tricuspid valve closes). The x descent occurs after the c wave during atrial relaxation, and the y descent occurs with tricuspid valve opening and blood flowing rapidly out of the atrium. These waves will be altered depending on outflow obstructions, which can result from arrhythmias, ischemia, valvular abnormalities, and pulmonary disease. Tricuspid stenosis results in large a waves. Atrial fibrillation results in discoordination of atrial contractions; thus, the a wave is lost. Cannon a waves are seen in atrial-ventricular dissociation, when the atria contract against a closed tricuspid valve. (See page 676: Central Venous and Pulmonary Artery Monitoring.)

30. **C.** CVP gives a good estimation of the volume status of the patient, especially if trends in the pressure are followed. If one has normal left and right ventricles and normal pulmonary physiology, the CVP gives a good estimation of LV filling pressure. This does not hold true if the right or left ventricle is ischemic, if valvular disease is present, or if there is pulmonary disease. Because CVP and PCWP both reflect intrapericardial pressures, they become similar during cardiac tamponade. (See page 676: Central Venous Pressure Monitoring.)

31. **B.** Svo_2 allows one to assess total body O_2 balance. It is dependent on cardiac output, O_2 saturation, and hemoglobin concentration. One can have a normal Svo_2 despite inadequate blood flow to an area of the body, because a small regional area of hypoperfusion will not significantly alter Svo_2. Intracardiac or intrapulmonary shunts will produce elevations of Svo_2 beyond normal (70%). The point at which the increase in the Svo_2 occurs can determine the anatomic site of the shunt. Cellular poisons and sepsis are other examples of situations in which an elevation in Svo_2 beyond normal can occur. (See page 676: Pulmonary Artery Monitoring.)

32. **E.** In most cases, PCWP and pulmonary diastolic pressure (PDP) are very similar (with PCWP being just slightly higher). This similarity allows one to estimate PCWP, which reflects LVEDP from the value of the PDP on a beat-to-beat basis and without the inherent risk that balloon inflation entails. There are several conditions in which the relationship between PDP and PCWP is altered, and using PDP in these cases will result in an underloaded ventricle. Most of these cases involve conditions of increased pulmonary pressures resulting from increased pulmonary resistance. This will be seen in chronic pulmonary disease, such as chronic obstructive pulmonary disease, idiopathic

pulmonary hypertension, and in acute situations such as pulmonary embolism, hypoxia, and acidosis. When confronted with patients having these conditions, PCWP should be sought to ensure accurate estimations of LVEDP. (See page 677: Pulmonary Vascular Resistance.)

33. **B.** In order to use a PAC to estimate LVEDP through the measurement of PCWP, one must position the PAC in the lungs at a site in which a continuous column of blood will be present from the tip of the catheter to the left atrium when the balloon is inflated. This condition occurs in West zone 3. A PAC positioned in West zone 2 will measure airway pressure during the respiratory cycle because, at peak inspiration, the alveolar pressure exceeds the capillary pressure. Conditions that increase West zones 2 and 1 (e.g., hypovolemia, positive end-expiratory pressure) can convert a properly placed PAC into an improperly placed PAC, rendering the PAC useless for PCWP monitoring. PAC in West zone 4 will be compressed by interstitial pressure, which is greater than left atrial pressure (LAP) and thus gives falsely elevated PCWP values. The following characteristics suggest that a PAC is not in West zone 3: PCWP > PAEDP (if no pulmonary hypertension is present), nonphasic PCWP tracing, and an inability to withdraw blood when wedged. The location of a PAC can be confirmed by a lateral chest radiograph to ascertain that the catheter tip is below the level of the left atrium. (See page 678: Alveolar-Pulmonary Artery Pressure Relationships.)

34. **A.** PCWP as an accurate estimation of LVEDP is predicated on normal LV compliance, the absence of aortic or mitral valve disease (aortic regurgitation, mitral stenosis, or mitral regurgitation), normal pulmonary airway pressures, normal size of pulmonary vascular bed, and normal pulmonary vascular resistance. Altering these assumptions will result in the inability to predict LV loading conditions with PCWP values. (See page 678: Intracardiac Factors.)

35. **A.** Pulmonary artery rupture is a rare but serious and possibly fatal complication of a PAC. The risk of rupture is increased in patients with pulmonary hypertension. Mortality following the rupture is aggravated further in patients who are heparinized or coagulopathic. (See page 678: Complications of Pulmonary Artery Catheter Monitoring.)

36. **A.** TEE gives the most accurate estimation of LV preload. It gives a very early indication of myocardial ischemia by its ability to detect wall motion abnormalities. By determining flows across the mitral valve or from the pulmonary veins, left ventricular and left arterial filling pressures can be calculated. TEE is not without its complications. Damage to the esophagus, hemodynamic instability, and dysrhythmias have been reported. (See page 681:

Transesophageal Echocardiography: Monitoring Applications.)

37. **A.** Cardiac output determinations by the thermodilution technique work by examining the temperature change resulting from a small injection of a solution that is colder than the patient. If the quantity and temperature of the injectate are known and the resulting temperature of the blood downstream is measured, one can determine the quantity of the blood required to have mixed with injectate to produce the measured temperature decrease. Conditions in which blood bypasses the downstream temperature measurement (i.e., shunts) will produce falsely elevated readings of cardiac output, because the computer assumes that a higher volume of blood diluted the injectate. A similar situation occurs in regurgitant lesions of the heart, because the injectate may oscillate in anterograde and retrograde manner during each cardiac cycle. This will effectively increase the volume into which the injectate has been diluted and will give an inaccurate overestimation of cardiac output. Aortic stenosis does not affect cardiac output determinations because it does not produce a shunt or affect the one-way movement of blood in the circulatory system. (See page 680: Indicator Dilution Applications.)

38. **A.** The ICP waveform is a pulsatile waveform that oscillates with the cardiac and respiratory cycles. The cranial cavity is a closed cavity filled with noncompliant substances; thus, introduction of additional substances into the cranial cavity, or the reduction of venous egress, produces an elevation in ICP. The cardiac cycle affects ICP in that the pulse volume adds additional volume into the intracranial cavity and thus raises pressure. Thoracic pressure also will be transmitted into the venous system and restrict the outflow of cerebral venous blood. The normal value of ICP is <15 mm Hg. Normal ICP does not translate to normal function, nor does abnormal ICP translate into abnormal function. (See page 683: Intracranial Pressure Monitoring.)

39. **B.** BIS monitoring integrates four different processed EEG. It displays its results in the form of a number from zero to 100. BIS values <60 predict the absence of consciousness. Using a BIS monitor allows for tighter control of anesthetic delivery and can facilitate faster emergence. BIS values do not reliably predict the absence of movement when noxiously stimulated. (See page 683: Electroencephalogram-Processing Electroencephalographic Data.)

40. **B.** The BIS monitor is a compilation of four processed EEGs. Each of the four processed EEGs is specific for a particular depth of anesthesia. These are ranked according to the particular EEG patterns being detected and reflect the number, between one and 100, being displayed on the monitor. The BIS monitor is accurate in predicting the depth of anesthesia.

Lower numbers reflect a sedated patient. A number <60 predicts the absence of consciousness. Studies have shown that it can reliably predict the level of consciousness, level of sedation, and probability of recall. It does not accurately predict the lack of movement with incision. (See page 683: Processing Electroencephalographic Data.)

41. **A.** Loss of SSEPs could arise from anatomic or physiologic causes. A disruption anywhere within the neural pathway (i.e., from the peripheral nerve to the somatosensory cortex) will result in loss of the SSEP. Physiologic perturbations also will lead to loss of SSEPs. Hypotension, hypoxia, or alterations in anesthetic depth will affect the quality of the SSEP. Because SSEPs are sensory in nature, they do not detect the effects at the ventral (motor) horn of the spinal cord. (See page 684: Evoked Potential Monitoring.)

42. **B.** SSEP monitors the function of the somatosensory pathway from the peripheral nerve to the somatosensory cortex. Loss of SSEP can result from anatomic issues (trauma, surgical excision), physiologic state (hypoxia, hypotension), or anesthetic depth. By keeping the latter two stable, any loss is suspected to be caused by surgical phenomena. SSEPs measure only sensory function. They do not give any indication regarding the function of the motor system and thus do not ensure an intact motor pathway postoperatively. For this reason, the wake-up test, which does monitor the motor pathway, is not a redundant test. (See page 684: Evoked Potential Monitoring.)

43. **C.** Convection is defined as the change in heat content resulting from the movement of air over the surface of the object. Conduction is defined as the change in heat content resulting from the object contact with another surface. Radiation is defined as the change in heat content resulting from absorption or emission of photons. Evaporation is defined as heat loss resulting from the vaporization of water. (See page 685: Temperature Monitoring.)

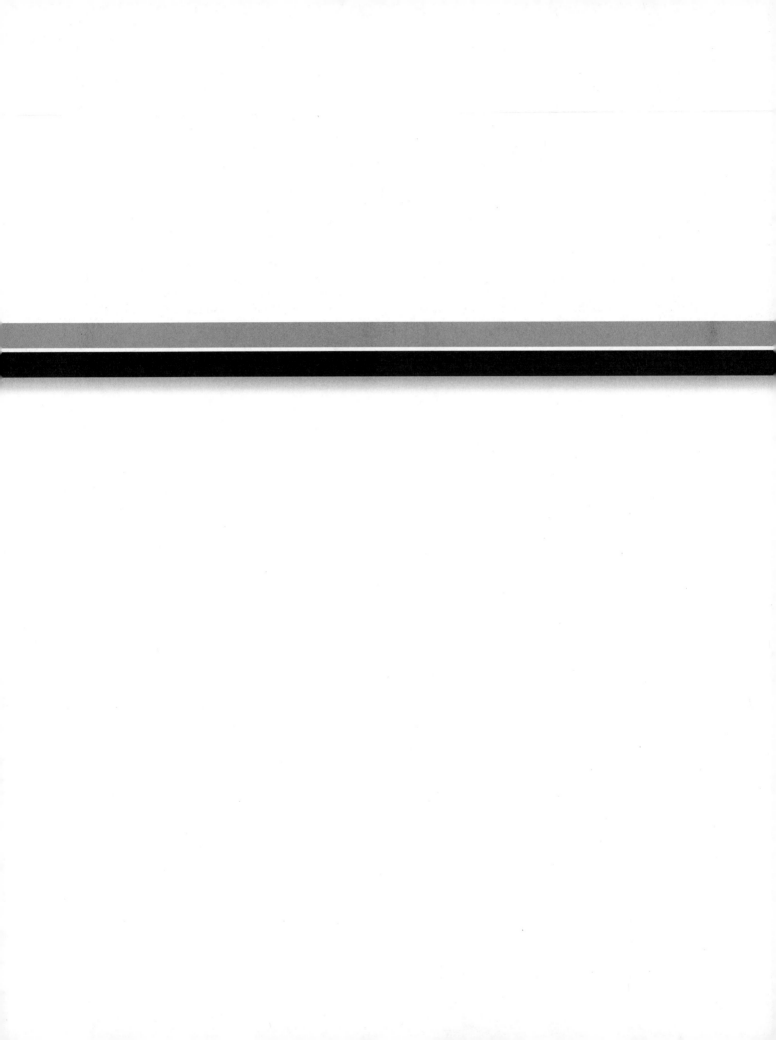

CHAPTER 25 ■ EPIDURAL AND SPINAL ANESTHESIA

1. All of the following statements regarding epidural anesthesia are true EXCEPT:

   A. It can be used to provide postoperative analgesia.
   B. It has been shown to decrease some postoperative complications.
   C. It may improve surgical outcome.
   D. It has become absolutely indicated as the standard of care for certain procedures.
   E. It has been shown to reduce intraoperative blood loss.

2. All of the following statements are true EXCEPT:

   A. The epidural space is bounded inferiorly by the intervertebral ligament.
   B. The interspinous ligament attaches to the ligamentum flavum anteriorly.
   C. The ligamentum nuchae continues inferiorly as the supraspinous ligament.
   D. Elastin is the primary component of the ligamentum flavum.
   E. The ligamentum flavum is thickest in the midline.

3. The epidural space:

   A. terminates cranially at C1
   B. communicates with the intervertebral space by way of the paravertebral foramina
   C. surrounds the vertebral canal
   D. contains a rich network of veins posteriorly
   E. becomes discontinuous upon injection of liquid

4. Which of the following statements regarding spinal needle insertion is TRUE?

   A. The first significant resistance encountered when advancing a needle using the paramedian approach is the interspinous ligament.
   B. If bone is repeatedly encountered at the same depth when the needle is advanced, the needle is likely walking down the inferior spinous process.

   C. The midline approach is preferred in patients with heavily calcified interspinous ligaments.
   D. Free flow of cerebrospinal fluid (CSF) following resolution of a paresthesia usually indicates that the needle is in good position.
   E. Penetration of the dura mater is more easily detected with a beveled needle.

5. The epidural test dose:

   A. if negative, confirms that the catheter is in the epidural space
   B. must be administered before giving a therapeutic dose
   C. may be omitted if aspiration of the catheter is negative for blood or CSF
   D. should have an increased concentration of epinephrine if the patient is taking beta-adrenergic blockers
   E. contains epinephrine, which, if given intravenously, typically produces an immediate increase in heart rate within 10 seconds

6. Rank the following local anesthetics in order of increasing duration for spinal anesthesia.

   A. Procaine, mepivacaine, tetracaine
   B. Lidocaine, mepivacaine, procaine
   C. Lidocaine, procaine, mepivacaine
   D. Procaine, bupivacaine, mepivacaine
   E. Tetracaine, procaine, bupivacaine

7. Spinal anesthesia duration is most prolonged when clonidine 100 μg is added to which of the following local anesthetics?

   A. Mepivacaine
   B. Lidocaine
   C. Tetracaine
   D. Procaine
   E. Bupivacaine

8. Rank the following local anesthetics in order of increasing duration for epidural anesthesia.

    A. Ropivacaine, bupivacaine, mepivacaine
    B. Etidocaine, mepivacaine, ropivacaine
    C. Chloroprocaine, etidocaine, mepivacaine
    D. Ropivacaine, chloroprocaine, mepivacaine
    E. Chloroprocaine, mepivacaine, etidocaine

9. All of the following statements regarding complications associated with epidural and spinal anesthesia are true EXCEPT:

    A. Use of fluid instead of air for loss of resistance during epidural anesthesia reduces the risk of headache upon accidental meningeal puncture.
    B. An epidural blood patch immediately relieves postdural puncture headache (PDPH) symptoms in approximately 99% of patients.
    C. Transient reduction in hearing acuity after spinal anesthesia is more common in female than in male patients.
    D. Back pain is more common following epidural anesthesia than after spinal anesthesia.
    E. Neurologic injury occurs in about 0.03 to 0.1% of all central neuraxial blocks.

10. All of the following statements regarding spinal or epidural anesthesia and spinal hematoma are true EXCEPT:

    A. Patients taking nonsteroidal anti-inflammatory drugs (NSAIDs) and receiving minidose heparin are not at increased risk.
    B. Patients treated with enoxaparin are at increased risk.
    C. Patients most commonly present with numbness or lower extremity weakness.
    D. Spinal hematoma occurs at an estimated incidence of less than one in 150,000.
    E. The removal of an epidural or an intrathecal catheter presents nearly as great a risk for spinal hematoma as its insertion.

11. Structures traversed by a properly placed needle in the subarachnoid space via the midline approach include all the following EXCEPT:

    A. interspinous ligament
    B. dura mater
    C. posterior longitudinal ligament
    D. supraspinous ligament
    E. ligamentum flavum

12. A patient receives a spinal anesthetic with a sensory level of T5. Which of the following is likely to occur?

    A. The small bowel will be dilated and relaxed.
    B. Glomerular filtration will be decreased by one-third.
    C. Vital capacity will be reduced by one-third.

D. The cardioaccelerator nerves will be unaffected.
E. Blood pressure will lower predominantly by decreasing venous return.

13. Which of the following has the lowest baricity?

    A. Lidocaine 5% in dextrose 7.5%
    B. A mixture obtained by mixing equal volumes of tetracaine 1% and water
    C. Bupivacaine 0.75% in dextrose 8.25%
    D. A mixture obtained by mixing equal volumes of tetracaine 1% and dextrose 10%
    E. Procaine 10%

14. At 37°C, the average density of CSF is ___ g/mL.

    A. 1.3
    B. 1.03
    C. 1.003
    D. 1.0003
    E. 0.03

15. Intravenous injection of a typical epidural test dose of an epinephrine-containing solution causes an average increase in heart rate of ___ beats/minute.

    A. 0
    B. 2
    C. 6
    D. 30
    E. 60

16. Which of the following statements concerning the addition of epinephrine to a local anesthetic solution during spinal anesthesia is TRUE?

    A. It is more effective at increasing the duration of lidocaine than is tetracaine.
    B. It is important for modulating the systemic blood level of local anesthetic.
    C. It may inhibit antinociceptive afferents in the spinal cord.
    D. It typically is administered in a concentration of 10 g/mL.
    E. It typically is administered in a concentration of 1:200,000.

17. Which of the following statements concerning the choice of local anesthetic solution for epidural use is TRUE?

    A. Agents of high anesthetic potency and duration of action necessarily have a slow onset.
    B. Etidocaine is an excellent choice for obstetric use because of wide sensory/motor discrimination.
    C. Ropivacaine has a time course similar to that of lidocaine.
    D. Prilocaine has less cardiovascular toxicity than does bupivacaine or etidocaine.
    E. Onset and duration of epidural anesthesia are most closely related to the volume of local anesthetic used.

18. The first function to be lost during the onset of spinal anesthesia is:

    A. touch
    B. motor power
    C. temperature sensation
    D. vibration
    E. autonomic activity

19. Which of the following statements concerning a decrease in blood pressure of 30% during spinal anesthesia is TRUE?

    A. It is primarily the result of arteriolar dilation.
    B. It should be treated with a modest head-up position to prevent further cephalad spread of the local anesthetic.
    C. It must be treated aggressively in all patients.
    D. It may be treated effectively with a venoselective constrictor.
    E. It indicates that the patient was hypovolemic before induction of spinal anesthesia.

20. All of the following statements about PDPHs are true EXCEPT:

    A. They frequently are unilateral.
    B. They are improved by recumbency.
    C. They usually are frontal or occipital.
    D. They may be accompanied by tinnitus and photophobia.
    E. They usually are self-limiting.

21. Measures to decrease the incidence of PDPH include all of the following EXCEPT:

    A. paramedian approach
    B. use of small-gauge spinal needles
    C. lowering the glucose concentration of the local anesthetic solution
    D. maintenance of the supine position for at least 12 hours postoperatively
    E. inserting the spinal needle bevel parallel to the dural fibers

22. Which of the following statements concerning high spinal anesthesia is TRUE?

    A. It is less common in parturients.
    B. It carries a high mortality rate.
    C. If it occurs, phrenic nerve paralysis is relatively short-lived.
    D. It is most likely to occur 30 minutes after the induction of spinal anesthesia.
    E. Apnea is always a consequence of ventilatory muscle paralysis.

23. Which of the following vertebrae has the most prominent spinous process?

    A. C5
    B. C2
    C. T1
    D. T12
    E. L5

For questions 24 to 36, choose A if 1, 2, and 3 are correct; B if 1 and 3; C if 2 and 4; D if 4; E if all.

24. Which of the following statements is/are TRUE?

    1. The vertebral canal is formed by two laminae anteriorly.
    2. The spinous process for C1 serves as a site for muscle and ligament attachments.
    3. Six sacral vertebrae are fused together to form the sacrum.
    4. The first cervical vertebra does not have a vertebral body.

25. Which of the following statements regarding vertebral anatomy is/are TRUE?

    1. The sacral cornu are located on either side of the sacral hiatus.
    2. The twelfth thoracic rib can be helpful in identifying the twelfth thoracic vertebrae.
    3. A horizontal line at the level of the iliac crests corresponds to the L4–L5 interspace.
    4. C5 is the most prominent spinous process encountered upon palpation of the posterior neck.

26. Which of the following statements is/are FALSE?

    1. The subdural space lies between the arachnoid mater and the pia mater.
    2. The dura mater fuses with the filum terminale at the level of the second sacral vertebrae.
    3. The plica medianis dorsalis is usually the structure responsible for inadequate spread of epidural anesthesia.
    4. At birth, the spinal cord ends at about the level of the third lumbar vertebra.

27. Which of the following statements regarding spinal needles is/are TRUE?

    1. The Quinke needle has a cutting edge.
    2. The Sprotte needle requires more insertion force than the Greene needle.
    3. Use of a stylet in a spinal needle may prevent formation of dermoid tumors in the subarachnoid space.
    4. The Whitacre needle has a "pencil-point" tip.

28. Combined spinal-epidural anesthesia (CSEA):

    1. has proved to be a technique without risk or limitation
    2. requires an epidural needle with a second lumen for the spinal needle
    3. has recently fallen out of favor as a viable anesthetic option
    4. may result in high subarachnoid concentrations of medication administered via the epidural catheter

29. Transient radicular irritation (TRI):

   1. is defined as pain and/or dysesthesia in the legs or buttocks after spinal anesthesia
   2. occurs more frequently in obese patients
   3. usually resolves within 72 hours
   4. occurs most frequently when bupivacaine is used

30. Anatomic features pertinent to the performance of neuraxial blockade include:

   1. In adults, the spinal cord ends at L1–L2.
   2. The angulation of the spinous processes of the thoracic vertebrae makes a paramedian approach preferable.
   3. In adults, the dural sac ends at S2.
   4. The largest interspace in the vertebral column is L2–L3.

31. The epidural space contains:

   1. CSF
   2. blood vessels
   3. unsheathed spinal roots
   4. adipose tissue

32. Factors that may worsen hypotension during epidural anesthesia include:

   1. epinephrine in the local anesthetic solution
   2. absorption of local anesthetic from the epidural space
   3. hypovolemia
   4. use of chloroprocaine

33. Important factors influencing the distribution of local anesthetics in the subarachnoid space include:

   1. density of the local anesthetic solution
   2. shape of the spinal canal
   3. position of the patient
   4. site of injection

34. Isobaric solutions injected at the L1 level are appropriate for spinal anesthesia for:

   1. cesarean section
   2. femoropopliteal bypass
   3. appendectomy
   4. repair of hip fracture

35. TRUE statement(s) about anatomy include:

   1. The ligamentum flavum is thickest in the midline, measuring 3 to 5 mm at the L2–L3 interspace of adults.
   2. Midline insertion of an epidural needle is least likely to result in unintended meningeal puncture.
   3. In the adult, the caudad tip of the spinal cord typically lies at the level of the first lumbar vertebrae.
   4. At birth, the spinal cord ends at about the level of the fifth lumber vertebra.

36. Spinal cord segments that contain the cell bodies of preganglionic sympathetic neurons include:

   1. T4
   2. C6
   3. T10
   4. S1

ANSWERS

---

1. **D.** There are no absolute indications for spinal or epidural anesthesia. Spinal and epidural anesthesia have been shown to blunt the stress response to surgery, decrease intraoperative blood loss, lower the incidence of postoperative thromboembolic events, and decrease morbidity and mortality in high-risk surgical patients. Also, both spinal and epidural techniques can be used to extend analgesia into the postoperative period or to provide analgesia to nonsurgical patients. (See page 691: Introduction.)

2. **A.** The epidural space is bounded inferiorly by the sacrococcygeal ligament covering the sacral hiatus. The interspinous ligament attaches between the spinous processes and blends anteriorly with the ligamentum flavum. Above T7, the supraspinous ligament continues as the ligamentum nuchae. The ligamentum flavum is a tough, wedge-shaped ligament composed of elastin. The ligamentum flavum is thickest in the midline, measuring 3 to 5 mm at the

L2–L3 interspace of adults. (See page 692: Ligaments.)

3. **C.** The epidural space is the space that lies between the spinal meninges and the sides of the vertebral canal. It is bounded cranially by the foramina magnum. The epidural space is not a closed space but communicates with the paravertebral space by way of the intervertebral foramina. The epidural space is composed of a series of discontinuous compartments that become continuous when the potential space separating the compartments is opened by injection of air or liquid. A rich network of valveless veins courses through the anterior and lateral portions of the epidural space, with few if any veins present in the posterior epidural space. (See page 693: Epidural Space.)

4. **D.** If a paresthesia occurs upon insertion of a spinal needle: immediately stop advancing the needle, remove the stylet, and look for CSF at the needle hub.

Obtaining CSF following resolution of a paresthesia indicates that the needle encountered a cauda equina nerve root in the subarachnoid space and the needle tip is in good position. Of course, one should not inject local anesthetic in the presence of a persistent paresthesia. The first significant resistance encountered using the paramedian approach should be the ligamentum flavum, because the interspinous ligament is bypassed. If bone is repeatedly encountered at the same depth when the needle is advanced, the needle is likely off the midline and walking along the vertebral lamina. The paramedian approach to the epidural and subarachnoid space is useful in situations where the patient's anatomy does not favor the midline approach (e.g., the inability to flex the spine or heavily calcified intraspinous ligaments). Penetration of the dura mater produces a subtle "pop" that is most easily detected with pencil-point needles. (See page 696: Midline Approach.)

5. **B.** Because of the risk of undetected intravenous or subarachnoid migration of the catheter, additional test doses must be administered before a therapeutic dose is given through the catheter. Aspiration of the catheter or needle to check for blood or CSF is helpful if positive, but the incidence of false-negative aspirations is too high to rely on this technique alone. The most common test dose is 3 mL of local anesthetic containing 5 μg/mL epinephrine. Intravascular injection of this dose of epinephrine typically produces an average heart rate increase of 30 beats/minute between 20 and 40 seconds after the injection. Heart rate increases may not be as evident in some patients taking beta-adrenergic blockers. In beta-blocked patients, systolic blood pressure increases of $\geq$20 mm Hg may be a more reliable indicator of intravascular injection. (See page 700: Epidural Test Dose.)

6. **A.** The principal determinant of spinal block duration is the local anesthetic drug used. Procaine is the shortest-acting local anesthetic for subarachnoid use. Lidocaine and mepivacaine are agents of intermediate duration, whereas bupivacaine and tetracaine are the longest-acting drugs currently available in the United States. (See page 704: Local Anesthetic.)

7. **C.** Tetracaine is the local anesthetic that is most dramatically prolonged by addition of adrenergic agonists. Clonidine prolongs tetracaine spinal block by 50 to 70%, with a larger effect occurring at lumbar dermatomes. (See page 704: Adrenergic Agonists.)

8. **E.** Chloroprocaine is the shortest-duration local anesthetic used for epidural anesthesia. Lidocaine and mepivacaine provide blocks of intermediate duration, and bupivacaine, ropivacaine, and etidocaine produce the longest-duration epidural block. (See page 704: Duration.)

9. **B.** Epidural blood patch is effective in relieving symptoms within 1 to 24 hours in 85 to 95% of patients; approximately 90% of patients in whom an initial blood patch fails will respond to a second blood patch. The use of fluid instead of air for loss of resistance during attempted epidural anesthesia does not alter the risk of accidental meningeal puncture, but it does markedly decrease the risk of subsequently developing PDPH. Compared with spinal anesthesia, back pain following epidural anesthesia is more common and of longer duration. It has been demonstrated that a 1- to 3-day transient mild decrease in hearing acuity is common after spinal anesthesia, with an incidence of roughly 40% and a 3:1 female-to-male predominance. Multiple large studies of spinal and epidural anesthesia report that neurologic injury occurs in approximately 0.03 to 0.1% of all central neuraxial blocks, although in most of these series the block was not clearly proven to be causative. (See page 711: Complications.)

10. **A.** Drugs not considered putting patients at increased risk of neuraxial bleeding and spinal hematoma formation when used alone may, in fact, increase the risk when they are combined. This may be the case when minidose unfractionated heparin and NSAIDs are used concurrently. Patients receiving fractionated low molecular weight heparin (e.g., enoxaparin) are considered to be at increased risk for spinal hematoma. Patients with spinal hematoma most commonly present with numbness or lower extremity weakness. Spinal hematoma is a rare but potentially devastating complication of spinal and epidural anesthesia, with an incidence estimated to be less than one in 150,000. The removal of an epidural or intrathecal catheter places the patient at nearly as great a risk of hematoma as catheter insertion. The timing of removal and anticoagulation should be coordinated. (See page 713: Complications: Spinal Hematoma.)

11. **C.** In the midline, the needle will penetrate skin, subcutaneous tissue, supraspinous ligament (superficial to the spinous processes), interspinous ligament (between the spinous processes), ligamentum flavum, epidural space, dura mater, and arachnoid membrane. The anterior and posterior longitudinal ligaments are anterior to the subarachnoid space, attaching to the anterior and posterior surfaces of the vertebral bodies. (See page 692: Anatomy: Ligaments.)

12. **E.** Spinal anesthesia to a level that affects the sympathetic nervous system (which originates from the intermediolateral cell column between T1 and L2) causes peripheral vasodilation (venodilation and arterial dilation). Blood pressure will decrease as a result of decreased venous return. The cardioaccelerator nerves arise from the T1–T4 dermatomes; they are affected by spinal anesthesia to T5 because the level of sympathetic blockade can be

two to six dermatomal levels higher than the sensory block. Renal blood flow and glomerular filtration rate tend to be maintained during spinal anesthesia, unless the mean blood pressure falls markedly. Spinal anesthesia causes contraction of the intestines and increased peristalsis because of unopposed vagal activity. High thoracic levels of spinal anesthesia have virtually no effect on resting ventilatory mechanics, but they compromise active exhalation. Intercostal paralysis interferes with the ability to cough and clear secretions. (See page 708: Cardiovascular Physiology: Spinal Anesthesia.)

13. **B.** Solutions of local anesthetic that have dextrose are hyperbaric. When an additive such as dextrose is not added, then density, and hence baricity, depend on the concentration (g%) of local anesthetic. Hence, 0.5% tetracaine has a lower baricity than 10% procaine. (See page 700: Block Height.)

14. **D.** The average density of CSF is 1.0003 g/mL at 37°C. (See page 700: Block Height.)

15. **D.** The most common test dose is 3 mL of local anesthetic containing 5 μg/mL epinephrine (1:200,000). Intravenous injection of this dose of epinephrine typically produces an average heart rate increase of 30 beats/minute between 20 and 40 seconds after injection. Heart rate increases may not be as evident in some patients taking beta-blockers; systolic blood pressure increases >20 mm Hg may be a more reliable indicator of intravascular injection in these patients. (See page 700: Epidural Test Dose.)

16. **C.** Epinephrine frequently is added to local anesthetic solutions to increase the duration of spinal anesthesia. This effect is believed to result, at least in part, from vasoconstriction of spinal cord and dural vessels. This leads to decreased vascular uptake of the local anesthetic. That it is more effective for tetracaine than for lidocaine or bupivacaine may be attributed to the finding that, of the three, tetracaine causes the greatest (and bupivacaine the least) vasoconstriction in spinal cord blood flow. Blood concentrations of local anesthetic during spinal anesthesia are not clinically significant; hence, epinephrine is not important for modulating the systemic levels of local anesthetic. Epinephrine and related agents may cause inhibition of antinociceptive afferents, an effect that is mediated by stimulation of alpha2 receptors in the spinal cord. The dose of epinephrine during spinal anesthesia usually is 0.2 to 0.3 mg (0.2–0.3 mL of 1:1000 solution). Lesser concentrations are used during epidural anesthesia, typically 1:200,000 (1 g/200,000 mL or 5 μg/mL). (See page 704: Adrenergic Agonists.)

17. **D.** Bupivacaine and etidocaine are highly potent, long-duration local anesthetics. The onset of bupivacaine epidural anesthesia is relatively slow (15–20 minutes), whereas the onset of etidocaine is more rapid. Bupivacaine has excellent sensory/motor discrimination; when used in obstetrics as a 0.125% solution, it can provide good sensory analgesia with minimal motor block. Etidocaine has relatively little sensory/motor discrimination and generally induces profound motor block. Prilocaine has less cardiovascular and central nervous system toxicities than lidocaine or bupivacaine, but it can cause methemoglobinemia when given in doses >600 mg. Ropivacaine has a time course similar to that of bupivacaine. Within limits, the onset and duration of epidural blockade are more closely related to the mass of drug rather than to variations in volume or concentration. (See page 704: Duration.)

18. **E.** The onset of block is fastest at sympathetic fibers. The level of sympathetic block may extend two to six dermatomes higher than loss of pinprick sensation and four to eight dermatomes higher than motor blockade. (See page 708: Differential Nerve Block.)

19. **D.** Hypotension during spinal anesthesia that is below that which blocks cardioaccelerator fibers is primarily caused by (1) venodilation leading to venous pooling and decreased cardiac output and (2) decreased systemic vascular resistance resulting from arterial dilation. The amount of hypotension is related to the level of the sympathectomy. Although the cephalad spread of a hyperbaric solution may be limited by placing the patient in a head-up position, this should not be done to treat existing hypotension, because it will further decrease venous return. A decrease in blood pressure of 20 to 30% usually is well tolerated, but selected patients with cardiac, renal, or cerebrovascular disease may require treatment. Potential treatments may include modest head-down position, vasoconstrictors, and fluid administration. (See page 711: Complications of Spinal and Epidural Anesthesia.)

20. **A.** PDPH is classically described as bilateral, in the occipital or frontal regions. It is worsened by the upright position, improved in the supine position, and may be accompanied by tinnitus and/or photophobia. Nearly all PDPHs resolve over time without invasive therapy; however, an epidural blood patch may be indicated when the symptoms are severe. (See page 711: Postdural Puncture Headache.)

21. **D.** The incidence of PDPH is increased in young patients, women, and pregnant patients. The paramedian approach results in less CSF leakage and thus decreases the chance for development of PDPH. Small-gauge needles and closed-tip needles are associated with a lower incidence of PDPH. Interestingly, there appears to be a direct relationship between the glucose concentration in the local anesthetic and the incidence of PDPH. Although bed rest is indicated in the treatment of PDPH, it does not decrease the likelihood of developing PDPH. (See page 711: Postdural Puncture Headache.)

22. C. Excessive spread of spinal anesthesia can occur in any patient, but parturients are most susceptible. It is most likely to occur shortly after induction of spinal anesthesia, but block height may be influenced for as long as 60 minutes after injection. When recognized early and treated with pressor support and ventilation, high spinal anesthesia should be merely an inconvenience, with no mortality. If phrenic nerve paralysis occurs, it usually is short-lived. Respiratory arrest may occur as a result of respiratory muscle paralysis or dysfunction of brainstem respiratory control centers. (See page 712: Total Spinal.)

23. C. The most prominent spinous process is T1. (See page 692: Anatomy: Vertebrae.)

24. D. With the exception of C1, the cervical, thoracic, and lumbar vertebrae consist of a body anteriorly, two pedicles that project posteriorly from the body, and two laminae that connect the pedicles. The first cervical vertebra differs from this typical structure in that it does not have a body or a spinous process. The five sacral vertebrae are fused together to form the wedge-shaped sacrum. (See page 692: Vertebrae.)

25. A. The sacral cornu are bony prominences on either side of the sacral hiatus and aid in identifying it. The spine of C7 is the first prominent spinous process encountered while running the hand down the back of the neck. The twelfth thoracic vertebrae can be identified by palpating the twelfth rib and tracing it back to its attachment to T12. A line drawn between the iliac crests crosses the body of L5 or the L4–L5 interspace. (See page 692: Vertebrae.)

26. B. Distally, the dura mater ends at approximately S2, where it fuses with the filum terminale. At birth, the spinal cord ends at about the level of the third lumbar vertebrae. In the adult, the caudal tip of the spinal cord typically lies at the level of the first lumbar vertebrae. The inner surface of the dura mater abuts the arachnoid mater. There is a potential space between these two membranes called the subdural space. The plica medianis dorsalis is thought to be a connective tissue band running from the dura mater to the ligamentum flavum. The plica medianis dorsalis does not appear to be clinically relevant with respect to clinical epidural anesthesia. (See page 693: Dura Mater.)

27. E. The Whitacre and Sprotte needle each has a pencil-point tip with a needle hole on the side of the shaft. The Greene and Quinke needles have beveled tips with cutting edges. Pencil-point needles require more force to insert than beveled-tip needles, but they provide a better tactile feel of the various tissues encountered as the needle is inserted. All spinal and epidural needles come with a tight-fitting stylet. The stylet prevents the needle from being plugged with skin or fat and dragging the skin into the epidural or subarachnoid spaces, where the skin may grow and form dermoid tumors. (See page 695: Needles.)

28. D. CSEA is growing in popularity because it combines the rapid-onset, dense block of spinal anesthesia with the flexibility afforded by an epidural catheter. Special epidural needles with a separate lumen to accommodate a spinal needle are available for CSEA. However, the technique is easily performed by first placing a standard epidural needle in the epidural space and then inserting an appropriately sized spinal needle through the shaft of the epidural needle into the subarachnoid space. A potential risk of CSEA is that the meningeal hole made by the spinal needle may allow dangerously high concentrations of subsequently administered epidural drugs to reach the subarachnoid space. (See page 700: Combined Spinal-Epidural Anesthesia.)

29. A. TRI is defined as pain and/or dysesthesia in the legs or buttocks after spinal anesthesia. All local anesthetics have been shown to cause TRI, although the risk appears to be greater with lidocaine than with other local anesthetics. Additional risk factors for TRI include surgery in the lithotomy position, outpatient status, and obesity. The pain usually resolves spontaneously within 72 hours. (See page 712: Transient Neurologic Symptoms.)

30. A. The largest interspace in the vertebral column is L5–S1, the site of the Taylor paramedian approach. In adults, the spinal cord ends at L1–L2 and the dural sac ends at S2. A line connecting the iliac crests most likely crosses L4 or the L4–L5 interspace. The angulation of the spinous processes of the thoracic vertebrae complicates a midline approach, thus making the paramedian approach preferable in this region. (See page 692: Anatomy.)

31. C. The epidural space is a potential space that normally is filled with loose connective tissue, fatty tissue, and blood vessels. CSF is in the subarachnoid space. The spinal roots appear to traverse the epidural space, but they maintain a thin sleeve of dura around them. (See page 693: Epidural Space.)

32. E. As with spinal anesthesia, epidural anesthesia has hemodynamic effects secondary to interruption of preganglionic sympathetic vasoconstrictor fibers. In addition, the relatively large doses of local anesthetic used are absorbed rapidly and may cause hypotension because of their negative inotropic and peripheral vasodilating effects. Epinephrine absorbed from the epidural space stimulates $beta_2$-receptors and leads to additional vasodilation and reduced diastolic blood pressure. The agents with more rapid onset, chloroprocaine and etidocaine, tend to produce greater hypotension because of rapid blockade of sympathetic fibers. Alternatively, high plasma concentrations of bupivacaine are more likely to cause myocardial depression. The hypotensive effects of

epidural anesthesia are exaggerated in hypovolemic patients. (See page 708: Cardiovascular Physiology.)

33. **E.** Many factors are considered to influence the spread of local anesthetic in CSF. The most important factors are the density of the local anesthetic solution, site of injection, shape of the spinal canal, and position of the patient (for hyperbaric and hypobaric solutions). (See page 700: Block Height.)

34. **C.** An isobaric solution tends to remain near the site of injection regardless of patient position (unless it is not truly isobaric). An isobaric injection in the lumbar region is appropriate for surgical procedures below the L1 dermatome (e.g., femoropopliteal bypass, repair of hip fracture). However, it is not appropriate for surgery at sites innervated by higher dermatomes. (See page 700: Block Height.)

35. **A.** The ligamentum flavum is thickest in the midline, measuring 3 to 5 mm at the L2–L3 interspace of adults. Midline insertion of an epidural needle is least likely to result in unintended meningeal puncture. In the adult, the caudad tip of the spinal cord typically lies at the level of the first lumbar vertebrae. However, in 10% of individuals, the spinal cord may extend to L3. At birth, the spinal cord ends at about the level of the third lumber vertebra. (See page 692: Anatomy.)

36. **B.** The intermediolateral gray matter of the T1–L2 spinal cord segments contains the cell bodies of the preganglionic sympathetic neurons. (See page 692: Spinal Cord.)

CHAPTER 26 ■ PERIPHERAL NERVE BLOCKADE

1. The highest systemic blood concentration of local anesthesia occurs after which of the following?

   A. Epidural anesthesia with pinprick level at T6
   B. Spinal anesthesia with pinprick level at T4
   C. Bier block anesthesia to left upper extremity
   D. Bilateral intercostal blocks at T6–T12
   E. Interscalene block to right shoulder

2. The absorption of local anesthetic drug and duration of anesthesia are related to all of the following EXCEPT:

   A. total dose of local anesthetic used
   B. use of epinephrine
   C. location of injection
   D. ester versus amide local anesthetic
   E. physical properties of the local anesthetic

3. Select the correct order of anesthetic techniques with respect to systemic blood concentration from highest to lowest.

   A. Spinal anesthesia, caudal, brachial plexus, intercostal block
   B. Intercostal, spinal anesthesia, brachial plexus, caudal block
   C. Intercostal, epidural, caudal, brachial plexus block
   D. Epidural, intercostal, caudal, spinal block
   E. Caudal, intercostal, brachial plexus, spinal block

4. All of the following concerning peripheral nerve blockade are true EXCEPT:

   A. Complaints of a "cramping" or "aching" sensation during injection may indicate intraneural injection.
   B. Use of a nerve stimulator with a variable amperage output and an insulated needle requires familiarity with anatomy.
   C. Obtaining a sensory paresthesia is an acceptable technique.
   D. Aspiration of blood or proximity of nerves to bones makes localization simpler.

   E. Ultrasound guidance to localize nerves is a simple technique to master.

5. All of the following statements are true EXCEPT:

   A. Toxicity from local anesthesia can occur 20 to 30 minutes following injection.
   B. Central nervous system excitation is a common hazard associated with high levels of local anesthetic.
   C. Local anesthetic toxicity is first manifested by hypertension and tachycardia.
   D. Contraindications to neuraxial blockade are infection at the site of injection and severe coagulopathy.
   E. Local anesthetic–induced myocardial depression may be manifested by bradycardia.

6. Which of the following statements concerning the trigeminal nerve is FALSE?

   A. It is a sensory and motor nerve innervating the face.
   B. There are four major branches of the trigeminal nerve exiting from the skull.
   C. The mandibular nerve is the largest branch and the only one to receive motor fibers.
   D. Most anesthetic applications of this nerves blockade can be performed by injection of the terminal branches of the nerve.
   E. The frontal branch bifurcates into the supratrochlear and supraorbital nerves.

7. All of the following statements concerning cervical plexus blockade are true EXCEPT:

   A. The cervical plexus consists solely of nerve fibers from C1 and C2.
   B. Blockade of the cervical plexus may involve only sensory nerves because of the separation of motor and sensory fibers early in their course.

C. Carotid endarterectomy may be performed under cervical plexus blockade.

D. Blockade of this plexus may provide adequate anesthesia for thyroid surgery or carotid endarterectomy.

E. Paresthesias usually are not necessary to perform adequate blockade of the cervical plexus.

8. Properly performed cervical plexus blockade may result in all of the following EXCEPT:

A. intravascular injection of local anesthetic with rapid onset of seizures

B. phrenic nerve paralysis

C. recurrent laryngeal nerve blockade

D. epidural or subarachnoid anesthesia

E. ipsilateral pneumothorax

9. Which of the following statements regarding sensory innervation of the airway is FALSE?

A. The nasal mucosa is innervated by fibers of the sphenopalatine ganglion.

B. The mucosa above the vocal cords is innervated by the superior laryngeal branch of the vagus nerve.

C. The mucosa below the vocal cords is innervated by the recurrent laryngeal branch of the vagus nerve.

D. The vocal cords are innervated by the trigeminal nerve.

E. The oral pharynx and supraglottic regions are innervated by the glossopharyngeal nerve.

10. Interscalene blockade is typically associated with all of the following EXCEPT:

A. anesthesia to the shoulder and upper arm

B. anesthesia of the ulnar border of the forearm

C. anesthesia of the musculocutaneous nerve

D. anesthesia to the radial and median nerves of the upper arm

E. possible Horner syndrome by spread to the sympathetic chain

11. The interscalene approach to the brachial plexus involves all of the following EXCEPT:

A. head positioning so that it is turned to the opposite side

B. palpation of the groove between the anterior and middle scalene muscle, which is located by having the patient tense the scalene muscles by raising the head slightly in the sniffing position

C. injection of 25 to 30 mL of local anesthetic

D. introduction of the needle perpendicular to the skin in all planes so that it is directed medially, cephalad, and slightly anteriorly

E. locating the cricoid cartilage

For questions 12 to 20, choose A if 1, 2, and 3 are correct; B if 1 and 3; C if 2 and 4; D if 4; E if all.

12. Complications of the interscalene approach to the brachial plexus may include:

1. puncture of the lung viscera and a pneumothorax

2. injection of local anesthesia into the epidural or subarachnoid space

3. intravascular injection of local anesthesia via the vertebral artery

4. ipsilateral Horner syndrome

13. Which of the following statements regarding the axillary approach to the brachial plexus is/are TRUE?

1. It carries the least chance of pneumothorax.

2. The musculocutaneous nerve is easily anesthetized.

3. Septa within the sheath may limit the spread of local anesthetic.

4. Injection at multiple sites in the axilla is not recommended because the axillary artery may be punctured.

14. Which of the following statements regarding intravenous regional anesthesia is/are TRUE?

1. The tourniquet should be inflated to 300 mm Hg or 2.5 times the patient's systolic blood pressure.

2. Lidocaine with epinephrine is the most commonly used anesthetic for this procedure.

3. If surgery is completed in 15 minutes, the tourniquet should be deflated and then reinflated to delay the sudden reabsorption of anesthetic.

4. Bupivacaine is the local anesthetic of choice in a patient with lidocaine allergy.

15. Intercostal blockade of T6–T12 results in which of the following?

1. It provides analgesia and motor relaxation for upper abdominal procedures.

2. It is useful in reducing pain associated with chest tube insertion or percutaneous biliary drainage procedures.

3. It has potential for local anesthesia toxicity, especially if performed bilaterally.

4. There is a high incidence of pneumothorax even when the anesthetic is performed by an experienced individual.

16. Which of the following statements regarding ilioinguinal/iliohypogastric nerve block is/are TRUE?

1. Anesthesia of the iliohypogastric nerve and ilioinguinal nerve is adequate for hernia repair.

2. The nerve roots from T12, L1, and L2 provide fibers to these two nerves.

3. The anteroinferior iliac spine provides the landmark for location of these two nerves.

4. Hematoma formation is a rare complication of this nerve block.

17. Which of the following statements regarding the stellate ganglion is/are TRUE?

1. Blockade of this ganglion results in sympathetic blockade of the upper extremity and head.

2. The ganglion is a large fusion of the first thoracic sympathetic ganglion, with the lower cervical ganglion on each side.
3. It lies lateral to the body of C7.
4. Chassaignac tubercle is a landmark identified during the blockade of this ganglion.

18. Which of the following is/are signs of a stellate ganglion blockade?

    1. Ptosis
    2. Miosis
    3. Anhidrosis
    4. Vasoconstriction

19. Which of the following statements regarding the celiac plexus is/are TRUE?

    1. Fibers from the celiac ganglion send postganglionic innervation to all intra-abdominal organs.

2. Neurolytic sympathetic blockade may provide relief of pain from malignancy of the pancreas, liver, or other upper abdominal organs.
3. Hypotension is the most common side effect of blockade of the celiac plexus.
4. Five milliliters of local anesthetic is required to block this plexus effectively.

20. Which of the following statements regarding an ankle block is/are TRUE?

    1. Three main peripheral nerves need to be blocked.
    2. The deep peroneal nerve is located in the deep plane of the anterior tibial artery.
    3. The sural nerve is the major sensory nerve to the sole of the foot.
    4. The deep peroneal nerve may be located by palpating the tendon of the extensor hallucis longus.

ANSWERS

1. **D.** The highest blood level of local anesthetic occurs after multiple intercostal nerve blocks. (See page 718: Local Anesthetic Drug Selection and Doses.)

2. **D.** The higher the dose of local anesthetic, the greater the amount of drug that is available for local effect. Use of epinephrine causes local vasoconstriction and therefore decreases the uptake of local anesthetic into the bloodstream. The relative absorption of local anesthetic is greatest after an intercostal nerve block. The physical properties of the local anesthetic will influence the absorption of the drug and the body's ability to break down the drug and excrete it. However, there is no difference in the absorption of the drug based upon the classification of the local anesthetic as an amide or ester. (See page 718: Local Anesthetic Drug Selection and Doses.)

3. **C.** The highest blood concentration occurs after an intercostal blockade, followed by epidural blockade, caudal blockade, and brachial plexus blockade. The lowest blood concentration occurs following a spinal blockade. (See page 718: Local Anesthetic Drug Selection and Doses.)

4. **E.** The traditional sign of successful localization of a nerve is eliciting a paresthesia. The patient will complain of an "electrical shock"–like sensation in the involved area. Complaints of "cramping" or "aching" sensation during injection is a sign of possible intraneural injection. Associated with this technique is a greater incidence of residual neuropathy in comparison with other techniques. Use of the nerve stimulator for localization of the nerve is an alternative technique. A nerve stimulator with variable amperage allows one to localize the nerve

without contacting it and may reduce the chance of nerve injury. When a low current is applied to a peripheral nerve, it will produce stimulation of the motor fibers. The closer it is in proximity to the nerve, the less amperage will be required to elicit the motor response. Familiarity with anatomy and technique is necessary to bring the needle in close proximity to the nerve. Transarterial localization of the brachial plexus is a technique for performing an axillary block. The axillary artery is transfixed, and the needle is passed through the artery. Local anesthetic is deposited on this side of the artery, and then the needle is withdrawn until it is brought back through the proximal wall. Additional local anesthetic is deposited here as well. Ultrasound guidance to localize nerves shows promise but requires complex equipment and experience. (See page 719: Nerve Localization.)

5. **C.** Local anesthetic toxicity is manifested by central nervous system excitation and myocardial depression. The myocardial depression may result in hypotension and bradycardia. Toxicity from local anesthetic may occur 20 to 30 minutes after injection, because this is the time of peak blood levels from slow absorption of high doses. Immediate symptoms are a result of intravascular local anesthetic injection. Contraindications to neuraxial blockade include severe coagulopathy and infection at the site of injection. (See page 720: Common Complications.)

6. **B.** The trigeminal nerve (fifth cranial nerve) is a sensory and motor nerve to the face. Its roots arise from the base of the pons, and it sends sensory branches to the large gasserian ganglion. There are three major branches of this nerve: the ophthalmic, maxillary, and mandibular. The ophthalmic branch

bifurcates to form the supratrochlear and supraorbital nerves. The maxillary branch is the middle branch and is a sensory nerve. The mandibular branch is the third and largest branch and is the only one with motor fibers. Blockade of the gasserian ganglion is used for treatment of disabling trigeminal neuralgia; however, it is very difficult to perform. Blockade of the three terminal branches is relatively simple. (See page 721: Specific Techniques: Trigeminal Nerve Blockade.)

7. **A.** The sensory fibers of the neck and posterior neck arise from nerve roots of C2, C3, and C4 nerves. The sensory fibers separate from the motor fibers early; therefore, isolated sensory blockade is possible. Cervical plexus blockade can be used for surgery on the neck, such as thyroidectomy and carotid endarterectomy. Occasionally, the thyroid gland may need supplemental local anesthesia, and the carotid bifurcation will need infiltration to block reflex hemodynamic changes. Paresthesias are not required to perform this procedure. (See page 723: Specific Techniques: Cervical Plexus Blockade.)

8. **E.** All of the following may be complications from cervical plexus blockade: intravascular injection into the vertebral artery, epidural or spinal anesthesia if the needle is advanced too far medially, phrenic nerve blockade, recurrent laryngeal nerve blockade, and vagal blockade. Ipsilateral pneumothorax should not occur. (See page 723: Specific Techniques: Cervical Plexus Blockade.)

9. **D.** Innervation of the nasal mucosa is by fibers of the sphenopalatine ganglion (a branch of the fifth cranial nerve). Sensory innervation of the oral pharynx and supraglottic regions is by the glossopharyngeal nerve. The larynx itself is innervated by the superior laryngeal branch of the vagus nerve in the area above the vocal cords. The recurrent laryngeal nerve provides innervation to the areas below the vocal cords. (See page 724: Airway Anesthesia.)

10. **B.** The interscalene approach to the brachial plexus at the level of C6 provides blockade for operations on the shoulder and upper arm procedures. It frequently spares C8 and T1 fibers and therefore does not provide adequate blockade to the ulnar border of the forearm. Nerve roots for the musculocutaneous, radial, and median nerves are adequately anesthetized. However, if a tourniquet is being used, a subcutaneous ring of anesthetic is required to block the superficial intercostobrachial fibers in the axilla. Horner syndrome may occur by spread of local anesthesia to the sympathetic chain. (See page 726: Upper Extremity: Brachial Plexus Blockade: Interscalene Approach.)

11. **D.** The patient is positioned supine with the head turned to the side opposite that to be blocked. The lateral border of the sternocleidomastoid muscle is identified. By tensing the scalene muscles, the groove between the anterior and middle scalene muscles may be palpated. The level of the cricoid cartilage is marked. A 22-gauge, 3.75-cm needle is introduced through the skin perpendicular to all planes at the level of the cricoid cartilage, such that it is directed medially, caudad, and slightly posterior. Approximately 25 to 30 mL of local anesthetic is required for adequate blockade. (See page 726: Upper Extremity: Brachial Plexus Blockade: Interscalene Approach.)

12. **E.** Complications from the interscalene approach to the brachial plexus are pneumothorax (if the needle is directed too inferiorly), spinal or epidural anesthesia (if the needle passes medially and enters the intervertebral foramina), intravascular injection into the vertebral artery (if the needle is too posterior, as the artery lies in its canal in the transverse process), and ipsilateral Horner syndrome (because of blockade of the sympathetic chain on the anterior vertebral body). Phrenic nerve blockade may occur as well. (See page 726: Upper Extremity: Brachial Plexus Blockade: Interscalene Approach.)

13. **B.** The axillary approach to the brachial plexus carries the least chance of pneumothorax. Fascial septa within the sheath may limit the spread of local anesthetic; therefore, injection of local anesthetic at multiple sites in the axilla is recommended. The musculocutaneous nerve departs from the sheath high in the axilla and may be spared with this technique. (See page 729: Brachial Plexus: Axillary Technique.)

14. **B.** Intravenous regional anesthesia (Bier block) is a form of regional anesthesia in which local anesthetic is injected into the upper extremity distal to an occluding tourniquet. The arm is elevated and exsanguinated by an elastic bandage. The tourniquet is inflated to 300 mm Hg or 2.5 times the patient's blood pressure. The radial pulse must be tested for occlusion. This may be done by palpation or by placement of the pulse oximeter on the extremity. Lidocaine 0.5% is the local anesthetic of choice, but it should not be used with epinephrine. Bupivacaine is not used because of its toxicity. Ideally, surgery lasting up to 1 hour may be performed by this procedure. However, the cannula may be left in place, and medication may be reinjected after 90 minutes. For surgical procedures between 20 and 40 minutes long, the tourniquet should be deflated, then reinflated, and then subsequently deflated, in an attempt to minimize sudden reabsorption of local anesthetic. (See page 730: Intravenous Regional Anesthesia.)

15. **A.** Intercostal blockade may provide both motor and sensory anesthesia of the abdomen and chest. This technique also is useful for reducing pain from chest tube insertion and percutaneous biliary drainage. It is advantageous over spinal or epidural blockade because there is no accompanying sympathetic blockade. Intercostal blockade results in the highest

blood concentration of local anesthetic and therefore has the greatest likelihood of toxicity from local anesthetic. The incidence of pneumothorax is rare in experienced hands. (See page 733: Intercostal Nerve Blockade.)

16. **D.** Ilioinguinal/iliohypogastric nerve blockade provides sensory anesthesia to the lower portion of the abdomen and groin. It is used for anesthesia for hernia repair, but blockade of these two nerves alone is inadequate for hernia repair. Subcutaneous infiltration is needed as well. These two nerves are easily located because of their anatomic relationship to the anterosuperior iliac spine. Nerve roots from L1 and sometimes T12 provide fibers to these two nerves. Hematoma formation is a rare complication of this block. (See page 735: Ilioinguinal Blockage.)

17. **E.** The stellate ganglion block allows separate blockade of the sympathetic fibers of the upper extremity and head. The ganglion is a fusion of the first thoracic sympathetic ganglion and the lower cervical ganglion on each side. It is located at the lateral border of the vertebral body of C7. The Chassaignac tubercle is the anterior tubercle of the transverse process of C6 vertebra. This landmark is used for locating the injection site for this block. (See page 736: Sympathetic Blockade: Stellate Ganglion.)

18. **A.** Signs of a stellate ganglion blockade are ptosis, miosis, and anhidrosis, which usually develop within 10 minutes of the blockade. Vasodilation of the arm also occurs. Nasal congestion is another common symptom associated with a stellate ganglion block.

(See page 736: Sympathetic Blockade: Stellate Ganglion.)

19. **A.** The celiac plexus is a sympathetic ganglion consisting of thoracic sympathetic ganglia fibers. This network of fibers is located at the level of the origin of the celiac artery. Fibers from this ganglion send postganglionic innervation to all the intra-abdominal organs and carry pain sensation from many intraperitoneal organs, such as the pancreas and liver. This block may provide relief of pain from malignancy of the pancreas, liver, or other upper abdominal organs. The most common complication of this block is hypotension. The nerve fibers of this ganglion are poorly localized; therefore, a large volume of local anesthetic (20–25 mL 0.75% lidocaine or 0.25% bupivacaine) is required the diffuse throughout the retroperitoneal space to reach all of the fibers of the ganglion. (See page 737: Celiac Plexus.)

20. **C.** Five peripheral nerves are anesthetized for an ankle block: the posterior tibial, sural, saphenous, deep peroneal, and superficial peroneal nerves. The posterior tibial nerve is the major nerve to the sole of the foot and is located just posterior to the posterior tibial artery. The sural nerve also innervates the sole of the foot. The saphenous nerve innervates the anterior surface of the foot; it is located medially. The deep peroneal nerve is located in the deep plane of the anterior tibial artery and can be located by identifying the anterior tibial artery or the tendon of the extensor hallucis longus. The superficial peroneal nerve is located along the skin crease between the anterior tibial artery and the lateral malleolus. (See page 743: Lower Extremity: Ankle Blockade.)

CHAPTER 27 ■ ANESTHESIA FOR NEUROSURGERY

For questions 1 to 11, choose the best answer.

1. Which of the following statements regarding synaptic transmission is TRUE?

   A. It is an all-or-none phenomenon.
   B. It is dependent on opening of calcium channels presynaptically.
   C. The combination of neurotransmitters with a receptor always causes depolarization of the postsynaptic membrane.
   D. Ligand-gated channels exist only on the presynaptic membrane.
   E. Gamma-aminobutyric acid (GABA) depolarizes the postsynaptic membrane.

2. Which of the following statements regarding brain metabolism is TRUE?

   A. The main substance used for energy production is glucose.
   B. The metabolic rate for O_2 consumption in an adult is the same as in children.
   C. The metabolic rate in adults is approximately 6 mL O_2/100 g of brain tissue per minute.
   D. The metabolic rate in children is approximately 1 mL O_2/100 g of brain tissue per minute.
   E. The metabolic rate in an elderly man is less than in a young man.

3. Which of the following statements regarding nitrous oxide (N_2O) is TRUE?

   A. N_2O increases cerebral blood flow (CBF).
   B. N_2O decreases intracranial pressure (ICP).
   C. N_2O decreases cerebral metabolic rate (CMR).
   D. Hypercapnia may blunt the effect of N_2O on ICP.
   E. Volatile anesthetics can counter the effect of N_2O on CBF.

4. Which of the following statements regarding the effects of barbiturates is FALSE?

   A. Barbiturates decrease CMR.
   B. At high doses, barbiturates can produce an isoelectric electroencephalogram (EEG).
   C. Barbiturates typically have no significant effect on mean arterial pressure (MAP).
   D. Barbiturates decrease ICP.
   E. Methohexital can activate seizure foci.

5. Which of the following statements regarding the effects of intravenous anesthetics is FALSE?

   A. Propofol reduces CMR.
   B. Benzodiazepines reduce CBF.
   C. Etomidate causes vasodilation.
   D. Morphine has either a minor or no effect on CMR.
   E. Ketamine can increase CBF.

6. Which of the following statements regarding evoked potentials is FALSE?

   A. A 20% reduction in amplitude in response to surgical maneuver is considered significant.
   B. Cortical evoked potentials are more vulnerable to anesthetic influence than brainstem evoked potentials.
   C. End-tidal concentrations of 0.5 minimum alveolar concentration (MAC) of inhalational agents provide satisfactory recording in neurologically intact patients.
   D. Volatile anesthetics cause dose-dependent increases in latency.
   E. For satisfactory intraoperative somatosensory evoked potential (SSEP) recordings, step changes in inhalational agent concentration must be avoided.

7. All of the following statements regarding the use of mannitol in neuroanesthesia are true EXCEPT:

   A. Its action begins 10 to 15 minutes after administration.
   B. Mannitol is effective when the brain-blood barrier is intact.

C. Mannitol causes vasodilation.

D. Mannitol may cause an initial increase in ICP.

E. Mannitol should always be administered quickly.

8. Which of the following statements regarding treatment of intracranial hypertension is FALSE?

A. Both mannitol and loop diuretics are used.

B. Corticosteroids may repair the blood-brain barrier.

C. For every 1 mm Hg change in $Paco_2$, CBF changes by 3 to 5 mL/100 g per minute.

D. The duration of effectiveness of hyperventilation may be as short as 4 to 6 hours.

E. When hyperventilation is used, the target $Paco_2$ is approximately 30 mm Hg.

9. Which of the following is most sensitive in detecting a venous air embolism?

A. End-tidal nitrogen

B. Precordial Doppler

C. Pulmonary artery catheter

D. Wheel-mill murmur

E. Transesophageal echocardiogram

10. The incidence of rebleeding following subarachnoid hemorrhage (SAH) is greatest within which of the following time periods?

A. 0 to 24 hours

B. 24 to 48 hours

C. 2 to 3 days

D. 3 to 4 days

E. 4 to 5 days

11. Which of the following statements regarding pathophysiologic changes during brain injury is TRUE?

A. During brain ischemia, intracellular sodium levels decrease.

B. The neurons in the penumbra are dead.

C. The mechanisms causing the neuronal damage are different for focal and global ischemia.

D. During ischemia, intracellular potassium levels increase.

E. Calcium influx resulting from brain trauma is a trigger for secondary damage.

For questions 12 to 31, choose A if 1, 2, and 3 are correct; B if 1 and 3; C if 2 and 4; D if 4; E if all are correct.

12. Which of the following statements regarding CBF is/are TRUE?

1. The brain receives approximately 15% of cardiac output.

2. Doubling the $Paco_2$ from 40 to 80 mm Hg doubles the CBF.

3. Reducing the $Paco_2$ from 40 to 20 mm Hg halves the CBF.

4. Changes in CBF resulting from changes in $Paco_2$ are minimal after 6 to 8 hours.

13. Which of the following statements regarding CBF is/are TRUE?

1. CBF undergoes autoregulation between MAP of 50 and 150 mm Hg.

2. Luxury flow is associated with a cerebral steal phenomenon.

3. Hypertensive patients demonstrate a right shift in autoregulation.

4. Inverse steal is associated with increased $Paco_2$.

14. TRUE statement(s) concerning the action potential include:

1. It results in a peak voltage of approximately +20 mV.

2. It is caused by slow increase in the sodium conduction.

3. It is generated by depolarization from the neuron past the threshold level.

4. Repolarization is a slow process.

15. TRUE statement(s) regarding cerebrospinal fluid (CSF) include:

1. CSF is primarily formed by choroid plexus.

2. CSF volume in the brain is 100 to 150 mL.

3. CSF is reabsorbed at a rate of 0.3 mL/minute.

4. CSF is completely replaced three to four times per day.

16. Which of the following statement(s) regarding ICP is/are TRUE?

1. Blood, CSF, and brain tissue all contribute to ICP.

2. Cerebral perfusion pressure is determined by ICP − central venous pressure (CVP).

3. ICP in humans is normally <10 mm Hg.

4. A small increase in intracranial volume will not greatly increase ICP because of compliance.

17. Which of the following statements regarding volatile anesthetics is/are TRUE?

1. Volatile anesthetics decrease CMR.

2. At equipotent doses, isoflurane reduces CMR more than does halothane.

3. Enflurane induces seizure activity in the presence of hypocapnia.

4. Desflurane is the inhalational agent of choice for patients with space-occupying lesions.

18. Which of the following contributes to the neural protective effect of barbiturates?

1. Blockage of sodium channels

2. Reduced calcium influx

3. Potentiation of GABA-mediated transmission

4. Inhibition of free radical formation

19. Which of the following statements regarding EEG monitoring is/are TRUE?

1. Induction of anesthesia usually produces an increase in alpha activity.

2. Complete electrical silence occurs at 15 to 20°C.
3. The EEG gives useful information regarding sensory pathway function.
4. Hypocarbia causes EEG slowing.

20. Which of the following statements regarding evoked potentials is/are TRUE?

    1. Opioids provide minimal change in SSEPs.
    2. Temperature fluctuation can alter SSEPs.
    3. Opioids produce little or no effect on brainstem auditory evoked potentials.
    4. Fluids to irrigate the brain can alter SSEPs.

21. Which of the following statements regarding ICP monitoring is/are TRUE?

    1. A subarachnoid bolt can be used to drain the CSF.
    2. Insertion of an intraventricular catheter facilitates accurate calculation of cerebral perfusion pressure.
    3. Intraventricular catheters are associated with a high infection rate.
    4. Infection is a major risk of subdural catheters.

22. Which of the following statements regarding neuroanesthesia is/are TRUE?

    1. Bolus administration of a large dose of atracurium may lower cerebral perfusion pressure.
    2. A total intravenous anesthetic technique may be useful when intracranial compliance is low.
    3. Succinylcholine may be the relaxant of choice when a rapid sequence induction is indicated.
    4. An alert, anxious patient may be premedicated.

23. Which of the following statements regarding posterior fossa surgery in the sitting position is/are TRUE?

    1. Jugular venous obstruction is a potential complication.
    2. It is associated with an increased risk of venous air embolism.
    3. Pneumocephalus is a frequent complication.
    4. Peripheral nerve injury may occur.

24. Which of the following statements regarding venous air embolism is/are TRUE?

    1. End-tidal nitrogen is a useful monitor of air embolism during general endotracheal anesthesia.
    2. To be maximally effective in detecting an air embolism, a Doppler ultrasonic transducer should be placed over the lower left sternal border.
    3. It causes increased pulmonary vascular resistance.
    4. The risk of paradoxical air embolism is 40%.

25. Complications of SAH and surgical treatment of cerebral aneurysm include:

    1. vasospasm
    2. hydrocephalus
    3. rebleeding
    4. intracranial hypotension

26. Which of the following statements regarding vasospasm following SAH is/are TRUE?

    1. It is clinically evident in 70% of patients.
    2. Vasospasm is a major cause of morbidity and mortality.
    3. The peak incidence occurs 2 weeks after the bleeding.
    4. Oxyhemoglobin has been implicated as a cause.

27. ECG changes associated with a ruptured cerebral aneurysm include:

    1. prolonged Q-T interval
    2. ST segment elevation
    3. ST segment depression
    4. Q waves

28. Which of the following regarding the Glasgow coma scale is/are TRUE?

    1. The maximum score is 15.
    2. Severe head injury is determined by a score of 8 or less.
    3. It evaluates motor function.
    4. Speech is not a part of the Glasgow coma scale.

29. Which of the following statements regarding the Cushing triad is/are TRUE?

    1. Arterial hypertension is a component.
    2. Tachycardia is a component.
    3. Intracranial hypertension is a component.
    4. Lowering systemic hypertension can improve cerebral perfusion.

30. Which of the following is/are components of inappropriate antidiuretic hormone secretion?

    1. Serum hypo-osmolality
    2. Hyponatremia
    3. Normal renal function
    4. Increased urinary sodium

31. Which of the following findings may occur in nonketotic hyperosmolar hyperglycemic coma?

    1. Glucosuria
    2. Decreased serum potassium
    3. Hypovolemia
    4. Increased serum sodium

ANSWERS

1. **B.** The release of neurotransmitter is initiated by an action potential while traveling down the axon of the presynaptic neuron, thus causing depolarization of the presynaptic terminal. This depolarization leads to opening of voltage-dependent calcium channels and entry of calcium from the extracellular fluid into the terminal. Binding of the neurotransmitter with the postsynaptic receptor results in opening of ligand-gated channels on the postsynaptic membrane. If the transmitter is excitatory, the membrane is depolarized. If it is inhibitory (e.g., GABA), the membrane is hyperpolarized and therefore less likely to generate an action potential. The result is a transient partial depolarization, or hyperpolarization, of the postsynaptic membrane. Synaptic transmission is not an all-or-none phenomenon. If the degree of depolarization is large enough to reach the firing level of the cell, a fully fledged action potential is generated. (See page 747: Synaptic Transmission.)

2. **A.** The main substance used for energy production in the brain is glucose. The overall metabolic rate for the brain of a young adult man is 3.5 mL O_2/100 g brain tissue per minute. This is virtually the same in elderly men. However, children have a higher metabolic rate of 5.2 mL O_2/100 g brain tissue per minute. (See page 748: Brain Metabolism.)

3. **A.** N_2O increases CBF and ICP. Barbiturates and hypocapnia in combination may prevent these increases. Volatile anesthetics may add to the increases in CBF obtained with N_2O. Evidence seems to indicate that a substantial increase in CMR can occur if N_2O is administered alone. (See page 752: Effects of Anesthetics and Other Adjunctive Drugs on Brain Physiology.)

4. **C.** Barbiturates decrease CMR and CBF. A major problem with barbiturates is that they can substantially reduce MAP. At high doses, thiopental can produce an isoelectric EEG and can decrease the CMR by 50%. Barbiturates also are effective in reducing elevated ICP. Methohexital can activate some seizure foci in patients with temporal lobe epilepsy. (See page 752: Effects of Anesthetics and Other Adjunctive Drugs on Brain Physiology.)

5. **C.** Etomidate, like the barbiturates, reduces CMR and CBF. In addition to the indirect effect of reduced cerebral metabolism on blood flow, etomidate is also a direct vasoconstrictor even before metabolism is suppressed. Propofol is a rapidly acting intravenous anesthetic that, like etomidate and barbiturates, reduces CMR and CBF. Benzodiazepines have been shown to reduce CMR and CBF; however, this effect is not as pronounced as that of barbiturates.

(See page 752: Effects of Anesthetics and Other Adjunctive Drugs on Brain Physiology.)

6. **A.** For SSEPs, a 50% reduction in amplitude from baseline in response to a specific surgical maneuver is considered to be a significant change warranting action to avert potential damage. Evoked potentials of cortical origin are more vulnerable to anesthetic influence than brainstem potentials. To obtain satisfactory intraoperative SSEP recordings, it is important to maintain constant anesthetic drug levels. Specifically, bolus administration of intravenous agents and step changes in inspired inhalational agent concentration must be avoided. High concentrations of volatile agents essentially eliminate cortical evoked potentials. However, an end-tidal volume concentration of 0.5 MAC of a volatile agent is compatible with satisfactory recordings in patients who are neurologically normal. In general, volatile agents cause a dose-dependent increase in latency and a decrease in amplitude of the SSEP. (See page 760: Anesthetic Considerations for Sensory Evoked Potential Recording.)

7. **E.** When mannitol is given as an intravenous infusion, its action begins in 10 to 15 minutes, and its effect lasts for approximately 2 hours. Mannitol is effective when the blood-brain barrier is intact. Because mannitol may initially increase ICP, it should be given slowly and in conjunction with maneuvers that decrease intracranial volume. Hypertonic agents such as mannitol should be administered cautiously in patients with pre-existing cardiovascular disease. In these patients, the transient increase in intravascular volume may precipitate left ventricular failure. Mannitol has been shown to cause vasodilation of vascular smooth muscle, which is dependent on dose and administration rate. (See page 768: Clinical Control of Intracranial Hypertension.)

8. **C.** Rapid brain dehydration and a lowered ICP can be produced by administering diuretics. The two diuretics that are used most commonly are the osmotic diuretic, mannitol, and the loop diuretic, furosemide. Corticosteroids reduce edema around brain tumors. However, steroids require many hours or days before a reduction in ICP becomes apparent. For every 1 mm Hg change in $PaCO_2$, CBF changes by 1 to 2 mL/100 g per minute. The duration of effectiveness of hyperventilation for lowering ICP may be as short as 4 to 6 hours, depending upon the pH of the CSF. The typical target $PaCO_2$ is 25 to 35 mm Hg. A $PaCO_2$ less than 25 to 30 mm Hg may be associated with ischemia resulting from extreme cerebral vasoconstriction. (See page 768: Clinical Control of Intracranial Hypertension.)

9. **E.**   The transesophageal echocardiogram is slightly more sensitive than precordial Doppler, but it is invasive and cumbersome. The transesophageal echocardiogram has the advantage of monitoring air in the right and left cardiac chambers and the aorta and thus can be used to detect both venous and arterial air embolism. (See page 773: Venous Air Embolism.)

10. **A.**   Rebleeding occurs most commonly during the first 24 hours following initial SAH. The chance of rebleeding is about 4% within the first day. After 48 hours it is 1.5% per day, with a cumulative rebleeding rate of 19% by the end of 2 weeks. (See page 777: Intracranial Aneurysm.)

11. **E.**   Ischemia can be either global or focal in nature. The mechanism leading to neuronal damage is probably similar for both. The penumbra receives collateral flow and is partially ischemic. In ischemic damage, intracellular levels of sodium and calcium increase, whereas intracellular potassium levels decrease. The high intracellular calcium level is thought to trigger a number of events that could lead to damage. (See page 751: Pathophysiology.)

12. **E.**   The brain receives approximately 15% of cardiac output, yet it makes up only 2% of total body weight. Increasing CO_2 levels causes vasodilation and increased blood flow. Doubling the CO_2 from 40 to 80 mm Hg doubles CBF. Reducing CO_2 from 40 to 20 mm Hg halves the flow. These changes are transient, and the blood flow returns to normal in 6 to 8 hours, even if the altered CO_2 levels are maintained. (See page 749: Cerebral Blood Flow.)

13. **A.**   Luxury flow caused by high CO_2 levels throughout the brain could "steal" blood from the areas that require extra O_2. Reducing CO_2 with hyperventilation (or the use of agents such as thiopental) would reduce blood flow to most areas of the brain; the vessels in the ischemic area would be maximally dilated because of low pH. This is called inverse steal. The CBF autoregulates with respect to pressure changes. In normotensive individuals, MAP can vary from 50 to 150 mm Hg, and CBF will be maintained constant because of an adjustment of cerebral vascular resistance. Patients who are hypertensive demonstrate a right-shift of autoregulation to a higher blood pressure. (See page 749: Cerebral Blood Flow.)

14. **B.**   The action potential is caused by a fast increase in the sodium conductance and a slower increase in the potassium conductance. When the neuron depolarizes past a threshold voltage level, an action potential is generated. The peak voltage of an action potential is approximately +20 mV. The voltage during the action potential returns rapidly to resting levels (repolarizes). (See page 747: Membrane Potential.)

15. **E.**   CSF is primarily formed in the choroid plexus of the cerebral ventricles. The CSF volume in the brain is approximately 150 mL; it is reabsorbed at a rate of 0.3 to 0.4 mL/minute·. This allows complete replacement of the CSF volume three or four times per day. (See page 749: Cerebrospinal Fluid.)

16. **B.**   Cerebral perfusion pressure is determined by the MAP–ICP. The ICP in humans is normally <10 mm Hg. Under normal circumstances, a small increase in intracranial volume will not greatly increase ICP because of the elastance of the components located in the cranium. An increase in ICP can be caused by increased CSF, increased CBF, or increased brain tissue volume (as caused by a tumor or edema). (See page 750: Intracranial Pressure.)

17. **A.**   The volatile anesthetics reduce the CMR; isoflurane reduces the metabolic rate to a greater extent than does halothane. Enflurane has been shown to induce seizure-type discharges, which are potentiated by hypocapnia. The main advantage of desflurane over isoflurane is a faster onset and a quicker recovery from anesthesia. Studies indicated that desflurane can cause a greater increase in ICP than isoflurane in patients with altered intracranial elastance. Therefore, it is not recommended for patients with space-occupying lesions. (See page 752: Effects of Anesthetics and Other Adjunctive Drugs on Brain Physiology.)

18. **E.**   Barbiturates exert a neural protective effect by lowering $CMRO_2$. They block sodium channels, reduce elevated ICP, reduce calcium influx, inhibit free radical formation, and potentiate GABA-mediated transmission. (See page 754: Brain Protection.)

19. **C.**   The EEG provides a monitor of global cerebral function, but not the function of a sensory pathway. Anesthetic inductions typically produce a decrease in alpha activity and an increase in beta activity. Hypocarbia produces a slowing of EEG activity. When the body temperature falls below 35°C, the EEG slows progressively, with electrical standstill occurring at 15 to 20°C. (See page 758: Electroencephalogram.)

20. **E.**   Opioids produce minimal changes in SSEP waveforms and have a minimal effect on brainstem auditory evoked potential recordings. Physiologic factors, such as temperature, systemic blood pressure, Pao_2, and $Paco_2$, can alter SSEPs and must be controlled during intraoperative recordings. Both hypothermia and hyperthermia alter all SSEPs. In addition, fluids used to irrigate the brain or spinal cord can cause marked changes in recordings despite normal core temperature measurements. (See page 760: Anesthetic Consideration for Sensory Evoked Potential Recording.)

21. **C.**   In contrast to an intraventricular catheter, a subdural-subarachnoid bolt does not require brain

tissue penetration and cannot be used to withdraw CSF and thereby lower ICP. The major complication of subdural device is infection. The intraventricular catheter allows CSF drainage and has a low infection rate; however, it does require penetration of brain tissue. (See page 763: Intracranial Pressure Monitoring.)

22. **E.** Alert, anxious patients can be given an anxiolytic before surgery, but no premedication should be given to obtunded or lethargic patients. Succinylcholine increases ICP and is not recommended for elective neurosurgical cases. It may be the agent of choice, however, if a rapid sequence induction is truly indicated. If the blood-brain barrier is disrupted, histamine release (as may result from a large bolus dose of atracurium, mivacurium, or curare) may cause vasodilation and may thus decrease cerebral perfusion pressure. (See page 768: Anesthetic Techniques and Drugs.)

23. **E.** The sitting position is used during posterior fossa surgery to facilitate surgical exposure. However, it is associated with numerous potential complications, including venous air embolism, peripheral nerve injuries, pneumocephalus, jugular venous obstruction, and quadriplegia. (See page 773: Venous Air Embolism.)

24. **B.** A patent foramen ovale exists in 20 to 30% of the population on autopsy studies. In the sitting position, a reported 50% of patients develop right atrial pressure that is greater than the left atrial pressure and thus have the potential for paradoxical air embolism. The calculated risk of paradoxical air embolism is approximately 5 to 10%. The precordial Doppler ultrasound transducer is the most sensitive noninvasive monitor for venous air embolism; it detects amounts of air as small as 0.25 mL. The transducer is positioned along the right parasternal border between the third and sixth intercostal spaces. The pulmonary artery pressure increases proportionately with the volume of air entering the pulmonary arteries. End-tidal nitrogen monitoring is specific for detecting air but is slightly less sensitive than a decrease in end-tidal CO_2 in detecting subclinical air embolism. (See page 773: Venous Air Embolism.)

25. **A.** There are several potential complications of SAH and the surgical treatments of aneurysms. The most important of these are rebleeding, vasospasm, intracranial hypertension, and hydrocephalus. (See page 777: Intracranial Aneurysm.)

26. **C.** Cerebral vasospasm is a major cause of morbidity and mortality in patients with SAH. Clinical vasospasm with ischemic deficit is observed in approximately 70% of patients, most often between days 4 to 12, with a peak at 6 to 7 days following SAH. There is evidence that vasospasm after SAH correlates with the amount of blood in the subarachnoid space. The component in the blood implicated in causing cerebral arterial vasospasm is oxyhemoglobin. Hypervolemia, hypertension, and hemodilution have become the mainstays of treatment for ischemic neurologic deficit caused by cerebral vasospasm. (See page 777: Intracranial Aneurysm.)

27. **E.** ECG changes associated with a ruptured cerebral aneurysm include ST segment depression or elevation, T-wave inversion or flattening, Q waves, prolonged Q-T intervals, and dysrhythmias. The ECG changes are not necessarily associated with increased operative morbidity and mortality. They usually resolve within 10 days following SAH and require no special treatment. (See page 777: Intracranial Aneurysm, Page 767: Perioperative Evaluation.)

28. **A.** Classification of severe head injuries are based on the Glasgow coma scale, which defines neurologic impairment in terms of eye opening, speech, and motor function. The total score that can be obtained is 15, and severe head injury is determined by a score of 8 or less persisting for 6 hours or more. (See page 782: Head Injury.)

29. **B.** In some patients, severe intracranial hypertension precipitates reflex arterial hypertension and bradycardia (Cushing triad). A reduction in systemic blood pressure in these patients can further aggravate cerebral ischemia by reducing cerebral perfusion pressure. (See page 782: Head Injury.)

30. **E.** The syndrome of inappropriate antidiuretic hormone secretion is associated with hyponatremia, serum and extracellular fluid hypo-osmolality, renal excretion of sodium, urine osmolality greater than serum osmolality, and normal renal and adrenal function. (See page 782: Head Injury.)

31. **E.** Diagnostic criteria for nonketotic hyperosmolar hyperglycemic coma are hyperglycemia, glucosuria, absence of ketosis, increased plasma osmolality, dehydration, and central nervous system dysfunction. Serum sodium may be high, normal, or low. (See page 782: Head Injury.)

CHAPTER 28 ■ RESPIRATORY FUNCTION IN ANESTHESIA

1. Which of the following statements regarding lung compliance is FALSE?

    A. Diseases that decrease lung compliance typically result in increased respiratory rates.
    B. Spontaneous respiratory rate is a poor indicator of lung compliance.
    C. Continuous positive airway pressure (CPAP) improves lung compliance and therefore lowers the work of breathing in patients with reduced compliance
    D. Diseases that increase lung compliance typically result in increased functional residual capacity (FRC).
    E. Significant increases in lung compliance can require the use of ventilatory muscles to exhale actively.

2. Which of the following statements regarding ventilation–perfusion (V/Q) matching is TRUE?

    A. West zone 1 can be best characterized as physiologic shunt.
    B. West zone 1 can be increased by increased pulmonary artery pressure (PPA).
    C. West zone 3 occurs above the level of the third rib in the sitting position.
    D. West zone 3 has PPA > pulmonary venous pressure (PPV) > alveolar pressure (PA) and therefore has perfusion in excess of ventilation.
    E. In west zone 1, pulmonary capillary wedge pressure (PCWP) is transmitted to the alveoli promoting alveolar collapse, resulting in no ventilation of this area.

3. FRC:

    A. is the maximal volume that can be exhaled in a single breath
    B. is increased by mechanical factors such as obesity or pregnancy

    C. can be used to quantify the degree of pulmonary restriction
    D. is significantly increased in the supine position
    E. is markedly reduced in patients with chronic obstructive pulmonary disease

4. Which of the following tests is most useful and cost effective in screening overall pulmonary function?

    A. The flow volume loop
    B. The CO_2 diffusing capacity of the lungs (DLCO)
    C. The maximum voluntary ventilation
    D. Spirometry measurements
    E. Blood gas analysis

5. Which of the following statements regarding postoperative pulmonary function is TRUE?

    A. The changes in postoperative pulmonary function are primarily obstructive.
    B. Postoperative spontaneous ventilation is characterized by the absence of sighs.
    C. Thoracic operations have a more severe impact on FRC than nonlaparoscopic upper abdominal operations.
    D. The normal postoperative respiratory rate is 12 to 13 breaths per minute.
    E. Intracranial procedures typically decrease FRC by 40 to 50%.

6. The maximum benefit from preoperative smoking cessation occurs at approximately:

    A. 24 hours
    B. 2 days
    C. 2 weeks
    D. 4 weeks
    E. 8 weeks

7. Which of the following statements regarding cigarette smoking and lung disease is FALSE?

A. Smoke increases mucus production and decreases ciliary motility.
B. Smoking leads to a decrease in proteolytic enzymes in the lung that directly cause damage to lung parenchyma.
C. Patients with chronic obstructive pulmonary disease (COPD) who smoke have up to a sixfold risk of developing postoperative pneumonia.
D. Normalization of mucociliary activity requires at least 2 to 3 weeks of abstinence from smoking.
E. Smokers' relative risk of postoperative pulmonary complications is doubled even in the absence of clinical pulmonary disease or abnormal pulmonary function tests.

8. All of the following strategies reduce the risk of postoperative pulmonary complications EXCEPT:

   A. anesthetic technique
   B. postoperative pain management
   C. incentive spirometry
   D. stir-up regimens
   E. intermittent CPAP by mask

For questions 9 to 15, choose A if 1, 2, and 3 are correct; B if 1 and 3; C if 2 and 4; D if 4; E if all.

9. Which of the following statements regarding the trachea is/are TRUE?

   1. In the supine position, the most likely place for aspirated material to fall is the right upper lobe.
   2. It is located 50% in the superior mediastinum and 50% in the inferior mediastinum.
   3. The tracheal bifurcation is usually at the level of T4.
   4. The trachea's fixed position in the inferior mediastinum serves as an important reference point.

10. Which of the following statements regarding bronchioles is/are TRUE?

    1. They are approximately 1 mm in diameter.
    2. They are the last segment of the conducting airways to contain cartilage.
    3. They have the highest proportion of smooth muscle in their walls.
    4. They can be involved in terminal gas exchange if recruited.

11. Which of the following characteristics regarding gas flow is/are true?

    1. With laminar gas flow, significant alveolar ventilation can occur even when tidal volume (V_t) is less than dead space.
    2. Density is the only physical gas property that is relevant under laminar gas flow conditions.
    3. Helium does not improve gas flow under laminar conditions.
    4. During turbulent flow, resistance decreases in proportion to flow rate.

12. The Hering-Breuer reflex:

    1. is blocked by bilateral vagotomy
    2. produces apnea in humans when CPAP exceeds 40 cm H_2O
    3. is a pulmonary stretch reflex that primarily is generated from the intercostal muscles but not the diaphragm
    4. is prominent in humans but not lower-order mammals

13. Which of the following result(s) in an enhanced CO_2 response (shift of CO_2 response curve upward and to the left)?

    1. Anxiety
    2. Metabolic acidosis
    3. Arterial hypoxemia
    4. Opioid antagonists in the absence of opioids

14. Inspiratory capacity:

    1. is defined as the greatest volume that can be inhaled from the resting expiratory level
    2. is commonly measured as part of routine pulmonary function testing
    3. can be a sensitive indicator of extrathoracic airway obstruction
    4. is less sensitive than expiratory measurements to extrathoracic obstruction.

15. Which of the following statements is/are TRUE?

    1. The direct effect of CO_2 on central chemoreceptors is responsible for >80% of the resultant increase in ventilatory response.
    2. A sudden decrease in the pressure of end-tidal CO_2 (PET_{CO_2}) in a mechanically ventilated patient most often is caused by pulmonary air embolism.
    3. Preoperative pulmonary function testing is important to predict the likelihood of postoperative pulmonary complications.
    4. Patients having intrathoracic operations are at a slightly lower risk of experiencing postoperative pulmonary complications than patients having abdominal operations.

ANSWERS

1. **B.** When lung compliance is small, larger changes in intrapleural pressure are needed to create the same Vt (i.e., one has to inhale harder to force the same volume of gas into the lungs). Thus, patients with low lung compliance typically breathe with a smaller Vt at more rapid rates. Spontaneous ventilatory rate is one of the most sensitive indices of lung compliance. CPAP will shift the vertical line to the right, thus allowing the patient to breathe on a steeper and more favorable portion of the volume-pressure curve. This results in a slower ventilatory rate with a larger Vt. Patients with diseases that increase lung compliance have larger than normal FRC (gas trapping) and pressure-volume curves that are shifted to the left and steeper. These patients expend less elastic work to inspire, but elastic recoil is reduced significantly. COPD and acute asthma are the most common examples of diseases with high lung compliance. If lung compliance and FRC are sufficiently high (elastic recoil is minimal), the patient must use ventilatory muscles to expire actively. (See page 793: Elastic Work.)

2. **D.** Zone 1 receives ventilation in the absence of perfusion and creates alveolar dead space ventilation. Normally, zone 1 areas exist only to a limited extent. However, in conditions of decreased Ppa, such as hypovolemic shock, zone 1 enlarges. Because Pa is approximately equal to atmospheric pressure, Ppa in Zone 1 is subatmospheric but necessarily greater than Ppv (Pa > Ppa > Ppv). Pa that is transmitted to the pulmonary capillaries promotes their collapse, with a consequent theoretical blood flow of zero to this lung region. Thus, Zone 1 receives ventilation in the absence of perfusion and creates alveolar dead space ventilation. Zone 3 occurs in the most gravity-dependent areas of the lung where Ppa > Ppv > Pa and blood flow is primarily governed by the Ppa to Ppv difference. Because gravity also increases Ppv, the pulmonary capillaries become distended. Thus, perfusion in zone 3 is lush, resulting in capillary perfusion in excess of ventilation, or physiologic shunt. The pressure difference between Ppa and Pa determines blood flow in zone 2. Ppv has little influence. Well-matched ventilation and perfusion occur in zone 2, which contains the majority of alveoli. (See page 800: Distribution of Blood Flow.)

3. **C.** FRC is the volume of gas remaining in the lungs at passive end expiration. Residual volume is that gas remaining within the lungs at the end of forced maximal expiration. The FRC also may be used to quantify the degree of pulmonary restriction. Disease processes that reduce FRC and lung compliance include acute lung injury, pulmonary edema, pulmonary fibrotic processes, and atelectasis. Mechanical factors also reduce FRC (e.g., pregnancy, obesity, and pleural effusion). The FRC decreases 10% when a healthy subject lies down. Ventilatory muscle weakness or paralysis also will decrease FRC. In contrast, patients with COPD have excessively compliant lungs that recoil less forcibly. Their lungs retain an abnormally large volume at the end of passive expiration, a phenomenon called gas trapping. (See page 804: Lung Volumes and Capacities.)

4. **D.** Although we have a host of pulmonary function tests from which to choose, spirometry is the most useful, cost-effective, and most commonly used test. (See page 807: Pulmonary Function Tests Summary.)

5. **B.** The changes in pulmonary function that occur postoperatively are primarily restrictive, with proportional decreases in all lung volumes and no change in airway resistance. This defect is generated by abdominal contents that impinge on and prevent normal movement of the diaphragm and an abnormal respiratory pattern that is shallow, rapid and devoid of sighs. The normal resting respiratory rate for adults is 12 breaths/minute, whereas the postoperative patient usually breathes approximately 20 breaths/minute. The operative site is one of the single most important determinants of the degree of pulmonary restriction and the risk of postoperative pulmonary complications. Nonlaparoscopic upper abdominal operations cause the most profound restrictive defect, precipitating a 40 to 50% decrease in FRC compared with preoperative levels, when conventional postoperative analgesia is employed. Lower abdominal and thoracic operations cause the next most severe change in pulmonary function, with decreases in FRC to 30% of preoperative levels. Most other operative sites, including intracranial, have approximately the same effect on FRC, with reductions to 15 to 20% of preoperative levels. (See page 810: Postoperative Pulmonary Function.)

6. **E.** Patients who smoke should be advised to stop smoking 2 months before elective operations to maximize the effect of smoking cessation or for at least 4 weeks to gain some benefit from improved mucociliary function. Normalization of mucociliary function requires 2 to 3 weeks of abstinence from smoking, during which time sputum increases. Several months of smoking abstinence are required to return sputum clearance to normal. If patients cannot stop smoking for these periods of time, they probably should be advised to stop smoking for at least 24 hours before the operation so that carboxyhemoglobin levels will approach normal. Smokers who decrease, but do not stop, cigarette consumption without the aid of nicotine replacement therapy continue to acquire equal amounts of nicotine from fewer cigarettes by changing their technique of

smoking to maximize nicotine intake. (See page 809: Effect of Cigarette Smoking on Pulmonary Function.)

7. **B.** Smoking affects pulmonary function in many ways. The irritant smoke decreases ciliary motility and increases sputum production. Thus, these patients have a high volume of sputum and decreased ability to clear it effectively. As smoking habits persist, airway reactivity and the development of obstructive disease become problematic. Studies of the pathogenesis of COPD suggest that smoking results in an excess of pulmonary proteolytic enzymes that directly cause damage to the lung parenchyma. Exposure to smoke increases synthesis and release of elastolytic enzymes from alveolar macrophages, cells instrumental in the genesis of COPD resulting from smoking.

Smoking is one of the main and most prevalent risk factors associated with postoperative morbidity. Patients with COPD who smoke have a twofold to a sixfold risk of developing postoperative pneumonia compared with nonsmokers. Further, smokers' relative risk of postoperative pulmonary complications is doubled, even if they do not have evidence of clinical pulmonary disease or abnormal pulmonary function. Normalization of mucociliary function requires 2 to 3 weeks of abstinence from smoking, during which time sputum increases. (See page 809: Effects of Cigarette Smoking on Pulmonary Function.)

8. **A.** There are several strategies by which it is possible to reduce risk of postoperative pulmonary complications: use of lung-expanding therapies postoperatively, choice of analgesia, and cessation of smoking. After upper abdominal operations, which are associated with the highest incidence of postoperative pulmonary complications, FRC recovers over 3 to 7 days. With the use of intermittent CPAP by mask, FRC will recover within 72 hours. Patients use incentive spirometers correctly only 10% of the time unless therapy is supervised. Stir-up regimens are as effective as incentive spirometry at preventing postoperative pulmonary complications, they are less expensive than supervised incentive spirometry, and thus they are preferred over incentive spirometry therapy. The choice of anesthetic technique for intraoperative anesthesia does not change the risk of postoperative pulmonary complications. However, the choice of postoperative analgesia strongly influences the risk of postoperative pulmonary complications. The advent of postoperative epidural analgesia, particularly for abdominal and thoracic operations, has markedly decreased the risk of postoperative pulmonary complications and appears to contribute to decreased length of stay in the hospital postoperatively. (See page 810: Postoperative Pulmonary Complications.)

9. **B.** The diameter of the right bronchus is generally greater than that of the left. In the adult, the right bronchus leaves the trachea at approximately 25 degrees from the tracheal axis, whereas the angle of the left bronchus is approximately 45 degrees. Thus, inadvertent endobronchial intubation or aspiration of foreign material is more likely to occur in the right lung than in the left. Furthermore, the right upper lobe bronchus dives almost directly posterior at approximately 90 degrees from the right main bronchus. Foreign bodies and fluid aspirated by a supine subject usually fall into the right upper lobe. In the adult, the trachea is a fibromuscular tube is approximately 10 to 12 cm long with an outside diameter of approximately 20 mm. The trachea enters the superior mediastinum and bifurcates at the sternal angle (the lower border of the fourth thoracic vertebral body). Normally, half of the trachea is intrathoracic, and the other half is extrathoracic. Both ends of the trachea are attached to mobile structures. Thus, the carina can move superiorly as much as 5 cm from its normal resting position. (See page 792: Conductive Airways.)

10. **B.** The bronchioles typically have diameters of 1 mm. They are devoid of cartilaginous support and have the highest proportion of smooth muscle in the wall. There are approximately three to four bronchiolar generations. The final bronchiolar generation is the terminal bronchiole, which is the last airway component that is not directly involved in gas exchange. (See page 792: Conductive Airways.)

11. **B.** A clinical implication of laminar flow in the airways is that significant alveolar ventilation can occur even when the Vt is less than anatomic dead space. This phenomenon is important in high-frequency ventilation. Viscosity is the only physical gas property that is relevant under conditions of laminar flow. Helium has a low density, but its viscosity is close to that of air. Therefore, helium will not improve gas flow that is laminar. Usually, flow is turbulent when there is critical airway narrowing or abnormally high airway resistance, thus making low density helium therapy useful. Resistance during laminar flow is inversely proportional to gas flow rate. Conversely, during turbulent flow, resistance increases in proportion to the flow rate. (See page 794: Resistance to Gas Flow.)

12. **B.** Golgi tendon organs (tendon spindles), which occur in series arrangements within ventilatory muscles, facilitate proprioception. The intercostal muscles are rich in tendon spindles, whereas the diaphragm has a limited number. Thus, the pulmonary stretch reflex primarily involves the intercostal muscles but not the diaphragm. When the lungs are full and the chest wall is stretched, these receptors send signals to the brainstem that inhibit further inspiration. In 1868, Hering and Breuer reported that lightly anesthetized, spontaneously breathing animals would cease or decrease ventilatory effort during sustained lung distention. This response was blocked by bilateral vagotomy. The Hering-Breuer reflex is prominent in lower-order

mammals, such as rabbits, but is only weakly present in humans. The Hering-Breuer reflex is sufficiently active in lower mammals, such that 5 cm H_2O CPAP will induce apnea. In humans, however, the reflex is only weakly present, as evidenced by the fact that humans will continue to breathe spontaneously with CPAP in excess of 40 cm H_2O. This inflation reflex is associated with inspiratory muscle inhibition, as documented by marked reductions in electrical activity of both the phrenic nerve and the diaphragmatic muscle itself. The second component of the Hering-Breuer reflex, the deflation reflex, produces increased ventilatory muscle activity following sustained lung deflation. (See page 797: Reflex Control of Ventilation.)

13. **A.**   Three clinical states result in a left shift and/or a steepened slope of the CO_2 response curve. These same three situations are the only causes of true hyperventilation (i.e., an increase in minute ventilation such that the decreased $Paco_2$ creates respiratory alkalemia). The three causes of hyperventilation (enhanced CO_2 response) are arterial hypoxemia, metabolic acidemia, and central etiologic factors. Examples of central etiologic factors that cause hyperventilation include drug administration, intracranial hypertension, hepatic cirrhosis, and nonspecific arousal states such as anxiety and fear. Aminophylline, salicylates, and norepinephrine stimulate ventilation independent of peripheral chemoreceptors. Opioid antagonists, given in the absence of opioids, do not stimulate ventilation. However, when they are given after opiate administration, they do reverse the effects of opioids on the CO_2 response curve. (See page 798: Quantitative Aspects of Chemical Control of Breathing.)

14. **B.**   The inspiratory capacity is the largest volume of gas that can be inspired from the resting expiratory level and frequently is decreased in the presence of significant extrathoracic airway obstruction. This measurement is one of the few simple tests that can detect extrathoracic airway obstruction. Most routine pulmonary function tests measure only exhaled flows and volumes, which are relatively unaffected by extrathoracic obstruction unless it is severe. Changes in the absolute volume of inspiratory capacity usually parallel changes in vital capacity. Expiratory reserve volume is not of great diagnostic value. (See page 804: Lung Volumes and Capacities.)

15. **D.**   Although the central response is the major factor in the regulation of breathing by CO_2, CO_2 has little direct stimulating effect on these chemosensitive areas. These receptors are primarily sensitive to changes in H^+ concentration. CO_2 has a potent but indirect effect by reacting with water to form carbonic acid, which dissociates into H^+ and bicarbonate ions. The $PETCO_2$ in ventilated patients varied linearly with the dead space to Vt ratio (Vd/Vt) and correlated poorly with $Paco_2$. Monitoring $PETCO_2$ gives far more information about ventilatory efficiency or dead space ventilation than it does about the absolute value of $Paco_2$. Anesthesiologists commonly measure $PETCO_2$ to detect venous air embolism during anesthesia. A lowered cardiac output alone, in the absence of venous air embolism, may sufficiently decrease pulmonary perfusion so that dead space ventilation increases and $PETCO_2$ falls. Thus, a depressed $PETCO_2$ is a sensitive but nonspecific monitor. The goals one hopes to achieve through preoperative pulmonary function testing would be to predict the likelihood of pulmonary complications, to obtain quantitative baseline information concerning pulmonary function, and to identify patients who may benefit from therapy to improve pulmonary function preoperatively. For patients who will have lung resection, pulmonary function testing does provide some predictive benefit. However, for other patients, the overwhelming evidence suggests that preoperative pulmonary function testing does not predict or assign risk for postoperative pulmonary complications. The operative site is the single most important determinant of both the degree of pulmonary restriction and postoperative pulmonary complications. Nonlaparoscopic upper abdominal operations increase the risk of postoperative pulmonary complications by at least twofold. Lower abdominal and intrathoracic operations are associated with slightly less risk, but still higher risk than extremity, intracranial, and head and neck operations. (See page 797: Central Chemoreceptors; page 802: and Assessment of Physiologic Dead Space; page 810: Postoperative Pulmonary Complications; page 807: Preoperative Pulmonary Assessment.)

CHAPTER 29 ■ ANESTHESIA FOR THORACIC SURGERY

1. The leading cause of cancer mortality in the United States and throughout the world is:

   A. lung cancer
   B. colorectal cancer
   C. breast cancer
   D. prostate cancer
   E. none of the above

2. The leading cause of cancer death in women in the United States is:

   A. lung cancer
   B. colorectal cancer
   C. breast cancer
   D. ovarian cancer
   E. none of the above

3. During a preanesthetic interview, you elicit the history of severe exertional dyspnea from an elderly man who smokes cigarettes. This implies:

   A. He is at increased risk of high-peak airway pressures on mechanical ventilation.
   B. Wet crackles will be heard at his lung bases on auscultation.
   C. Preoperative flow volume loops will demonstrate a restrictive pattern.
   D. He has a severely diminished respiratory reserve and is at high risk of postoperative ventilatory support.
   E. He will require mechanical ventilatory tidal volumes of 15 to 20 mL/kg.

4. Acute lung injury, an early form of acute respiratory distress syndrome, is sometimes seen postoperatively after thoracic surgery. Risk factors for acute lung injury after chest surgery include:

   A. alcohol abuse
   B. planned pneumonectomy
   C. high intraoperative ventilatory pressures

   D. excessive amounts of fluid administration
   E. all of the above

5. Choose the FALSE statement regarding the physical examination of a patient undergoing thoracic surgery.

   A. Deviation of the trachea indicates potentially difficult intubation.
   B. Clubbing often is seen in patients with a left-to-right shunt.
   C. If cyanosis is present, the patient's Pao_2 level is typically <55 mm Hg.
   D. The compliance of the pulmonary circulation is reduced in patients with chronic obstructive pulmonary disease.
   E. A narrowly split second heart sound is a sign of pulmonary hypertension.

6. Which of the following can increase pulmonary vascular resistance?

   A. Systemic acidemia
   B. Septicemia
   C. Systemic hypoxia
   D. Positive end-expiratory pressure (PEEP)
   E. All of the above

7. Choose the FALSE statement regarding flow volume loops.

   A. Small airway resistance is best displayed at expiration between 25% and 75% of vital capacity.
   B. Lung volume is displayed on the horizontal axis.
   C. Patients with restrictive lung disease have a decreased maximum midexpiratory flow rate.
   D. The flow volume loop displays essentially the same information as the spirometer.
   E. Effort-dependent areas of the loop determine large airway patency.

8. All of the following statements regarding the treatment of wheezing are true EXCEPT:

   A. Ipratropium bromide causes bronchodilation by increasing 3'5'-cyclic guanosine monophosphate levels.
   B. Aminophylline should be used cautiously in patients with myocardial ischemia.
   C. Cromolyn sodium is of little value in the treatment of an acute wheezing episode.
   D. Steroids decrease mucosal edema and prevent the release of bronchoconstricting substances.
   E. beta-Agonist aerosols cause bronchodilation by increasing 3'5'-cyclic adenosine monophosphate levels.

9. The following are true regarding intraoperative monitoring during thoracic surgery EXCEPT:

   A. A permanent ischemic complication can occur after placement of a radial artery catheter in a patient with normal Allen test results.
   B. The central venous pressure (CVP) is helpful in determining right ventricular performance.
   C. A central line placed in the external jugular vein often kinks after patient positioning.
   D. The CVP has been shown to have a poor correlation with left atrial pressure in patients with pulmonary disease.
   E. Patients with chronic obstructive pulmonary disease presenting for lung resection usually have a left-sided heart strain pattern on the electrocardiogram.

10. Pulmonary artery catheters:

    A. are most often directed to the right lower lobe
    B. should lie in the nondependent lung when one-lung ventilation is used
    C. yield accurate data only when they are placed in West zone 1 or 2
    D. yield inaccurate data when placed in the dependent lung
    E. can cause a left bundle branch block

11. A patient is found to have a pulmonary artery rupture. Which of the following statements is TRUE?

    A. Pulmonary artery perforation usually presents as chest and back pain.
    B. The bleeding usually occurs from the left side.
    C. Lung resection may be necessary.
    D. Pulmonary artery rupture is more common in younger patients.
    E. It occurs more commonly in men.

12. Which of the following is TRUE regarding the diffusing capacity for carbon monoxide (DLCO)?

    A. A preoperative DLCO less than 60% of predicted indicates high risk of mortality after lung resection.
    B. DLCO testing is of little clinical use.
    C. DLCO correlates well with forced expiratory volume in 1 second (FEV_1).
    D. It is impaired by interstitial lung disease.
    E. Predicted postoperative diffusing capacity percent is a poor predictor of mortality after lung resection.

13. With respect to the intraoperative use of transesophageal echocardiography (TEE), which of the following statements is FALSE?

    A. TEE is useful for detecting ventricular dysfunction.
    B. Peripheral and central lung tumors are equally easy to locate with TEE.
    C. TEE can be used to detect pulmonary artery compression by a mediastinal tumor.
    D. TEE can help determine whether cardiopulmonary bypass is necessary for tumor resection.
    E. Aortic dissection can be diagnosed by TEE.

14. All of the following statements regarding pulse oximetry are true EXCEPT:

    A. Absorbance of light occurs at 660 and 940 nm.
    B. The presence of dyshemoglobins can affect values.
    C. Pulse oximeters are accurate over the range of 20 to 100% saturation.
    D. Pulse oximeters are a noninvasive means of assessing oxygenation.
    E. The presence of a low cardiac output can affect values.

15. Which of the following statements is TRUE regarding changes seen when a patient is positioned in the lateral decubitus position?

    A. Blood flow to the nondependent lung is significantly greater than it is to the dependent lung.
    B. The distribution of blood flow is turned by 180 degrees compared with the supine position.
    C. An awake, spontaneously breathing patient, will demonstrate poor ventilation–perfusion matching in the dependent lung.
    D. Controlled ventilation is required to ensure gas exchange and adequate ventilation when a thoracotomy is performed.
    E. The nondependent hemidiaphragm is displaced higher into the chest.

16. A patient undergoing a right thoracotomy with one-lung ventilation is given vecuronium bromide and is placed in the left lateral decubitus position. The following statements are true EXCEPT:

    A. Thirty-five percent of the cardiac output participates in gas exchange in the left lung.
    B. Hypoxic pulmonary vasoconstriction reduces blood flow to the nondependent hypoxic lung by 50%.
    C. The patient's functional residual capacity is reduced by receiving vecuronium bromide.
    D. One-lung ventilation causes a right-to-left shunt in the nonventilated lung.

E. Atelectasis can inhibit optimal ventilation to the dependent lung.

17. When positioning the double-lumen tube:

    A. Insertion through the vocal cords is performed with the distal curvature facing laterally.
    B. The tube should be advanced until moderate resistance is encountered.
    C. The Miller laryngoscope blade yields a much easier tube insertion than does a Macintosh laryngoscope blade.
    D. The stylet should be removed after the tube is rotated 90 degrees.
    E. A left-sided tube should be rotated 90 degrees to the right after the tip passes through the vocal cords.

18. All the following are absolute indications for one-lung ventilation EXCEPT:

    A. pneumonectomy
    B. massive hemorrhage
    C. bronchopleural fistula
    D. unilateral abscess
    E. bronchopulmonary lavage

19. When checking the position of the double-lumen tube, all of the following are true EXCEPT:

    A. Use of an underwater seal is a good method to verify separation before bronchopulmonary lavage.
    B. Inflation of the bronchial cuff rarely requires >2 mL of air.
    C. Selective capnography can be used to ensure correct placement.
    D. The pediatric bronchoscope should be passed through the tracheal lumen first.
    E. If breath sounds are not equal after the tracheal cuff is inflated, the tube should be advanced 2 to 3 cm.

20. All of the following inhibit hypoxic pulmonary vasoconstriction EXCEPT:

    A. propofol
    B. pulmonary embolism
    C. epinephrine
    D. mitral stenosis
    E. infection

21. All of the following are true regarding patients with mediastinal masses EXCEPT:

    A. Local anesthesia is an anesthetic option for biopsy.
    B. Airway obstruction on induction of anesthesia may be relieved with neuromuscular blocking agents.
    C. Hypotension on induction of anesthesia may be secondary to cardiac compression.
    D. Mediastinal masses may coexist with superior vena cava syndrome.
    E. Passage of a rigid bronchoscope beyond the obstruction may be lifesaving.

22. Mediastinoscopy:

    A. commonly occludes the left radial pulse
    B. may be associated with right hemiparesis
    C. may cause injury to the superior laryngeal nerve
    D. is a procedure with potential for life-threatening hemorrhage
    E. must be performed with the patient under general anesthesia

23. Regarding lung volume reduction surgery, all of the following are true EXCEPT:

    A. This procedure is necessary in patients with end-stage emphysema.
    B. Ventilation can usually be decreased after the chest is open.
    C. Nitrous oxide should be avoided.
    D. Pneumothorax may be difficult to diagnose.
    E. Patients have a greater amount of functional lung tissue after surgery.

24. Which of the following statements regarding bronchopulmonary lavage is TRUE?

    A. The cuff seal of an endobronchial tube should be adjusted so that no leak is present at 50 cm H_2O.
    B. Most patients require 3 days of mechanical ventilation following lavage.
    C. The patient is turned so the lavage side is uppermost.
    D. Once lung separation is achieved while the patient is under general anesthesia, the patient is allowed to regain consciousness for the procedure.
    E. The onset of rales in the ventilated lung indicates heart failure.

For questions 25 to 38, choose A if 1, 2, and 3 are correct; B if 1 and 3; C if 2 and 4; D if 4; and E if all.

25. The goals of performing pulmonary function tests (PFTs) in a patient scheduled for lung resection for treatment of a malignancy are:

    1. to establishing the maximum amount of resectable lung tissue
    2. to identify the patient needing postoperative ventilatory support
    3. to evaluate the benefits of bronchodilators in reversing existing airway obstruction
    4. to evaluate whether increased inspired O_2 concentration increases ventilation and therefore work of breathing

26. Which of the following sympathomimetic drugs are beta$_2$-selective and produce minimal cardiac effect from beta$_1$-stimulation?

    1. Albuterol
    2. Terbutaline
    3. Metaproterenol
    4. Epinephrine

27. Respiratory changes that occur after lower abdominal surgery include:

    1. Total lung capacity decreases to the same extent after abdominal surgery as after extremity surgery.
    2. Tidal volume is decreased for approximately 2 weeks.
    3. Pulmonary compliance increases.
    4. Vital capacity decreases by 25%.

28. Which of the following statements about preoperative testing of pulmonary function is/are TRUE?

    1. A 15% improvement in PFT results after bronchodilator therapy is an indication for preoperative bronchodilator administration.
    2. Spirometry and arterial blood gases are the first studies performed in the evaluation of patients considered for pneumonectomy.
    3. A preoperative $Paco_2$ level of >50 mm Hg is an indication for split lung function testing.
    4. A mean pulmonary artery pressure of >40 mm Hg after balloon occlusion indicates that the patient likely will not tolerate pneumonectomy.

29. Which of the following statements regarding pulmonary evaluation for lung resectability is/are TRUE?

    1. A vital capacity of at least three times the tidal volume is necessary for an effective cough.
    2. A vital capacity of <50% of predicted capacity is an indicator of increased risk.
    3. An FEV_1 of <800 mL in a 70-kg patient is an absolute contraindication to lung resection.
    4. A ratio of residual volume to total lung capacity of 10% is consistent with a high risk for pulmonary resection.

30. Which of the following statements concerning smoking is/are TRUE?

    1. Smoking decreases forced vital capacity and maximum midexpiratory flow rate.
    2. Cessation of smoking for 48 hours before surgery shifts the oxyhemoglobin curve to the left.
    3. Most of the beneficial effects of smoking cessation do not occur before 2 to 3 months.
    4. Smoking increases mucociliary transport.

31. Which of the following statements concerning oxygenation and ventilation is/are TRUE?

    1. An esophageal or precordial stethoscope ensures adequate oxygenation.
    2. The alveolar dead space affects the arterial-alveolar CO_2 gradient.
    3. Hypercarbia usually is a greater problem than systemic hypoxia during one-lung ventilation.
    4. CO_2 readings can help indicate correct double-lumen tube placement.

32. Which of the following statements regarding bronchial blockers is/are TRUE?

    1. They are effective in maintaining lung isolation despite surgical manipulation.
    2. A Univent tube is useful when postoperative ventilation is required.
    3. Placement of an endobronchial catheter into the bronchus should be performed blindly.
    4. Bronchial blockers may be used in children younger than 12 years.

33. During one-lung ventilation:

    1. Tidal volumes should be adjusted to 10 to 12 mL/kg.
    2. Continuous positive airway pressure to the nondependent lung increases arterial O_2 concentration.
    3. Hyperventilation can lead to a decreased Pao_2 level.
    4. Use of an inspired O_2 concentration of 100% may increase shunting.

34. Hypoxic pulmonary vasoconstriction:

    1. is increased in the presence of potent inhaled anesthetics
    2. is indirectly inhibited by hypothermia
    3. is inhibited by ibuprofen
    4. is activated by collapse of the nondependent lung

35. Rigid bronchoscopy is the procedure of choice for:

    1. assessing vascular tumors of the lower airway
    2. securing an airway in a difficult intubation
    3. bronchoscopy in small children
    4. evaluation of upper lobe lesions

36. Which of the following statements regarding myasthenia gravis is/are TRUE?

    1. Examination of pupillary size can differentiate between myasthenic and cholinergic crisis.
    2. These patients are very sensitive to depolarizing muscle relaxants and are resistant to nondepolarizing muscle relaxants.
    3. Thymectomy is considered to be the treatment of choice in most patients with generalized myasthenia gravis.
    4. This condition is associated with a markedly decreased release of acetylcholine from nerve terminals.

37. Which of the following statements regarding cryoanalgesia is/are TRUE?

    1. A cryoprobe is generally placed on the skin.
    2. Hypoesthesia in the scar is a common late finding.
    3. Conduction is interrupted for approximately 1 to 2 weeks.
    4. It is not used routinely for thoracotomy.

38. Which of the following statements regarding video-assisted thoracic surgery (VATS) is/are TRUE?

1. CO_2 may be insufflated into the pleural cavity.
2. Continuous positive air pressure can interfere with the surgical procedure.
3. The need for one-lung ventilation is greater for VATS than for open thoracotomy.
4. It may take 30 minutes for complete lung collapse.

ANSWERS

1. **A.** Lung cancer was the cause of death for 600,000 people in the world in 1995. Lung cancer was also responsible for the deaths of 160,440 people in 2004 in the United States; this number comprised 28% of all cancer deaths. In comparison, the combined mortality from colorectal, breast, and prostate cancer in the United States was 127,210. (See page 813: Key Points.)

2. **A.** Lung cancer has recently surpassed breast cancer as the leading cause of cancer death in women in the United States. More than 50% more women in the United States will die of lung cancer than of breast cancer. (See page 813: Key Points.)

3. **D.** During any preanesthetic assessment, it is important to ask about dyspnea. Dyspnea is a sensation of shortness of breath, which occurs when a patient's requirement for ventilation is greater than the patient's ability to respond to that demand. When the anesthetist quantitates the degree of physical activity required to produce the sensation of dyspnea, certain postoperative predictions can be made. Once a patient complains of dyspnea produced by minimal exertion, the ventilatory reserve is implicitly significantly diminished, and the FEV_1 is predicted to be less than 1500 mL. It is not unusual for these patients to need postoperative ventilatory support. (See page 814: Preoperative Evaluation.)

4. **E.** Patients with a preoperative history of alcohol abuse have been identified as being at increased risk of acute lung injury after thoracic surgery. Patients who undergo pneumonectomy, who are exposed to high airway pressures on mechanical ventilation, or who receive an excessive amount of fluid relative to their needs have also been identified as being at increased risk of acute lung injury. (See page 814: Risk Factors for Acute Lung Injury.)

5. **B.** Clubbing is seen frequently in patients with congenital heart disease associated with a right-to-left shunt, in patients with chronic lung disease, or in those with malignancies. If cyanosis is present, the arterial saturation is 80% or less, which correlates with a Pao_2 level of 50 to 52 mm Hg. Displacement of the trachea should alert the anesthesiologist to the potential for difficult intubation. Patients with chronic obstructive pulmonary disease have reduced compliance of the pulmonary capillary bed. A narrowly split second heart sound is a sign of pulmonary hypertension. (See page 814: Physical Examination.)

6. **E.** Systemic acidosis, sepsis, hypoxemia, and PEEP can increase pulmonary vascular resistance; this increase in pulmonary vascular resistance can place the patient at risk of right ventricular failure. This risk of right ventricular failure is further increased if the patient had been suffering from chronic obstructive pulmonary disease characterized by distention of the pulmonary capillary bed with decreased compliance in response to increased pulmonary blood flow. (See page 815: Evaluation of the Cardiovascular System.)

7. **C.** In patients with restrictive lung disease, the maximum midexpiratory flow rate is usually normal, whereas total lung capacity is reduced. Lung volume is displayed on the horizontal axis of a flow volume curve, and flow is displayed on the vertical axis. The shape and peak of flow rates during expiration at high volumes are effort dependent and indicate the patency of the larger airways. Effort-independent expiration occurs at low lung volumes and usually reflects smaller airway resistance. The best measurement for small airway disease is a maximum midexpiratory flow rate of 25 to 75% of vital capacity. The flow volume loop essentially displays the same information as the spirometer but is more convenient for measurement of specific flow rates. (See page 816: Flow Volume Loops.)

8. **A.** Ipratropium bromide blocks the formation of 3′5′-cyclic guanosine monophosphate and therefore has a bronchodilatory effect. The balance between 3′5′-cyclic adenosine monophosphate (which produces bronchodilation) and 3′5′-cyclic guanosine monophosphate (which produces bronchoconstriction) determines the state of contraction of the bronchial smooth muscle. Aminophylline may cause ventricular dysrhythmias and thus should be used cautiously when treating patients who have cardiac disease. Steroids decrease mucosal edema and prevent the release of bronchoconstricting substances. Cromolyn sodium stabilizes the mast cells and inhibits degranulation and histamine release. It is useful in the prevention of bronchospastic attacks but is of little value in the treatment of an acute exacerbation. (See page 818: Wheezing and Bronchodilation.)

9. **E.** Patients presenting for lung surgery often have right-sided heart strain evident on the electrocardiogram. A CVP catheter reflects blood volume, right ventricular performance, and venous tone. The major disadvantage of using the external jugular vein for placement of a CVP is that the catheter may kink when the patient is turned laterally. The CVP has been shown to have poor correlation with the left atrial pressure in patients with pulmonary disease. A negative Allen test does not guarantee that an ischemic injury will not occur after placement of a radial artery catheter. (See page 819: Intraoperative Monitoring.)

10. **A.** The tip of a flow-directed pulmonary artery catheter usually will end up in the right lower lobe, because this is the area of highest pulmonary blood flow. A pulmonary artery catheter lying in a West zone 1 or 2 region yields inaccurate hemodynamic measurements. During thoracotomy with one-lung ventilation, a catheter in the dependent lung should produce accurate hemodynamic measurements. Right bundle branch block is a potential complication of pulmonary artery catheterization. (See page 820: Pulmonary Artery Catheterization.)

11. **C.** If bleeding after pulmonary artery rupture continues, surgical exploration and lung resection may be necessary. The bleeding often comes from the right side because that is where the pulmonary artery catheter usually is positioned. Populations at risk include women and the elderly. Risk factors for this complication include hypothermia, pulmonary hypertension, and anticoagulation. Pulmonary artery perforation most commonly manifests as hemoptysis. (See page 820: Pulmonary Artery Catheterization.)

12. **D.** Gas exchange ability by the lungs can be evaluated by testing the DLCO. This parameter is impaired in such disorders as interstitial lung disease. If the tested DLCO is less than 40%, there is an increased risk of postoperative respiratory complications and mortality following lung resection surgery. Little relationship exists between predicted postoperative DLCO and predicted postoperative FEV_1. Predicted postoperative diffusing capacity percent is the strongest single predictor of risk of complications and mortality after lung resection. (See page 817: Diffusing Capacity for Carbon Monoxide.)

13. **B.** TEE can consistently locate central lung tumors, whereas peripheral lung tumors are located only 30% of the time. TEE is a useful intraoperative monitor for ventricular function, valvular function, and wall motion abnormalities. TEE can help determine when cardiopulmonary bypass is necessary for mediastinal tumor resection. TEE can also show mediastinal tumors compressing the pulmonary artery. (See page 820: Transesophageal Echocardiography.)

14. **C.** Pulse oximeters, now a standard of care for noninvasive monitoring of oxygenation, are fairly accurate in estimating oxygenation over the range of 60 to 100%. A sensor containing two light-emitting diodes (LEDs) and one photodetector is placed on the fingertip or ear lobe. The LEDs emit light at 660 and 940 nm, and absorbance is measured by a photodetector. Accuracy may be affected by dyshemoglobins, dyes, hypothermia, and low cardiac output. (See page 820: Monitoring of Oxygenation and Ventilation.)

15. **D.** Controlled positive-pressure ventilation is the only way to provide adequate ventilation and to guarantee gas exchange during a thoracotomy. In the lateral decubitus position, the distribution of blood flow and ventilation is similar to that in the upright position, but turned by 90 degrees. Good ventilation–perfusion matching at the level of the dependent lung results in adequate oxygenation in the awake, spontaneously breathing patient. The dependent hemidiaphragm is pushed higher into the chest by the abdominal contents than is the nondependent diaphragm. (See page 821: Lateral Position, Awake, Breathing Spontaneous, Chest Closed.)

16. **A.** Before the initiation of one-lung anesthesia, the average percentage of cardiac output participating in gas exchange is 45% in the nondependent lung and 55% in the dependent lung. After the initiation of one-lung anesthesia, hypoxic pulmonary vasoconstriction reduces the blood flow to the nondependent lung by 50%. The functional residual capacity and the total lung volume decrease during one-lung ventilation. There are several reasons for this, including general anesthesia, paralysis, pressure from the abdominal contents, compression by the weight of mediastinal structures, and suboptimal positioning on the operating table. Atelectasis is one cause of suboptimal ventilation to the dependent lung. (See page 823: One-Lung Ventilation, Anesthetized, Paralyzed, Chest Open.)

17. **B.** Advancement of a double-lumen tube should be stopped when moderate resistance to further passage is encountered, which indicates that the tube tip has been seated in the stem bronchus. The Macintosh laryngoscope blade is preferred for intubation with a double-lumen tube because it provides the largest area through which to pass the tube. The insertion of the tube between the vocal cords is performed with the distal concave curvature facing anteriorly. It is important to remove the stylet before rotating or advancing the tube further, to avoid tracheal or bronchial lacerations. After the tip of the tube passes the vocal cords, the stylet is removed. A right-sided tube then is rotated 90 degrees to the right; a left-sided tube is rotated 90 degrees to the left. (See page 826: Positioning Double-Lumen Tubes.)

18. **A.**   In clinical practice, a double-lumen tube is used commonly for lobectomy or pneumonectomy; however, these are relative indications for lung separation. Separation of the lungs to prevent spillage of pus or blood from an infected or bleeding source is an absolute indication for one-lung ventilation. Bronchopleural or bronchocutaneous fistulae represent low-resistance escape pathways for the tidal volume delivered by positive-pressure ventilation. These are both absolute indications for one-lung ventilation. During bronchopulmonary lavage, an effective separation of the lungs is mandatory to avoid accidental spillage of fluid from the lavaged lung to the nondependent ventilated lung. (See page 824: Absolute Indications for One-Lung Ventilation.)

19. **E.**   If breath sounds are not equal after the tracheal cuff is inflated, the double-lumen tube is likely too far down. Withdrawing the tube by 2 or 3 cm usually restores equal breath sounds. Inflation of the bronchial cuff rarely requires >2 mL of air. The bronchoscope usually is introduced first through the tracheal lumen. The carina is visualized, and bronchial cuff herniation should not be seen. Common methods of ensuring the correct placement of a double-lumen tube include fluoroscopy, chest radiography, selective capnography, and the use of an underwater seal. If the bronchial cuff is not inflated and positive-pressure ventilation is applied to the bronchial lumen of the double-lumen tube, gas will leak past the bronchial cuff and will return to the tracheal lumen. If the tracheal lumen is connected to an underwater seal system, gas will be seen bubbling up through the water. The bronchial cuff then can be gradually inflated until no gas bubbles are seen. (See page 826: Positioning Double-Lumen Tubes.)

20. **A.**   Propofol, in doses of 6 to 12 mg/ kg per hour, does not abolish hypoxic pulmonary vasoconstriction during one-lung ventilation in human patients. Factors associated with an increase in pulmonary artery pressure antagonize the effects of increased resistance caused by hypoxic pulmonary vasoconstriction and result in increased flow to the hypoxic region. Indirect inhibitors of hypoxic pulmonary vasoconstriction include mitral stenosis, thromboembolism, and vasopressors such as epinephrine. Direct inhibitors of hypoxic pulmonary vasoconstriction include infection and vasodilator drugs. (See page 836: Effects of Anesthetics and Hypoxic Pulmonary Vasoconstriction.)

21. **B.**   When a patient has a mediastinal mass and there is concern that airway obstruction may occur during anesthetic induction, an awake fiber-optic intubation is the technique of choice. Spontaneous respiration should be maintained, because muscle paralysis may result in airway compression and may worsen the obstruction. Ventilatory difficulties may be relieved by passing the rigid bronchoscope beyond the obstruction under direct laryngoscopy or by changing the position of the patient. Mediastinal masses can cause superior vena cava syndrome. Cardiac compression may become apparent after the induction of anesthesia. (See page 840: Diagnostic Procedures for Mediastinal Masses.)

22. **D.**   Mediastinoscopy is a means for assessing spread of lung carcinoma. Hemorrhage is a real risk and may be life-threatening. Pressure on the innominate artery by the mediastinoscope has been thought to cause transient left hemiparesis; therefore, it is recommended that blood pressure be monitored in the left arm and that the right radial pulse be monitored continuously. A decrease in the right radial pulse would be an indication for repositioning the mediastinoscope. Recurrent laryngeal nerve injury may occur either secondary to damage by the mediastinoscope or by tumor involvement. If both recurrent laryngeal nerves are damaged, upper airway obstruction may result. Mediastinoscopy may be performed using local anesthesia. (See page 841: Mediastinoscopy.)

23. **B.**   Extensive bullae represent end-stage emphysematous destruction of the lung. Once the chest is open during lung volume reduction surgery, more of the tidal volume may enter the compliant bullae, which are no longer limited by chest wall integrity, and an increase in ventilation is needed until the bullae are resected. Nitrous oxide should be avoided, because it can cause expansion of the bullae. The diagnosis of pneumothorax may be made by a unilateral decrease in breath sounds (which may be difficult to distinguish in a patient with bullous disease). Unlike most cases of pulmonary resection, patients following bullectomy are left with a greater amount of functional lung tissue than was previously available to them, and the mechanics of respiration are improved. (See page 844: Lung Cysts and Bullae.)

24. **A.**   During bronchopulmonary lavage, the cuff seal should be checked to maintain perfect separation of lungs at a pressure of 50 cm H_2O to prevent leakage of lavage fluid. A stethoscope should be placed over the ventilated lung to check for rales that may indicate leakage of lavage fluid into this lung. Once the trachea is intubated, the patient is turned so the side to be treated is lowermost, and the double-lumen tube position and seal are checked once again. After a further period of ventilation, most patients can be extubated in the operating room. (See page 847: Bronchopulmonary Lavage.)

25. **A.**   Preoperative PFTs allow the surgeon and anesthetist to determine the maximum amount of resectable lung before the patient would become a pulmonary cripple. If the amount of planned resection would cause significant morbidity, then reconsideration of the surgical plan may be in order. PFTs also allow one to plan for postoperative ventilatory support after lung resection. Preoperative

PFTs also evaluate whether the patient exhibits airway obstruction and whether that obstruction reverses completely or in part after bronchodilator therapy. (See page 815: Pulmonary Function Testing and Evaluation for Lung Resectability.)

26. **A.** Albuterol, terbutaline, and metaproterenol are $beta_2$-selective sympathomimetic drugs that have little effect on $beta_1$-receptors (cardiac receptors). They are used to increase intracellular cyclic adenosine monophosphate concentrations in bronchial smooth muscle and thereby produce bronchodilation. Epinephrine stimulates both $beta_1$- and $beta_2$-receptors. (See page 819: Sympathomimetic Drugs.)

27. **C.** Tidal volume decreases by 20% within 24 hours after surgery and gradually returns to normal after 2 weeks. Vital capacity is decreased by 25 to 50% within 1 to 2 days after surgery and generally returns to normal after 1 to 2 weeks. Pulmonary compliance decreases by 33% with similar reductions in functional residual capacity. Total lung capacity decreases after abdominal surgery but not after extremity surgery. (See page 815: Effects of Anesthesia and Surgery on Lung Volume.)

28. **E.** A 15% improvement in PFT results may be considered a positive response to bronchodilator therapy and an indication that this should be initiated preoperatively. The postoperative stress on the right ventricle and remaining pulmonary vascular bed can be simulated by occluding the pulmonary artery of the lung to be resected using a balloon-tip pulmonary artery catheter. If the mean pulmonary artery pressure increases to >40 mm Hg, it is unlikely that the patient will be able to tolerate pneumonectomy without developing respiratory failure or cor pulmonale postoperatively. If the PaO_2 level is >46 mm Hg in a patient considered for lung resection, split lung function testing should be done to estimate the exact contribution of the resected portion of the lung to ventilation and/or perfusion. (See page 816: Spirometry.)

29. **A.** A vital capacity of at least three times the tidal volume is necessary for an effective cough. An FEV_1 of <800 mL in a 70-kg patient probably is incompatible with life and is an absolute contraindication to lung resection. A vital capacity of <50% of predicted, or <2 L, is an indicator of increased risk. A ratio of residual volume to total lung capacity of >50% is indicative of a high-risk patient for pulmonary resection. (See page 816: Spirometry.)

30. **B.** Most of the beneficial effects of smoking cessation, such as improvement in ciliary function, improvement in closing volume, increased maximum midexpiratory flow rate, and reduction in sputum, usually occur 2 to 3 months following the smoking cessation. Smoking increases airway irritability, decreases mucociliary transport, and increases secretions. Smoking also decreases forced vital capacity. Smoking cessation 48 hours before surgery has been shown to decrease the level of carboxyhemoglobin and to shift the oxyhemoglobin dissociation curve to the right, thus increasing O_2 availability. (See page 817: Smoking.)

31. **C.** Normally, there is a small arterial-alveolar CO_2 gradient of approximately 4 to 6 mm Hg that is dependent on the alveolar dead space. The capnogram waveform is helpful in diagnosing airway obstruction, incomplete relaxation, and the position of the double-lumen tube. An esophageal or precordial stethoscope does not guarantee adequate oxygenation. During one-lung ventilation, systemic hypoxia usually is a greater problem than is hypercarbia. This is because CO_2 is 20 times more diffusible than O_2; arterial CO_2 concentration is more dependent on ventilation, whereas arterial O_2 concentration is more dependent on perfusion. (See page 820: Monitoring of Oxygenation and Ventilation.)

32. **C.** The Univent tube may be helpful for cases in which changing the double-lumen tube to a single-lumen tube may be difficult (e.g., following bilateral lung transplantation). It is a single-lumen endotracheal tube with a movable endobronchial blocker. The bronchial blocker technique can be useful in achieving selective ventilation in adults and in children younger than 12 years, and it should be placed via bronchoscopic guidance. These tubes are not used very commonly because they are easily displaced. Displacement of the bronchial blocker necessitates a pause in surgery while it is replaced under bronchoscopic guidance. (See page 824: Methods of Lung Separation.)

33. **E.** During one-lung ventilation, the dependent lung should be ventilated with a tidal volume of 10 to 12 mL/kg. The single most effective maneuver to increase arterial O_2 concentration during one-lung ventilation is the application of continuous positive airway pressure to the nondependent lung. It is important not to hyperventilate the patient's lungs because hypocapnia will increase vascular resistance in the dependent lung, inhibit nondependent lung hypoxic pulmonary vasoconstriction, increase the shunt, and therefore decrease PaO_2 concentration. A high inspired O_2 concentration may cause absorption atelectasis and may potentially increase the degree of shunt because of alveolar collapse. (See page 831: Inspired Oxygen Fraction.)

34. **C.** Normally, collapse of the nonventilated, nondependent lung results in the activation of reflex hypoxic pulmonary vasoconstriction. Some indirect inhibitors of hypoxic pulmonary vasoconstriction include volume overload, thromboembolism, and hypothermia. Hypoxic pulmonary vasoconstriction is

depressed in a dose-dependent manner by all potent inhaled anesthetics. It has been suggested that prostaglandins have a role in hypoxic pulmonary vasoconstriction inhibition. Prostaglandin inhibitors have been investigated as potentiators. Ibuprofen, a cyclo-oxygenase inhibitor, has been found to potentiate hypoxic pulmonary vasoconstriction. (See page 835: Hypoxic Pulmonary Vasoconstriction.)

35. **B.**   The rigid bronchoscope is the instrument of choice for removal of foreign bodies, control of massive hemoptysis, assessment of vascular tumors, bronchoscopy in small children, and resection of endobronchial lesions. Flexible bronchoscopy is useful in evaluating upper lobe lesions and in securing an airway in difficult intubations. (See page 837: Anesthesia for Diagnostic Procedures.)

36. **B.**   The distinction between a myasthenic crisis and a cholinergic crisis may be made using a Tensilon test or by examining pupillary size (which will be large in a myasthenic crisis, but small during a cholinergic crisis). Thymectomy now is considered the treatment of choice in most patients with myasthenia gravis. Patients with myasthenia gravis are sensitive to the nondepolarizing relaxants and are resistant to succinylcholine. The basic abnormality in myasthenia gravis is a decrease in the number of postsynaptic acetylcholine receptors at the end plates of the affected muscles. Myasthenia gravis is an autoimmune disorder, and most affected patients have circulating antibodies to the acetylcholine receptors. (See page 847: Myasthenia Gravis.)

37. **C.**   A cryoprobe is generally placed directly on the nerve to disrupt the axon. Hypoesthesia in the scar is a common late finding. In this way, conduction to the nerve is interrupted until the nerve regenerates over the next 1 to 6 months. Cryoanalgesia is not used routinely for thoracotomy. (See page 850: Postoperative Pain Control.)

38. **E.**   During VATS, CO_2 may be insufflated into the pleural cavity to help visualization by the surgeon. Continuous positive air pressure can interfere with the surgical procedure and is used only as a last resort in VATS. The need for one-lung ventilation is greater with VATS than with open thoracotomy because it is not possible to retract the lung during VATS, although it is possible during open thoracotomy. It may take 30 minutes for complete lung collapse; thus, the operated lung should be deflated as soon as possible following tracheal intubation and positioning of the double-lumen tube. (See page 842: Video-Assisted Thoracoscopic Surgery.)

CHAPTER 30 ■ CARDIOVASCULAR ANATOMY AND PHYSIOLOGY

1. All of the following statements regarding cardiac valvular anatomy are true EXCEPT:

   A. Tricuspid valvular area is normally 8 to 11 cm^2.
   B. Pulmonary valvular area is roughly 4 cm^2.
   C. Mitral valvular area is normally 6 to 8 cm^2.
   D. Aortic valvular area is normally 3 to 4 cm^2.
   E. Severe mitral stenosis typically occurs at a valvular area of 4 cm^2.

2. Which statement regarding coronary circulation is FALSE?

   A. The left coronary artery gives rise to the left anterior descending artery and the circumflex artery.
   B. Occlusive disease to the left anterior descending artery cause ischemic electrocardiogram (ECG) changes in leads V$_3$, V$_4$, and V$_5$.
   C. The majority of blood supply to the atrioventricular node (AVN) and common bundle of His is by the septal perforating branches of the left anterior descending artery.
   D. Occlusive disease to the right coronary artery results in ischemic ECG changes in leads II, III, and aV$_F$.
   E. The sinus node is supplied by the right coronary artery.

3. Coronary sinus drainage includes all of the following EXCEPT:

   A. great cardiac vein
   B. middle cardiac vein
   C. thebesian veins
   D. posterior left ventricular vein
   E. oblique vein of Marshall

4. The sinoatrial (SA) node is located:

   A. in the floor of the right atrium, near the junction of the inferior vena cava
   B. in the septum of the right atrium, near the fossa ovalis
   C. in the wall of the right atrium, near the junction of the superior vena cava
   D. in the floor of the right atrium, near the ostium of the coronary sinus
   E. in the superior edge of the membranous interventricular septum

5. Regarding cardiac neural regulation, which of the following is FALSE?

   A. Sympathetic innervation arises from the stellate ganglion and caudal cervical sympathetic trunks via the right dorsal medial and dorsal lateral cardiac nerves.
   B. The right and left coronary cardiac nerves and the left lateral cardiac nerve are the major cardiac parasympathetic supply.
   C. Afferent nerves from the heart ascend via the vagus nerve and the spinal cord to the brain.
   D. The left atrium has more parasympathetic fibers than the SA node.
   E. Alpha$_1$-, alpha$_2$-, beta$_1$-, and beta$_2$-adrenergic receptors are located throughout the heart; with the percentage of beta$_1$ being roughly three to five times more prevalent than beta$_2$.

6. The x descent:

   A. is produced by atrial systole, coinciding with the P wave on ECG
   B. results from the increasing intra-atrial pressure during atrial diastole
   C. results from isovolumetric ventricular contraction, the period between closure of the atrioventricular valves and opening of the aortic and pulmonary valves
   D. results from the opening of the atrioventricular valves, along with ventricular relaxation
   E. results from forward blood flow and decreasing atrial pressure at the initiation of ventricular ejection

7. Which of the following is FALSE?

   A. Pacemaker cells in the unexcited state are maintained at a resting potential of −80 mV by the inward rectifier current.
   B. During fast sodium influx, the transmembrane potential reverses from −80 mV to +20 to +30 mV, corresponding to phase 1 of the cardiac pacemaker cell action potential.
   C. Phase 4 depolarization in the SA node is responsible for cardiac automaticity.
   D. The absolute refractory period of cardiac cell depolarization ends at a point coinciding with the beginning of the T wave on ECG.
   E. Automaticity decreases in order from SA node, to AVN, His bundle, proximal Purkinje fibers, and distal Purkinje fibers.

8. Cardiac output is the product of heart rate and stroke volume. Several factors that affect cardiac output are preload, afterload, heart rate, contractility, and ventricular compliance. All of the following statements are true EXCEPT:

   A. Cardiac index (cardiac output divided by body surface area) is normally 2.5 to 3.5 L/m^2 per minute.
   B. Preload is determined by blood volume, venous tone, ventricular compliance, ventricular afterload, and myocardial contractility.
   C. Left ventricular afterload depends on left ventricular geometry (shape, size, radius), aortic impedance, aortic wall stiffness, aortic blood mass, and blood viscosity.
   D. Cardiac output is increased at heart rates of greater than 160 beats/minute by increasing the extent and velocity of shortening of myocardial fibers and increased dP/dT.
   E. Increased contractility increases the ejection fraction if end-systolic volume decreases while end-diastolic volume remains the same.

9. Which of the pressure volume loops below describes mitral stenosis?

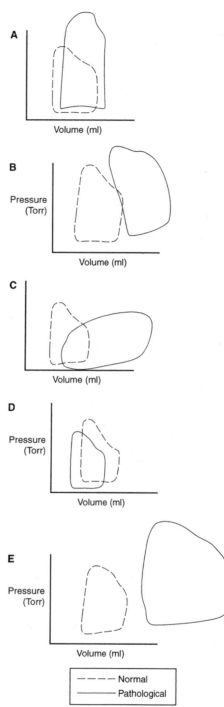

10. All of the following statements regarding peripheral circulation are true EXCEPT:

    A. The brachial artery can be punctured during attempted cannulation of the basilic vein.
    B. Circle of Willis is formed by junction of the posterior communicating arteries, the vertebral arteries, and the external carotid arteries.

C. The celiac artery is a direct branch of the abdominal aorta.

D. The greater saphenous vein overlies the medial malleolus.

E. The bronchial veins drain into the superior vena cava through the azygos system.

For questions 11 to 18, choose A if 1, 2, and 3 are correct; B if 1 and 3; C if 2 and 4; D if 4; and E if all are correct.

11. The Bezold-Jarisch reflex:

1. is transmitted via nonmyelinated C fibers resulting from stimulation of left ventricular mechanoreceptors

2. may be seen in response to reperfusion of previous ischemic myocardium

3. is in response to noxious stimuli to the ventricular wall

4. results in decreased parasympathetic tone leading to tachycardia, hypertension, and coronary artery vasoconstriction

12. Which of the following statements is/are TRUE?

1. Parasympathetic stimulation to the heart decreases heart rate via muscarinic receptors, decreasing adrenergic receptor activation through G-protein–mediated pathways.

2. Sympathetic stimulation occurs via $alpha_1$-, $beta_1$-, and $beta_2$-receptors through G-protein–mediated pathways.

3. Chronotropic and inotropic effects of $beta_1$ activation result from increased numbers of calcium channels available for activation.

4. Sympathetic stimulation to the heart is via the stellate ganglia, with the right stellate having more chronotropic effect and the left stellate having more inotropic effect.

13. Which of the following statements is/are TRUE?

1. Coronary arterial blood flow is determined by the duration of diastole, as well as the difference between aortic diastolic pressure and left ventricular end-diastolic pressure.

2. Right coronary artery flow occurs only during diastole.

3. The critical closure or critical flow pressure for coronary flow is 20 mm Hg.

4. During periods of high oxygen demand, the myocardium can increase oxygen extraction by 20 to 25%.

14. Concerning coronary autoregulation, which of the following statements is/are correct?

1. Myocardial oxygen tension, acting through mediators such as adenosine, is a primary determinant of autoregulation.

2. Autoregulation varies between different myocardial layers.

3. Arteriolar vasodilation, which occurs to maintain coronary flow in stenotic vessels, is exhausted when the stenosis is >90%.

4. "Coronary steal" occurs when pharmacologic vasodilation causes increased flow in normal arteries and away from stenotic arteries.

15. Which of the following statements is/are correct?

1. The preferred source of energy in myocardium is glucose.

2. At rest, per minute, myocardial oxygen consumption is 8 to 10 mL O_2/100 g of myocardium.

3. Wall tension is measured according to Fick law.

4. Normal myocardial oxygen extraction is 60 to 70% and changes little with myocardial work because of decreased coronary vascular resistance.

16. Which of the following statements regarding peripheral circulatory physiology is/are TRUE?

1. In a normal arterial system, mean pressure remains constant, whereas pulse pressure and systolic pressure increase as blood moves peripherally.

2. Pulsus paradoxus is the arterial pressure fluctuation with inspiration.

3. Central control of blood pressure occurs in the nucleus solitarius, the caudal ventrolateral medulla, and the rostral ventrolateral medulla.

4. Sympathetic nervous system control of blood pressure is primarily through norepinephrine acting at $beta_2$-receptors.

17. Which of the following statements regarding specific peripheral circulations is/are TRUE?

1. Renal blood flow is autoregulated to maintain glomerular filtration.

2. Hypoxic pulmonary vasoconstriction is decreased by respiratory alkalosis.

3. The major site of resistance to portal flow is postsinusoidal.

4. Normal compensatory increases in venous tone resulting from decreased blood volume, posture change, or positive airway pressure are intact during anesthesia.

18. When comparing myocardial supply with its demand, the following statement(s) is/are CORRECT:

1. The oxygen supply is dependent upon the diameter of the coronary arteries, left ventricular end-diastolic pressure, aortic diastolic pressure, and arterial oxygen content.

2. Coronary blood flow is influenced by intramyocardial pressure, heart rate, and blood viscosity.

3. The coronary perfusion pressure is the difference between the aortic diastolic pressure and left ventricular end-diastolic pressure.

4. Acidosis, hyperthermia, and increased 2,3-diphosphoglycerate (2,3-DPG) affect the myocardial oxygen supply.

ANSWERS

1. **E.** The tricuspid valve is a trileaflet valve (anterior, posterior, and medial) 8 to 11 cm^2 in area. The pulmonary valve is a trileaflet valve (right, left, and anterior) of about 4 cm^2 in area. The mitral valve is a bileaflet valve (anteromedial and posterolateral) of 6 to 8 cm^2. Severe mitral stenosis occurs at areas of <1 cm^2. The aortic valve is a trileaflet valve with right and left (or coronary) leaflets and a posterior (noncoronary) leaflet. (See page 857: Anatomy.)

2. **C.** In most patients, the right coronary artery supplies the sinus node, the AVN, and common bundle of His. The left anterior descending artery supplies the AVN and common bundle of His in approximately 10% of hearts. The left anterior descending artery supplies the anterior left ventricle, which is reflected in ECG leads V$_3$ to V$_5$. The circumflex artery supplies the posterior left ventricle, which is reflected in ECG leads I and aV$_L$. The right coronary artery supplies the inferior and diaphragmatic portions of the heart, as reflected in ECG leads II, III, and aV$_F$. (See page 858: Coronary Circulation.)

3. **C.** The thebesian veins traverse the myocardium and drain into various cardiac chambers. The thebesian venous drainage, along with the bronchial and pleural venous drainage, contributes to the normal 1 to 3% arteriovenous shunt. The great, middle, posterior left ventricular veins, and the oblique vein of Marshall (vein of the left atrium) all drain into the coronary sinus. (See page 859: Peripheral Venous Circulation.)

4. **C.** The SA node arises in the right atrium near the junction of the superior vena cava and communicates with the AVN via the internodal conduction system. The AVN is located in the floor of the right atrium near the coronary sinus ostium and sends fibers to the superior edge of the membranous interventricular septum, the origination of the bundle of His. The conduction system bifurcates into right and left bundle branches and terminates in the Purkinje fiber network. (See page 859: Cardiac Conduction System.)

5. **D.** The highest concentrations of parasympathetic nerves are in the SA node, followed by the AVN, the right atrium, and the left atrium and ventricles. In the heart, the proportion of beta$_1$- to beta$_2$-receptors in the right atrium is 74 to 26%, respectively. The ventricles show a beta$_1$ to beta$_2$ difference of 86 to 14%, respectively. (See page 859: Cardiac Receptors.)

6. **E.** The a wave is produced by atrial systole, coinciding with the P wave on ECG. The v wave results from the increasing intra-atrial pressure during atrial diastole. The c wave results from isovolumetric ventricular contraction, the period between closure of the atrioventricular valves and opening of the aortic and pulmonary valves. The y descent results from the opening of the atrioventricular valves, along with

ventricular relaxation. The x descent results from forward blood flow and decreasing atrial pressure at the initiation of ventricular ejection. (See page 861: Cardiac Cycle.)

7. **B.** Rapid sodium influx is responsible for phase 0 of cardiac cell depolarization. Phase 1 is caused by partial repolarization as a result of potassium efflux. Slow calcium influx and sodium efflux lead to phase 2 (or plateau). Phase 3 (or repolarization) is the result of continued potassium efflux and closure of calcium and sodium channels. Phase 4 is initiated following achievement of resting membrane potential and reflects slow depolarization resulting from slow potassium efflux; this is responsible for the automaticity of cardiac cells. (See page 864: Cardiac Electrophysiology.)

8. **D.** Although cardiac output does increase with increased heart rate, this increase becomes limited at heart rates of >160 beats/minute. The rapid filling phase of diastole occurs in the first half-second of diastole. If diastole is shortened by increased heart rate, then ventricular filling will be reduced; this will ultimately decrease cardiac output. Ejection fraction is determined by the equation EF = EDV − ESV/EDV (where EF is ejection fraction, EDV is end-diastolic volume, and ESV is end-systolic volume). With increased contractility, end-systolic volume will decrease. If end-diastolic volume is unchanged, this will result in increased ejection fraction. (See page 869: Cardiac Output.)

9. **D.** Pressure volume loops provide an indication of ventricular compliance and contractility. Figure D shows the effects of mitral stenosis, namely, decreased volume ejected, resulting from decreased filling during diastole. Figure A shows aortic stenosis. Figure B shows acute aortic regurgitation. Figure C shows mitral regurgitation. Figure E shows chronic aortic regurgitation. (See page 872: Pressure Volume Loops.)

10. **B.** The cerebral circulation consists of the anterior communicating arteries, the internal carotid arteries, the posterior communicating arteries, and the vertebral arteries. Together these vessels form the circle of Willis. The external carotid arteries supply the face and neck but not the brain. In the upper extremity, the brachial artery is beneath the basilic vein; it may be punctured during attempted basilic vein cannulation in the antecubital fossa. The abdominal branches of the aorta include the superior mesenteric, inferior mesenteric, and celiac arteries, principally supplying the gastrointestinal tract. The greater saphenous vein, overlying the medial malleolus, is frequently used as a conduit during aortocoronary bypass grafting. Bronchial veins from the extrapulmonary portions of the proximal

tracheobronchial tree drain via the azygos and hemiazygos veins into the superior vena cava. (See page 859: Peripheral Venous Circulation.)

11. **A.** The Bezold-Jarisch reflex is initiated by left ventricular mechanoreceptors secondary to noxious ventricular stimuli. It results in increased parasympathetic activity causing bradycardia, hypotension, and coronary artery vasodilation. Examples of stimuli include ischemia and reperfusion following ischemia (i.e., nitrate or heparin therapy, thrombolytic therapy, or coronary artery bypass graft). (See page 861: Coronary Arteriography and page 878: Table 30-9: Cardiovascular Reflexes.)

12. **E.** Parasympathetic stimulation to the heart decreases heart rate via muscarinic receptors, thus decreasing adrenergic receptor activation through G-protein–mediated pathways. Sympathetic stimulation occurs via alpha$_1$-, beta$_1$-, and beta$_2$-receptors through G-protein–mediated pathways. Chronotropic and inotropic effects of beta$_1$-activation results from increased numbers of calcium channels available for activation. Sympathetic stimulation to the heart is via the stellate ganglia, with the right stellate having more chronotropic effect and the left stellate having more inotropic effect. (See page 867: Physiology of the Cardiac Nerves.)

13. **B.** Coronary flow occurs during diastole for the left ventricle and during both diastole and systole in the right ventricle. The major determinants of coronary flow are aortic diastolic pressure and left ventricular end-diastolic pressure. When intraventricular pressures exceed 20 mm Hg, critical flow pressure is exceeded, and coronary flow ceases. Because of high oxygen consumption in myocardium, extraction is high, resulting in the lowest venous P$_{O_2}$ concentration anywhere in the body (coronary sinus P$_{O_2}$ equals 18–20% or 18–30% saturated). Thus, increased O$_2$ demand can be supplied only by increased flow and not by increasing extraction. (See page 877: Coronary Circulatory Physiology.)

14. **E.** Myocardial oxygen tension, acting through mediators such as adenosine, is a primary determinant of autoregulation. Autoregulation varies among the different myocardial layers. Arteriolar vasodilation, which occurs to maintain coronary flow in stenotic vessels, is exhausted when the stenosis is >90%. "Coronary steal" occurs when pharmacologic vasodilation causes increased flow in normal arteries and away from stenotic arteries. (See page 868: Coronary Autoregulation.)

15. **C.** The preferred sources of energy in the myocardium are lactate and fatty acids. Glucose is used as a primary energy source only during hypoxia or with high glucose or insulin levels. Wall tension is measured using Laplace law: $T = Pr/2h$ (where T is wall tension, P is interventricular pressure, r is cardiac radius, and h is ventricular muscle thickness). At rest, myocardial oxygen consumption is 8–10 mL/100 gm of myocardium/minute. Normal myocardial oxygen extraction is 60–70% (See page 876: Myocardial Metabolism.)

16. **A.** The arterial pressure waveform is dependent on pressure wave velocity, pulse duration, and length of tube. In small, nondistensible peripheral arteries, the pulse waves travel very fast and are reflected centrally equally fast. This produces a larger systolic waveform and increases the pulse pressure, although mean pressure is unchanged. Factors affecting blood pressure are central and autonomic factors, as well as hormonal mechanisms (antidiuretic hormone, renin-angiotensin system, and atrial natriuretic peptide). Sympathetic control is via norepinephrine, acting at alpha$_1$-receptors causing vasoconstriction, and epinephrine acting at alpha$_2$-receptors causing vasodilation. Pulsus paradoxus is the increased pressure drop that occurs with inspiration. Normally, a decrease of 6 mm Hg occurs in arterial pressure with inspiration. However, with pericardial tamponade, this pressure drop is even greater. Three medullary centers, the nucleus tractus solitarius, the caudal ventrolateral medulla, and the rostral ventrolateral medulla, are important in blood pressure control. (See page 877: Arterial Pulses and Blood Pressure.)

17. **A.** Renal blood flow is high to meet the metabolic demands of sodium reabsorption by the kidney and is autoregulated. Hypoxic pulmonary vasoconstriction is enhanced by metabolic acidosis, with no change resulting from respiratory acidosis. Both metabolic alkalosis and respiratory alkalosis decrease hypoxic pulmonary vasoconstriction. The major site of resistance to portal flow is postsinusoidal. Normal compensatory venous responses are abolished with autonomic neuropathy or during anesthesia. Thus, alterations to venous return caused by positive-pressure ventilation, change in posture, or decreased blood volume go uncompensated. (See page 881: Specific Peripheral Circulations.)

18. **E.** A balance must always exist between oxygen consumption (demand) and myocardial oxygen supply if ischemia is to be avoided. Myocardial oxygen supply is dependent upon the diameter of the coronary arteries, left ventricular end-diastolic pressure, aortic diastolic pressure, and arterial oxygen content. In the normal heart, the coronary perfusion pressure is the difference between the aortic diastolic pressure and the left ventricular end-diastolic pressure. Myocardial blood flow is determined by the blood pressure at the coronary ostia, arteriolar tone, intramyocardial pressure or extravascular resistance, coronary occlusive disease, heart rate, coronary collateral development, and blood viscosity. Myocardial oxygen supply is also affected by the level of arterial oxygenation. Oxygen content resulting from changes in Pa$_{O_2}$, hemoglobin, DPG, pH, Pc$_{O_2}$, or temperature can affect the oxyhemoglobin dissociation curve and can be important in patients with obstructive lung disease or severe anemia. (See page 876: Myocardial Supply-Demand Ratio.)

CHAPTER 31 ■ ANESTHESIA FOR CARDIAC SURGERY

1. The area of the myocardium most at risk for ischemia is the:

   A. right ventricle
   B. apex of the left ventricle
   C. interventricular septum
   D. portion of the right atrium containing the sinoatrial node
   E. subendocardial region of the left ventricle

2. The principal determinants of myocardial oxygen demand are:

   A. wall tension and contractility
   B. systemic vascular resistance and heart rate
   C. mean arterial blood pressure and heart rate
   D. preload and afterload
   E. mean arterial blood pressure and systemic vascular resistance

3. Under normal conditions, approximately what is the oxygen saturation of blood entering the coronary sinus?

   A. 10%
   B. 25%
   C. 50%
   D. 75%
   E. 90%

4. Regarding perfusion of the left ventricular subendocardium, which one of the following statements is most accurate?

   A. It occurs mostly during systole.
   B. It occurs mostly during diastole.
   C. It increases with an increase in left ventricular end-diastolic pressure.
   D. It is unaffected by heart rate.
   E. It decreases with an increase in aortic diastolic pressure.

5. The normal area of the aortic valve is:

   A. 0.2 to 0.4 mm^2
   B. 2 to 4 mm^2
   C. 0.2 to 0.4 cm^2
   D. 4 to 8 cm
   E. 2 to 4 cm^2

6. Which of the following conditions best describes a physiologic change associated with mitral stenosis?

   A. Left ventricular outflow obstruction
   B. Left ventricular dysfunction resulting from chronic pressure overload
   C. Left ventricular dysfunction resulting from chronic volume overload
   D. Decreased right ventricular pressure
   E. Increased left atrial pressure and concomitant right ventricular hypertrophy

7. An advantage of membrane over bubble oxygenators in cardiopulmonary bypass circuits is:

   A. The uptake of inhaled anesthetics is more predictable with membrane oxygenators.
   B. There is less trauma to blood constituents.
   C. Pulsatile flow is possible with the use of a membrane oxygenator.
   D. Membrane oxygenators offer a cost advantage over bubble oxygenators.
   E. Carbon dioxide exchange is significantly more effective.

8. The most common test employed to evaluate the adequacy of anticoagulation for cardiopulmonary bypass is:

   A. heparin concentration assay
   B. antithrombin III index
   C. activated partial thromboplastin time
   D. activated clotting time
   E. prothrombin time

9. Advantages of centrifugal versus roller pumps cardiopulmonary bypass machines include all of the following EXCEPT:

   A. less blood trauma
   B. less risk of air emboli
   C. elimination of tubing wear and the risk of plastic microemboli
   D. ability to deliver pulsatile blood flow
   E. reduction in line pressures

10. For each degree centigrade decrease in body temperature, metabolic rate is decreased by approximately:

    A. 1%
    B. 2%
    C. 4%
    D. 8%
    E. 10%

11. Nitric oxide dilates pulmonary vascular beds via:

    A. production of cyclic adenosine monophosphate (cAMP)
    B. inhibition of cAMP
    C. production of cyclic guanosine monophosphate (cGMP)
    D. inhibition of cGMP
    E. none of the above

12. A patient with previously normal left ventricular function is undergoing elective coronary artery bypass grafting. Immediately following separation from cardiopulmonary bypass, the following measurements are noted: a blood pressure via radial intra-arterial catheter of 78/52 mm Hg, a heart rate of 94 beats/minute, a pulmonary artery pressure of 28/18 mm Hg, and a cardiac index of 2.7. The most prudent initial intervention would be:

    A. direct measurement of intra-aortic pressures to verify radial artery correlation
    B. the addition of a phenylephrine infusion to provide alpha-receptor–mediated vasoconstriction
    C. the addition of an epinephrine infusion to provide both inotropic support and alpha-receptor–mediated vasoconstriction
    D. an intra-aortic volume infusion using pulmonary capillary wedge pressures as a guide to the adequacy of left ventricular filling
    E. a trial of atrial pacing after placement of epicardial leads

13. The most frequent cause(s) of perioperative neurologic complications following coronary artery bypass grafting is/are:

    A. changes in carotid artery flow dynamics during aortic cross-clamping
    B. low-flow states in patients with pre-existing cerebral vascular disease
    C. emboli
    D. intraoperative hemodilution

    E. ischemia to watershed regions of the brain during the rewarming phase of cardiopulmonary bypass

14. Of the following anesthetic techniques for cardiac surgery, the one associated with the best outcome in terms of perioperative morbidity is:

    A. a predominantly opioid-based anesthetic in conjunction with benzodiazepines
    B. a "balanced" anesthetic technique using opioid analgesics combined with potent inhalation agents titrated for varying degrees of stimulation
    C. continuous high-dose sufentanil infusion
    D. a predominantly potent inhalation agent–based technique with epidural catheter placement for postoperative analgesia
    E. none of the above

15. In the immediate postcardiopulmonary bypass period, milrinone may be particularly useful in the treatment of right ventricular failure secondary to high pulmonary vascular resistance because:

    A. The positive chronotropic effect of milrinone results in improved cardiac output from the noncompliant right ventricle.
    B. Milrinone improves right ventricular contractility while decreasing pulmonary vascular resistance.
    C. Milrinone decreases preload to the right ventricle by decreasing resistance in venous capacitance vessels.
    D. The improvement in left ventricular performance afforded by milrinone in turn decreases right ventricular afterload.
    E. All of the above

16. The most common cause of persistent bleeding following heparin reversal in the cardiac surgical patient is:

    A. heparin rebound
    B. hypothermia
    C. reduced platelet count and/or function
    D. diminished capillary integrity
    E. inactivation of antithrombin III

For questions 17 to 31, choose A if 1, 2, and 3 are correct; B if 1 and 3; C if 2 and 4; D if 4; and E if all.

17. Nitroglycerin is a useful agent in the treatment of myocardial ischemia in that it:

    1. is a coronary arterial dilator
    2. reduces venous return
    3. may reverse acute coronary vasospasm
    4. reduces heart rate via baroreceptor mechanisms

18. A 48-year-old man with a history of severe hypertrophic cardiomyopathy is undergoing general anesthesia for elective total knee arthroplasty. A precipitous fall in cardiac output is noted just before the skin incision. His vital signs include a blood pressure of 172/88 mm Hg and a heart rate of

104 beats/minute. Which of the following interventions is/are most likely to improve cardiac output?

1. Administration of an inotropic agent
2. Administration of a volatile anesthetic agent
3. Titration of a vasodilator to decrease afterload
4. Administration of esmolol to decrease heart rate

19. Which of the following conditions may be associated with segmental wall motion abnormalities on transesophageal echocardiogram?

1. Myocardial ischemia
2. Hypovolemia
3. Myocardial infarction
4. Left bundle branch block

20. Which of the following statements regarding stroke following coronary artery bypass graft surgery with is/are TRUE?

1. Stroke occurs in approximately 5 to 10% of patients.
2. Diabetes is an independent risk factor.
3. Excessive warming during and following cardiopulmonary bypass may increase the likelihood of its occurrence.
4. Stroke is most commonly the result of perioperative hypoperfusion injury.

21. Physiologic effects of nitroglycerin include:

1. systemic venodilation
2. decreased afterload
3. coronary artery dilation
4. cyanide production

22. Pharmacologic agents with coronary artery dilator properties include:

1. nifedipine
2. nitroglycerin
3. diltiazem
4. magnesium

23. Which of the following statements regarding cardiac valvular structure and pathology is/are TRUE?

1. The normal aortic valve is composed of three leaflets.
2. The normal mitral value consists of three leaflets.
3. Mitral valve stenosis is most commonly of rheumatic origin.
4. Chordae tendineae connected to the papillary muscles help prevent prolapse of the aortic valve leaflets into the left ventricle during systole.

24. Mechanisms by which heparin exerts its anticoagulant effect include:

1. activation of factor XIIa
2. direct inhibition of factor II
3. inhibition of kallikrein
4. potentiation of antithrombin III

25. Which of the following statements about cardiac tamponade is/are TRUE?

1. Clinical signs and symptoms include paradoxical pulse, tachycardia, and hypotension.
2. Stroke volume increases.
3. Cardiac output becomes rate dependent.
4. Compression of the left ventricular is usually most severe.

26. Which of the following statements regarding the normal function of an intra-aortic balloon pump is/are TRUE?

1. It is designed to reduce afterload.
2. It is designed to increase diastolic blood pressure.
3. When properly inserted, the distal tip lies just below the subclavian.
4. The balloon is designed to deflate during diastole.

27. Techniques commonly employed for perioperative blood conservation during cardiac surgery include:

1. red blood cell scavenging
2. perioperative administration of antifibrinolytic agents
3. intraoperative autologous hemodilution
4. nonpulsatile flow during cardiopulmonary bypass

28. TRUE statements regarding intraoperative electrocardiographic monitoring include:

1. Lead II can be monitored to detect ischemia in the inferior wall of the left ventricle, as well as to assist in the detection of cardiac arrhythmias.
2. Lead V_5 will aid in the detection of ischemia to the anterior wall of the left ventricle.
3. Lead V_5 is monitored to detect ischemia in regions of the myocardium supplied by the left anterior descending coronary artery.
4. Ischemia of the lateral wall of the left ventricle is detected by monitoring leads I and aVL.

29. Relatively strong indications for the perioperative placement of a pulmonary artery catheter in the patient undergoing cardiac surgery include:

1. procedures in which continuous retrograde cardioplegia is to be employed during cardiopulmonary bypass
2. a patient with moderate to severe pulmonary hypertension
3. access to central circulation for the infusion of vasoactive drugs
4. assistance in the management of the patient with impaired left ventricular function

30. Examples of congenital cardiac lesions in which cyanosis develops as a result of obstruction to pulmonary flow include:

1. patent ductus arteriosus
2. ventricular septal defect

3. coarctation of the aorta
4. tetralogy of Fallot

31. Which of the following statements regarding amrinone and milrinone is/are TRUE?

1. They are phosphodiesterase inhibitors.
2. They increase myocardial contractility.
3. They decrease pulmonary vascular resistance.
4. They increase systemic vascular resistance.

ANSWERS

---

1. **E.**   Although zones of ischemic myocardium result from inadequate coronary blood flow through the vessels supplying those regions, the area of myocardium most vulnerable to ischemia is the subendocardial region of the left ventricle. This is not only because of a greater metabolic requirement in the presence of greater systolic shortening but also because subendocardial blood flow is restricted during systole. (See page 887: Coronary Blood Flow.)

2. **A.**   Wall tension and contractility are the principal determinants of myocardial oxygen demand. Wall tension is, in turn, directly proportional to intracavitary pressure and ventricular radius and is inversely proportional to the thickness of the ventricular wall. Therefore, myocardial oxygen demand can be reduced by interventions that prevent or treat ventricular distention and reduce contractility. (See page 887: Coronary Artery Disease: Myocardial Oxygen Demand.)

3. **C.**   Oxygen extraction in the coronary circulation is extremely efficient; blood entering the coronary sinus is typically about 50% saturated. Although extraction can be increased somewhat in response to stress, the principal mechanism by which oxygen supply is increased in response to increased oxygen demand is via an increase in coronary blood flow. (See page 887: Coronary Artery Disease: Myocardial Oxygen Supply.)

4. **B.**   The left ventricular subendocardium is one of the areas of the heart most vulnerable to ischemia because of its high metabolic requirements. Perfusion of the subendocardial tissue of the left ventricle takes place mostly during diastole; this is in contrast to perfusion of the right ventricle, which occurs principally during systole. Perfusion pressure is defined as the difference between aortic diastolic pressure and left ventricular end-diastolic pressure. An increase in aortic diastolic pressure will therefore increase perfusion, whereas an increase in left ventricular end-diastolic pressure will decrease perfusion. In so far as changes in heart rate affect diastolic time, changes in heart rate do cause changes in perfusion. (See page 887: Coronary Artery Disease: Coronary Blood Flow.)

5. **E.**   The normal aortic valve diameter is 1.9 to 2.3 cm, and the normal aortic valve area is 2 to 4 cm². Aortic stenosis is classified based on the degree of narrowing of the aortic valve area. Aortic stenosis is considered critical when the area of the aortic valve is <0.8 cm². Patients with this degree of aortic stenosis are almost always symptomatic, and surgical correction is indicated. (See page 898: Valvular Heart Disease: Aortic Stenosis.)

6. **E.**   In mitral stenosis, left atrial pressure elevation is a consequence of a narrowed mitral orifice. This increased pressure is transmitted back through the pulmonary circulation, leading to right ventricular hypertrophy. Conversely, the left ventricle is not subject to pressure or volume overload, and normal function generally is preserved. (See page 903: Mitral Stenosis.)

7. **B.**   Studies comparing the two types of oxygenators reveal less trauma to blood constituents with membrane oxygenators. Hemolysis and the resultant release of red cell debris are potential problems associated with bubble oxygenators. Likewise, a decrease in platelet activity, resulting from platelet destruction, increased aggregation, and adherence to the oxygenator, may lead to impairment of postoperative hemostasis. (See page 910: Oxygenators.)

8. **D.**   The activated clotting time indicates the time required for thrombus formation after a sample of whole blood is mixed with a clotting accelerator. A value of >400 seconds generally is believed to reflect a degree of anticoagulation adequate for cardiopulmonary bypass. (See page 911: Anticoagulation.)

9. **D.**   Centrifugal cardiopulmonary bypass machines operate by a magnetically controlled impeller and an electric motor and are rapidly replacing the older roller pump systems. Advantages of the centrifugal system include less trauma to blood entering the system, lower line pressures, reduced risk of air emboli, and elimination of tubing wear and plastic emboli resulting from tubing compression (spallation). Neither roller pumps nor centrifugal pumps can deliver physiologically significant pulsatile blood flow. (See page 908: Cardiopulmonary Bypass: Pumps.)

10. **D.** For each degree centigrade reduction in body temperature, there is a reduction of 8% in the metabolic rate. (See page 908: Cardiopulmonary Bypass: Heat Exchanger.)

11. **C.** Nitric oxide exerts most of its effects by stimulating the guanylyl cyclase enzyme, leading to increased production of cGMP. In turn, cGMP stimulates phosphodiesterases, which relax vascular smooth muscle promoting vasodilation. (See page 908: Cardiopulmonary Bypass.)

12. **A.** Although frequently accurate, radial artery pressure may be as much as 30 mm Hg lower than central aortic pressure following cardiopulmonary bypass. Peripheral vasodilation during rewarming is thought to be the cause of the discrepancy, which may be readily detected by direct transduction of intra-aortic pressure via the operative field. This aortic-radial pressure gradient usually dissipates within 45 minutes of separation from bypass. (See page 915: Arterial Blood Pressure.)

13. **C.** Although the incidence of stroke after coronary artery bypass grafting is approximately 3%, the incidence of subtle cognitive deficits elicited by postoperative neuropsychiatric testing is much higher (60–70%). The origin of perioperative neurologic insults is believed to be primarily embolic. Macroemboli, such as atheroma and particulate matter, account for most overt perioperative strokes. Microemboli (air, platelet aggregates) are likely responsible for the subtle cognitive changes seen after coronary artery bypass grafting. Most neuropsychiatric deficits improve over the initial 2 to 6 months following cardiac surgery, although significant numbers of patients (13–39%) exhibit residual impairment. (See page 916: Central Nervous System Function and Complications.)

14. **E.** Two large outcome studies by Tuman et al. and by Slogoff and Keats reinforced the premise that the choice of anesthetic per se has no effect on outcome in patients undergoing cardiac surgery. More important is the ability of the anesthesiologist to preserve compensatory cardiovascular mechanisms while preventing perioperative episodes of myocardial ischemia. In that no data exist to document the superiority of any one anesthetic technique for cardiac surgery, it becomes apparent that the proper management of the anesthetic is more important than the technique employed. (See page 916: Selection of Anesthetic Drugs.)

15. **B.** A phosphodiesterase III inhibitor, milrinone, acts via a non–beta-receptor pathway to effect a decrease in pulmonary vascular resistance while improving left and right heart contractility. Such interventions are the treatments of choice in conditions of right ventricular failure secondary to high pulmonary vascular resistance, whereas overdistention of the ventricle is carefully avoided. (See page 920: Discontinuation of Cardiopulmonary Bypass.)

16. **C.** The usual causes of persistent oozing following heparin neutralization include inadequate surgical hemostasis and reduced platelet count and/or function, although insufficient doses of protamine, dilution of clotting factors, and, rarely, "heparin rebound" may be contributing factors. Thrombocytopenia and diminished platelet function are frequent consequences of extracorporeal circulation, resulting from platelet activation and destruction when in contact with the bypass circuit. (See page 924: Postbypass Bleeding.)

17. **A.** Nitroglycerin is a modest coronary arterial dilator and as such is the drug of choice for the acute treatment of coronary artery vasospasm. The reduction in venous return afforded by the venodilatory effect of nitroglycerin leads to a lessening in myocardial wall tension and thus to a reduction in myocardial oxygen demand. The use of nitroglycerin may result in reflex tachycardia caused by a sudden decrease in venous return. (See page 897: Nitrates.)

18. **C.** The anesthetic management of hypertrophic cardiomyopathy is directed at maintaining ventricular filling and minimizing the factors predisposing to variable outflow obstruction. In this case, the myocardial depression afforded by a volatile agent may be desirable, as would be a decrease in heart rate. Similarly, inotropic agents may compound the problem. Vasodilators do not improve the outflow obstruction and may result in precipitous drops in systemic arterial pressures. (See page 901: Hypertrophic Cardiomyopathy.)

19. **E.** Segmental wall motion abnormalities are most commonly associated with myocardial ischemia or infarction. However, other conditions can also cause segmental wall motion abnormalities. Among these conditions are pacing, bundle branch blocks, myocarditis, tachycardia, and hypovolemia. In addition, nonischemic myocardium in proximity to ischemic or infarcted tissue may appear to have abnormal wall motion ("tethering phenomenon"). (See page 889: Ischemia.)

20. **A.** The incidence of stroke after coronary artery bypass graft surgery is approximately 3%. Patients of advanced age (>70 years) and those with diabetes, peripheral vascular disease, pre-existing cerebrovascular disease, history of stroke, and/or atheromatous plaque in the ascending aorta are at increased risk of postoperative stroke. In addition, operative factors such as prolonged duration of bypass and excessive rewarming during and after bypass increase the risk of neurologic complications. (See page 913: Preoperative Evaluation: Central Nervous System Function and Complications.)

21. **A.** Nitroglycerin is a systemic venodilator. In addition, at higher doses, nitroglycerin also dilates systemic arterial beds. Therefore, it both reduces preload (by decreasing venous return) and reduces afterload (by decreasing systemic arterial pressure). Nitroglycerin is the drug of choice in the treatment of coronary vasospasm because it is also an effective dilator of the coronary arterial bed, including stenosed arteries and collateral beds. Despite its clinical utility, nitroglycerin may also cause methemoglobinemia, especially in patients with deficiencies of methemoglobin reductase. Sodium nitroprusside, not nitroglycerin, can produce cyanide and thiocyanate upon metabolism, thus posing the risk of toxicity during prolonged infusions or following administration of relatively large quantities over short time periods. (See page 887: Coronary Artery Disease: Treatment of Ischemia.)

22. **E.** Nifedipine and diltiazem are calcium channel blockers that dilate coronary arteries and are used as antianginal agents in the prevention of coronary vasospasm. Nitroglycerin also has coronary artery dilating properties, associated with the production of nitric oxide. Magnesium is another coronary artery vasodilator, which has been used to reduce infarct size and to minimize reperfusion injury in the setting of acute ischemia. (See page 887: Coronary Artery Disease: Treatment of Ischemia.)

23. **B.** The normal aortic valve consists of three leaflets, whereas the normal mitral valve is composed of two leaflets. Rheumatic fever is by far the most common cause of mitral stenosis. Chordae tendineae connected to the papillary muscles help prevent prolapse of the mitral valve leaflets. (See page 898: Valvular Heart Disease.)

24. **C.** Heparin is a polyionic mucopolysaccharide extracted from bovine lung or porcine intestinal mucosa. Binding of heparin to antithrombin III greatly increases its intrinsic thrombin inhibitory properties, thereby preventing the formation of fibrinous clots. In addition, heparin binds directly to factor II (thrombin), thus inhibiting its action. Aprotinin is an antifibrinolytic agent and protease inhibitor that delays activation of the intrinsic coagulation cascade via inhibition of factor XIIa. In addition, it inhibits kallikrein and other serine proteases such as plasmin. It is used during cardiopulmonary bypass to reduce blood loss, improve platelet function, and reduce the systemic inflammatory response to cardiopulmonary bypass. (See page 908: Cardiopulmonary Bypass: Anticoagulation.)

25. **B.** Cardiac tamponade involves an elevation in intrapericardial pressure, which impairs venous return and may cause cardiac chamber collapse. Under this circumstance, the chambers with the lowest intracardiac pressures (atria and right ventricle during diastole) are most at risk of collapse. Stroke volume in cardiac tamponade is relatively fixed; hence, cardiac output becomes dependent on heart rate. (See page 926: Postoperative Considerations.)

26. **A.** The intra-aortic balloon pump uses a synchronized counterpulsation method to improve myocardial function by decreasing myocardial oxygen demand and increasing myocardial oxygen supply. The device is most commonly inserted into the femoral artery and advanced so the distal tip lies just below the subclavian artery and the proximal end is above the renal arteries. The balloon inflates during diastole, thereby increasing aortic diastolic pressure and improving coronary perfusion as well as facilitating forward flow. During the subsequent systole, the balloon deflates, reducing systemic afterload and facilitating left ventricular ejection. (See page 913: Preoperative Evaluation: Intraaortic Balloon Pump.)

27. **A.** Antifibrinolytic agents such as tranexamic acid, epsilon-aminocaproic acid, and aprotinin have been shown to decrease blood loss in high-risk patients undergoing cardiac surgery. Such agents act to inhibit the fibrinolytic cascade triggered by the effects of extracorporeal circulation. Intraoperative hemodilution achieved by the removal of autologous blood provides a safe source of whole blood for reinfusion while being spared the damaging effects of the bypass circuit. (See page 912: Blood Conservation in Cardiac Surgery.)

28. **E.** Simultaneous monitoring of multiple electrocardiographic leads improves the sensitivity of ischemia detection while aiding in its localization. Leads II, III, and aVF are the most sensitive to ischemic changes in the inferior ventricular wall, typically supplied by the right coronary artery. Lead V_5 is commonly used to monitor the anterior wall of the left ventricle (left anterior descending artery), whereas leads I and aVL provide the greatest information concerning the lateral left ventricular wall (left circumflex artery). (See page 915: Monitoring.)

29. **C.** Although indications for the placement of a pulmonary catheter vary among institutions, those conditions in which left ventricular filling pressures cannot be reliably predicted by transduced right atrial pressures generally predicate pulmonary artery catheter placement. These conditions include pulmonary hypertension, left ventricular dysfunction or decreased compliance, and valvular dysfunction. Other indications include operations requiring prolonged operative time or combined procedures (valve replacement plus coronary grafting). (See page 915: Monitoring.)

30. **D.** In patients with tetralogy of Fallot, right ventricular outflow obstruction exists that may lead to cyanosis as a result of decreased pulmonary flow. The presence of a ventricular septal defect complicates the problem by providing a path of preferential flow in

the setting of decreased systemic vascular resistance. Ventricular septal defects and patent ductus arteriosus result in increased pulmonary blood flow from volume overload, whereas coarctation of the aorta results in left ventricular pressure overload. (See page 927: Table 31.26.)

31. **A.** Amrinone and milrinone are two drugs in a class of phosphodiesterase III inhibitors. These agents are very effective at decreasing pulmonary vascular resistance and increasing myocardial contractility. They are also systematic arterial vasodilators and therefore reduce left ventricular afterload, reducing myocardial work. (See page 913: Preoperative Evaluation: Discontinuation of Cardiopulmonary Bypass.)

CHAPTER 32 ■ ANESTHESIA FOR VASCULAR SURGERY

1. The most effective medical therapy for atherosclerotic peripheral vascular disease is:

   A. dipyridamole
   B. urokinase
   C. warfarin (Coumadin)
   D. aspirin
   E. smoking cessation

2. In patients presenting for vascular surgery, the incidence of significant coronary artery disease (stenosis >70%) detected by angiography in patients without any clinical symptoms of coronary stenosis is:

   A. <1%
   B. 11%
   C. 37%
   D. 78%
   E. >90%

3. For patients undergoing vascular surgery, when is myocardial ischemia most likely to occur?

   A. Preoperatively
   B. During the induction of anesthesia
   C. Intraoperatively, before revascularization
   D. In the immediate postoperative period
   E. From 48 to 72 hours postoperatively

4. Which of the following monitoring modalities is most sensitive in the detection of intraoperative myocardial ischemia?

   A. Simultaneous electrocardiographic ST segment analysis in leads II and V$_5$
   B. Hemodynamic data derived from a pulmonary artery catheter
   C. Transesophageal echocardiography
   D. Intraoperative cardiac isoenzyme determinations
   E. Continuous cardiac output monitoring

5. Most neurologic deficits following carotid endarterectomy are thought to result from:

   A. concomitant contralateral carotid stenosis
   B. prolonged carotid artery cross-clamp in the absence of shunt use
   C. thromboembolism
   D. perioperative vasospasm
   E. inadequate intraoperative carotid artery perfusion pressure

6. Each of the following are potential postoperative complications specific to carotid endarterectomy EXCEPT:

   A. hypertension
   B. bradycardia
   C. neurologic deficits
   D. respiratory insufficiency
   E. renal insufficiency

7. Distal ischemia as a consequence of aortic surgery generally results from:

   A. prolonged aortic occlusion
   B. inadequate distal runoff
   C. thrombosis resulting from inadequate anticoagulation
   D. postperfusion vasospasm
   E. atheroemboli

8. All of the following are advantages of prosthetic grafts over native vein grafts in peripheral vascular bypass procedures EXCEPT:

   A. Prosthetic grafts may be used in situations in which adequate native vein segments are unavailable.
   B. Prosthetic grafts have significantly higher patency rates than vein grafts.
   C. Bypasses using prosthetic grafts can be performed more quickly.
   D. Greater technical expertise is required for saphenous vein grafting.

E. Bypasses using prosthetic grafts necessitate less dissection and fewer incisions than native vein grafts.

9. The most important factor shown to be of clinical importance in preserving renal function during aortic cross-clamping is:

A. lisinopril
B. fenoldopam
C. dopamine
D. preoperative intravascular status
E. mannitol

For questions 10 to 20, choose A if 1, 2, and 3 are correct; B if 1 and 3; C if 2 and 4; D if 4; and E if all.

10. Strategies that have been shown to reduce the incidence of myocardial ischemia in patients undergoing vascular surgery include:

1. treatment of tachycardia with beta-adrenergic blocking agents
2. prevention of hypothermia
3. correction of anemia (hematocrit of <28)
4. prophylactic infusions of nitroglycerin

11. Which of the following statements regarding carotid artery occlusive disease is/are TRUE?

1. It is rarely bilateral.
2. Plaques most often develop at the lateral aspect of the carotid bifurcation.
3. Patients who present with transient ischemic attacks have a 40% risk of stroke during the subsequent year.
4. The most common cause is atherosclerosis.

12. Methods that have been employed to determine the need for shunt placement during carotid endarterectomy include:

1. intraoperative electroencephalogram evaluation
2. xenon-gated measurements of cerebral blood flow
3. transcranial Doppler techniques
4. somatosensory-evoked potential (SSEP) monitoring

13. Factors that may contribute to systemic hypotension or organ dysfunction following aortic occlusion and subsequent reperfusion include:

1. metabolic acidosis
2. reactive hyperemia
3. oxygen-derived free radicals
4. endotoxemia

14. Which of the following statements regarding the artery of Adamkiewicz is/are FALSE?

1. It is responsible for >85% of the spinal cord blood supply.
2. It originates between L1 and L2 in 10% of patients.

3. It is the sole source of arterial flow to the posterior portions of the spinal cord.
4. It originates between T8 and T12 in 75% of patients.

15. Which of the following measures have demonstrated definitive utility in the prevention of spinal cord ischemia associated with aortic occlusion during vascular procedures?

1. Early use of sodium bicarbonate
2. Maintenance of normal cardiac function
3. Cerebrospinal fluid drainage
4. Brief aortic cross-clamp times

16. In comparing surgical approaches for either occlusive or aneurysmal abdominal aortic disease, advantages of a retroperitoneal over a traditional transabdominal approach include:

1. fewer postoperative pulmonary complications
2. lower incidence of ileus and small bowel obstruction
3. shorter intensive care and overall hospital stays
4. decreased long-term incisional pain

17. Surgical techniques employed during occlusion of the thoracic aorta to decompress the heart and allow some degree of distal perfusion include:

1. placement of an aortic shunt
2. normovolemic hemodilution
3. placement of an ex vivo axillofemoral bypass graft
4. segmental surgical repair

18. Which of the following statements regarding renal function after aortic reconstruction procedures is/are TRUE?

1. Procedures involving infrarenal aortic occlusion do not adversely affect renal function.
2. Dopamine has been shown to be highly effective in preventing renal failure.
3. Intraoperative urine output is a reasonable predictor of postoperative renal function.
4. The best measures to prevent perioperative renal compromise are maintenance of adequate intravascular volume and maintenance of myocardial function.

19. Potential advantage(s) of regional anesthetic techniques over general anesthesia for lower extremity vascular bypass procedures include(s):

1. avoidance of hyperdynamic responses to tracheal intubation and extubation
2. reduced postoperative hypercoagulability and graft thrombosis
3. reduced incidence of postoperative respiratory complications
4. a reduction in perioperative cardiac complications

20. During an endovascular repair of an aortic aneurysm, the following potential incidents or complications could occur:

1. potential renal impairment secondary to intravenous dye

2. aneurysm rupture
3. graft migration
4. electrolyte abnormalities

ANSWERS

---

1. **E.** Although antiplatelet medications such as aspirin may retard the progression of atherosclerosis and associated cardiovascular events, cessation of smoking is by far the most effective form of medical therapy. This emphasizes the dramatic impact of tobacco abuse on the progression of atherosclerotic disease. Smoking cessation rates are approximately 25% after major surgery. Despite the low success rates, the benefits of smoking cessation are so great that such programs may be cost-effective. Systemic anticoagulation and thrombolytic agents are generally reserved for cases of acute ischemia. (See page 935: Medical Therapy for Atherosclerosis.)

2. **C.** Hertzer et al. performed coronary angiography in 1,000 consecutive patients slated to undergo vascular surgery and identified significant coronary artery stenosis (>70% occlusion) in 37% of patients who had no symptoms of coronary disease. These data indicate a high index of suspicion for coronary artery stenosis in patients presenting for vascular surgery, even in the absence of a prior history of cardiac disease. (See page 938: Coronary Artery Disease in Patients with Peripheral Vascular Disease.)

3. **D.** Patients undergoing vascular surgery are most likely to exhibit myocardial ischemia in the immediate postoperative period as a result of factors such as pain and adrenergic stress, hypercoagulability, and increased oxygen consumption associated with hypothermia and shivering. Landesburg et al. discovered that patients experienced twice as many episodes of myocardial ischemia after vascular surgery than preoperatively or intraoperatively. In fact, perioperative Holter monitoring indicates that the intraoperative period may be the time with the lowest incidence of ischemia. (See page 943: Detection of Perioperative Myocardial Ischemia.)

4. **C.** Data have shown that mechanical dysfunction of the myocardium occurs before surface electrocardiography changes during episodes of ischemia, a finding that supports the utility of echocardiography in the detection of intraoperative ischemia. It has been observed that new regional wall motion abnormalities (by transesophageal echocardiography) were more sensitive than electrocardiographic ST segment changes in detecting intraoperative ischemia. (See page 943: Detection of Perioperative Myocardial Ischemia.)

5. **C.** Although maintenance of adequate carotid artery perfusion pressure is an anesthetic goal during carotid endarterectomy, most studies indicate that as many as 65 to 95% of all neurologic deficits after carotid endartectomy may result from thromboembolic events. These may occur during surgical manipulation of the diseased vessel or in association with shunt placement. An embolism-related stroke rate of at least 0.7% has been reported in association with shunt placement, although no convincing data exist to indicate that routine shunt insertion reduces the incidence of postoperative neurologic deficits. (See page 948: Monitoring and Preserving Neurologic Integrity.)

6. **E.** Common problems arising after carotid endarterectomy include the onset of new neurologic dysfunction, hemodynamic instability during emergence from general anesthesia, and respiratory insufficiency. Blood pressure abnormalities are common after carotid endarterectomy; hypertension is more common than hypotension. Severe hypertension seems to occur more often in patients with poorly controlled preoperative hypertension. (See page 946: Carotid Endarterectomy.)

7. **E.** Although heparin is routinely administered before aortic occlusion to reduce the risk of thrombus formation, it is recognized that distal ischemic events following aortic surgery are generally the result of dislodgment of atheroemboli from the diseased aorta. It is believed by some that in the absence of major distal occlusive disease, systemic heparinization may be unnecessary when repairing abdominal aortic aneurysms. (See page 958: Surgical Procedures for Aortic Reconstruction.)

8. **B.** Prosthetic bypasses can be performed with less dissection than saphenous vein bypasses, which require multiple incisions for vein harvest. However, prosthetic grafts have significantly lower long-term patency rates. (See page 967: Lower Extremity Revascularization.)

9. **D.** Renal protection is still a controversial topic, with no therapies proven to yield superior outcome.

Many different methods of renal protection have been advocated, most of them centering on improving renal blood flow or glomerular flow. These include dopamine, fenoldopam, angiotensin-converting enzyme inhibitors, prostaglandins, vasodilators, isovolemic hemodilution, furosemide, and mannitol. Outcomes have not been shown to improve with any of these techniques. One of the most important factors for preventing postoperative renal failure remains good hydration (as the most important factor for maintaining renal blood flow) during clamping and post-clamp release. (See page 963: Protecting the Spinal Cord and Visceral Organs.)

10. **A.**   In high-risk patients undergoing noncardiac surgery, there was an increased incidence of myocardial ischemia associated with anemia (hematocrit level of <28) and hypothermia (presumably resulting from increased oxygen consumption accompanying postoperative shivering). Although the perioperative treatment of tachycardia with beta-adrenergic blocking agents has proven efficacious in the prevention of myocardial ischemia, the use of prophylactic infusions of intravenous nitroglycerin has not been shown to reduce the incidence of ischemic episodes in patients with known or suspected coronary artery disease who are undergoing noncardiac surgery. (See page 943: Management of Perioperative Myocardial Ischemia and Infarction in Vascular Patients.)

11. **C.**   The most common cause of carotid occlusive disease is atherosclerotic plaque, which usually develops at the lateral aspect of the carotid bifurcation. It is bilateral in approximately 50% of cases. The natural history of patients who present with transient ischemic attacks resulting from carotid occlusive disease is an approximate 10% risk of stroke during the ensuing year. (See page 946: Carotid Endarterectomy.)

12. **E.**   Surgeons who perform shunt procedures selectively use a monitor of cerebral perfusion to identify appropriate subjects for shunt insertion. Methods employed include carotid SSEP monitoring, intraoperative electroencephalograms, and direct monitoring of cerebral blood flow (e.g., xenon-gated flow measurements). However, none of these techniques has been shown to improve neurologic outcomes significantly in patients undergoing carotid vascular surgery. (See page 948: Monitoring and Preserving Neurologic Integrity.)

13. **E.**   Hypoxia to tissues distal to aortic occlusion leads to anaerobic metabolism and resultant acidosis. In addition, oxygen-derived free radicals, prostaglandins, cytokines, and other vasoactive mediators are produced, and this may result in hypotension and organ dysfunction when reperfusion occurs. Among the many factors described are renin, angiotensin, epinephrine, norepinephrine, prostacyclin, endothelin, prostaglandin F_1, thromboxane A_2 and B_2, lactate, potassium, oxygen-derived free radicals, platelet activators, cytokines, and activated complement (C3 and C4). Reactive hyperemia following reperfusion of ischemic vascular beds contributes to systemic hypotension resulting from a redistribution of blood flow. Hypoxic insult to intestines during aortic occlusion and the associated increase in gut permeability may produce endotoxemia. (See page 958: Humoral and Coagulation Profiles.)

14. **B.**   The blood supply to the thoracolumbar spinal cord (from T8 to the conus terminalis) is derived in large part by the major radicular artery known as the artery of Adamkiewicz. It arises from the left side in 60% of cases. In 75% of patients, it joins the anterior spinal artery between T8 and T12; it arises between L1 and L2 in 10% of patients. Although much of the blood flow in the anterior spinal artery is dependent on the artery of Adamkiewicz, the posterior portions of the spinal cord are supplied by the paired posterior spinal arteries, derived in part from the vertebral system. These arteries account for approximately 25% of spinal cord blood flow. (See page 955: Pathophysiology of Aortic Occlusion and Reperfusion.)

15. **C.**   Spinal cord ischemia with resultant paraplegia is a devastating complication of aortic occlusion and occurs in 1 to 11% of procedures involving the distal descending thoracic aorta. Although attempts to improve spinal cord perfusion pressure through cerebrospinal fluid drainage and hyperventilation have been undertaken, the only definitive methods in the prevention of spinal cord ischemia are rapid surgery and the maintenance of normal cardiac function. (See page 955: Pathophysiology of Aortic Occlusion and Reperfusion.)

16. **A.**   In a randomized, prospective trial comparing the traditional transabdominal approach with the retroperitoneal approach for elective infrarenal aortic reconstruction, the retroperitoneal approach was associated with a lower incidence of ileus and small bowel obstruction, shorter stays in the hospital and intensive care unit, and lower hospital costs. There was no difference in postoperative pulmonary complications, however, and the retroperitoneal approach was accompanied by an increase in long-term incisional pain. (See page 958: Surgical Procedures for Aortic Reconstruction.)

17. **B.**   The placement of aortic (Gott) shunts, the use of temporary ex vivo axillofemoral bypass grafts, and partial bypass techniques all have been employed as a means to decompress the heart and provide distal perfusion in the face of thoracic aortic occlusion. These techniques attenuate the hemodynamic response to aortic unclamping, reduce reperfusion acidosis, and possibly ameliorate the hormonal and metabolic aberrations associated with aortic occlusion.

Although segmental, sequential surgical repair may minimize the duration of ischemia to any given vascular bed, it does not allow for decompression or distal perfusion during periods of occlusion. (See page 963: Protecting the Spinal Cord and Visceral Organs.)

18. **D.** The development of acute renal failure following aortic reconstruction is associated with a mortality rate of >30%. Although it is more common in patients requiring supraceliac aortic occlusion, infrarenal occlusion is not without risk, as evidenced by data indicating that infrarenal aortic cross-clamping decreased renal blood flow by 38%, increased renal vascular resistance by 75%, and redistributed blood flow from the renal cortex. Indeed, infrarenal aortic reconstruction may be associated with a 3% incidence of renal failure. Previous data have shown that intraoperative urine output is a poor indicator of postoperative renal function. The best predictor of postoperative renal failure is preoperative renal function. Although various strategies, including administration of mannitol, furosemide, and low-dose dopamine, have been employed to increase renal blood flow and promote diuresis, none has been shown conclusively to prevent renal failure. Maintenance of adequate intravascular volume and maintenance of myocardial function are the most successful preventative measures. (See page 963: Protecting the Spinal Cord and Visceral Organs.)

19. **A.** It is a widely held belief that regional anesthetic techniques are associated with fewer postoperative respiratory complications than are general anesthetic techniques. Data indicate that regional techniques may reduce postoperative hypercoagulability and graft thrombosis in patients undergoing lower extremity vascular bypass procedures. A reduction in cardiac complications is often cited as a reason for the avoidance of general anesthesia. Although some studies have suggested a possible reduction of cardiac complications, this remains unsubstantiated. (See page 968: Anesthetic Management of Elective Lower Extremity Revascularization.)

20. **E.** The technique for implantation of endovascular aortic grafts generally requires bilateral common femoral artery or iliac artery cutdown in the supine position. Preimplantation angiography is required to identify the vasculature. Dye loads may be considerable (100–250 mL). Major complications in endovascular stent grafting have included aneurysm rupture during the time of graft implantation, renal insufficiency secondary to contrast use and the late complications including migration of the graft with late aneurysmal rupture. (See page 961: Endovascular Surgery for Aortic Aneurysms.)

CHAPTER 33 ■ ANESTHESIA AND THE EYE

For questions 1 to 9, choose the best answer.

1. When considering the anatomy of the eye, all of the following statements are correct EXCEPT:

   A. Sphenoid and zygomatic bones are integral part of the orbit.
   B. Blood supply to the eye is achieved by means of both internal and external carotid arteries.
   C. The eye is composed of three layers: sclera, uveal tract, and retina.
   D. The trochlear nerve supplies the lateral rectus muscle.
   E. The motor innervation of the eye and its adnexa are supplied by the oculomotor, trochlear, abducens, and facial nerves.

2. Which of the following statements about aqueous humor is TRUE?

   A. It is entirely formed in the posterior chamber.
   B. The formation process entails an active transport of sodium and bicarbonate.
   C. Aqueous humor is iso-osmolar to plasma.
   D. Carbonic anhydrase has an active role in the active secretion in the posterior chamber.
   E. Obstruction of venous return to the right side of the heart does not affect intraocular pressure (IOP).

3. Which of the following statements with respect to IOP is FALSE?

   A. IOP normally varies between 10 and 22 mm Hg.
   B. IOP is equal to intracranial pressure.
   C. IOP becomes atmospheric if the eye cavity has been entered.
   D. The major control of IOP is exerted by the fluid content.
   E. Coughing can increase IOP by as much as 40 mm Hg.

4. Which statement regarding the relationship between IOP and glaucoma is FALSE?

   A. IOP above 22 mm Hg is considered abnormal.
   B. IOP is influenced by both external pressure on the eye and obstruction of venous return.
   C. Open-angle glaucoma results from sclerosis in the trabecular system and responds to epinephrine and selective beta-blockers.
   D. Closed-angle glaucoma is an acute process that responds well to atropine.
   E. Laryngoscopy and tracheal intubation may elevate IOP.

5. Which of the following statements regarding neuromuscular blocking drugs is FALSE?

   A. In contrast to depolarizing drugs, nondepolarizing neuromuscular blocking drugs lower IOP.
   B. Succinylcholine causes an average increase in IOP of approximately 8 mm Hg.
   C. No technique consistently and completely blocks the ocular hypertensive response to succinylcholine administration.
   D. Succinylcholine should be used only with extreme reluctance in ocular surgery because of the high probability of causing eye injury.
   E. Succinylcholine causes an increase in IOP that dissipates within minutes.

6. Decreased IOP is associated with all of the following EXCEPT:

   A. sevoflurane
   B. elevated body temperature
   C. trimethaphan
   D. sorbitol
   E. glycerin

7. Which of the following statements regarding the oculocardiac reflex is FALSE?

A. It can be triggered by pressure on the globe or a retrobulbar block.

B. If the oculocardiac reflex occurs, surgery can continue if the patient has been premedicated with an anticholinergic agent.

C. This reflex can end in serious cardiac complications including cardiac arrest.

D. Atropine premedication can have an abortive action on this effect.

E. The oculocardiac reflex dissipates within seconds after cessation of eye manipulation.

8. Which of the following statements is TRUE?

A. Treatment of glaucoma with echothiophate poses minimal implications for general anesthesia.

B. Intraocular acetylcholine administration can be associated with bronchospasm.

C. Cocaine used alone for topical anesthesia in ocular surgery sensitizes the heart to endogenous catecholamines.

D. Cyclopentolate administration is associated with miosis.

E. Intraocular sulfur hexafluoride administration requires minimal changes in the general anesthetic technique.

9. True statements regarding ocular injuries during general anesthesia include all of the following EXCEPT:

A. Clear goggles should be worn to protect the eyes from injury from argon laser.

B. Hibiclens solution can result in corneal damage.

C. Corneal abrasion is the most common ocular complication of general anesthesia.

D. Venous retinal hemorrhages are usually self-limiting and resolve completely within a few months.

E. Retinal infarction may result from pressure exerted by an anesthetic face mask.

10. Related concerns regarding sympathomimetics and beta-blockers used for intraocular surgery include all of the following EXCEPT:

A. Adrenergic agents are associated with mydriasis.

B. Epinephrine administered in the anterior chamber causes systemic effects (e.g., tachycardia) in more than 20% of patients.

C. Phenylephrine in a concentration of 10% administered locally has been associated with cardiac dysrhythmias and ischemia.

D. Timolol can cause bronchospasm.

E. Topical beta-blockers should be used with caution in patients with congestive heart failure.

11. Differences between a retrobulbar and peribulbar block include all of the following EXCEPT:

A. The oculocardiac reflex occurs with both the retrobulbar block and the peribulbar block.

B. The peribulbar block requires larger doses of local anesthetic.

C. The onset of action for peribulbar block is quicker.

D. There are no reported cases of brainstem anesthesia with peribulbar block.

E. The approach for peribulbar block includes two sites: inferotemporal and superonasal.

For questions 12 and 13, choose A if 1, 2, and 3 are correct; B if 1 and 3 are correct; C if 2 and 4 are correct; D if only 4 is correct; and E if all are correct.

12. A 27-year-old man is brought to the emergency room after sustaining a motor vehicle accident. Massive bleeding and visible damage to the right orbit are noticed during assessment. Surgical intervention is mandatory. Which of the following statements is/are TRUE?

1. Succinylcholine can be safely used to secure the airway.

2. Awake intubation is an acceptable alternative for securing the airway.

3. Additional injuries have to be included in the anesthesia assessment (cranial fractures, airway injury, etc.)

4. Retrobulbar block offers the advantage of local anesthesia without the need of airway manipulation, which could trigger increases in the IOP.

13. A 4-month-old baby boy is scheduled for elective strabismus corrective surgery. Which of the following is/are of concern for the anesthesiologist?

1. Strabismus can be acquired secondary to cataracts.

2. The risk of nausea and vomiting can be attenuated with a combination of serotonin (5-HT) inhibitors, dopamine inhibitors, and/or corticosteroids.

3. Laryngeal mask airway can be safely used if there are no risk factors for aspiration.

4. Pretreatment with atropine is contraindicated.

ANSWERS

---

1. **D.**   The walls of the orbit are composed of the following bones: frontal, zygomatic, greater wing of the sphenoid, maxilla, palatine, lacrimal, and ethmoid.

Blood supply to the eye and orbit is by means of branches of both the internal and external carotid arteries. Venous drainage of the orbit is accomplished through the multiple anastomoses of the superior and inferior ophthalmic veins. Venous drainage of the eye is achieved mainly through the central retinal vein. All these veins empty directly into the cavernous sinus. The covering of the eye is composed of three layers: sclera, uveal tract, and retina. The sensory and motor innervations of the eye and its adnexa are as follows: a branch of the oculomotor nerve supplies a motor root to the ciliary ganglion, which in turn supplies the sphincter of the pupil and the ciliary muscle; the trochlear nerve supplies the superior oblique muscle; the abducens nerve supplies the lateral rectus muscle; and the facial nerve supplies the frontalis and the upper lid orbicularis, and the lower branch supplies the orbicularis of the lower lid. (See page 975: Ocular Anatomy.)

2. **B.**   Two-thirds of the aqueous humor is formed in the posterior chamber by the ciliary body in an active secretory process involving both the carbonic anhydrase and the cytochrome oxidase systems. The remaining one-third is formed by passive filtration of aqueous humor from the vessels on the anterior surface of the iris. At the ciliary epithelium, sodium is actively transported into the aqueous humor in the posterior chamber. Bicarbonate and chloride ions passively follow the sodium ions. This active mechanism causes the osmotic pressure of the aqueous to be many times greater than that of plasma. Aqueous humor flows from the posterior chamber through the pupillary aperture into the anterior chamber, and then the aqueous flows into the peripheral segment of the anterior chamber and exits the eye through the trabecular network, the Schlemm canal, and the episcleral venous system. A network of connecting venous channels eventually leads to the superior vena cava and the right atrium. Thus, obstruction of venous return at any point from the eye to the right side of the heart impedes aqueous drainage, elevating IOP accordingly. (See page 976: Ocular Physiology.)

3. **B.**   IOP exceeds not only tissue pressure by 2 to 3 mm Hg, but also intracranial pressure by as much as 7 to 8 mm Hg. IOP normally varies between 10 and 22 mm Hg. If the eye cavity has been entered, IOP becomes atmospheric. A major control of IOP is exerted by the fluid content, particularly the aqueous humor. Straining, vomiting, or coughing can increase IOP by as much as 40 mm Hg. (See page 976: Maintenance of Intraocular Pressure.)

4. **D.**   IOP normally varies between 10 and 21.7 mm Hg and is considered abnormal above 22 mm Hg. Three main factors influence IOP: external pressure on the eye by the contraction of the orbicularis oculi muscle and the tone of the extraocular muscles, venous congestion of orbital veins (as may occur with vomiting and coughing), and changes in intraocular contents (lens, vitreous, intraocular tumor, blood, or aqueous humor). Laryngoscopy and tracheal intubation may also elevate IOP, even without any visible reaction to intubation, although the effect is exaggerated when the patient coughs. Topical anesthetization of the larynx may attenuate the hypertensive response to laryngoscopy, but it does not reliably prevent associated increases in IOP. With open-angle glaucoma, the elevated IOP exists with an anatomically open anterior chamber angle; it is thought that sclerosis of trabecular tissue results in impaired aqueous filtration and drainage. Treatment consists of medication to produce miosis and trabecular stretching. Closed-angle glaucoma is characterized by movement of the peripheral iris into direct contact with the posterior corneal surface, thus mechanically obstructing aqueous outflow. Atropine premedication in the dose range used clinically has no effect on IOP in either open-angle or closed-angle glaucoma. (See page 976: Maintenance of Intraocular Pressure.)

5. **D.**   Neuromuscular blocking drugs have both direct and indirect actions on IOP. If paralysis of the respiratory muscles is accompanied by alveolar hypoventilation, the latter secondary effect may supervene to increase IOP. In contrast to nondepolarizing drugs, the depolarizing drug succinylcholine elevates IOP by an average of 8 mm Hg. Changes in extraocular muscle tone do not contribute significantly to the increase in IOP observed after succinylcholine administration. Various methods have been advocated to prevent succinylcholine-induced elevations in IOP. Although some attenuation of the increase results, no technique consistently and completely blocks the ocular hypertensive response. The efficacy of pretreatment with nondepolarizing drugs is controversial. Succinylcholine, if unaccompanied by pretreatment with a nondepolarizing neuromuscular blocking drug, is relatively contraindicated in patients with penetrating ocular wounds and should not be given for the first time after the eye has been opened. Nonetheless, it no longer is valid to recommend that succinylcholine be used only with extreme reluctance in ocular surgery. Clearly, any succinylcholine-induced increment in IOP is usually dissipated before surgery is started. (See page 979: Neuromuscular Blocking Drugs.)

6. **B.**   Hypoventilation, as well as administration of carbon dioxide, elevates IOP. Virtually all central nervous system depressants, including neuroleptics, opioids, and induction agents (e.g., barbiturates, etomidate, and propofol), lower IOP. Inhalation anesthetics purportedly cause dose-related decreases in IOP. Hypothermia lowers IOP. On initial consideration, hypothermia may be expected to raise IOP because of the associated increase in viscosity of aqueous humor. However, hypothermia is linked with decreased formation of aqueous humor and with vasoconstriction; hence, the net result is a reduction in IOP. Ganglionic blockers such as trimethaphan

significantly lower IOP in normal subjects, despite mydriasis. Intravenous administration of hypertonic solutions such as dextran, urea, mannitol, and sorbitol elevate plasma osmotic pressure, thereby decreasing aqueous humor formation and reducing IOP. Glycerin decreases IOP, although it is less predictable than mannitol. (See page 978: Effects of Anesthesia and Adjuvant Drugs on Intraocular Pressure.)

7. **B.** The oculocardiac reflex is triggered by pressure on the globe and by traction on the extraocular muscles, the conjunctiva, or the orbital structures. The reflex may also be elicited by performance of a retrobulbar block. Although the most common manifestation of the oculocardiac reflex is sinus bradycardia, a wide spectrum of cardiac dysrhythmias may occur, including junctional rhythm, ectopic atrial rhythm, atrioventricular blockade, ventricular bigeminy, multifocal premature ventricular contractions, wandering pacemaker, idioventricular rhythm, asystole, and ventricular tachycardia. Hypercarbia and hypoxemia are thought to augment the incidence and the severity of the oculocardiac reflex. The most common manifestation of this reflex is bradycardia. The afferent limb is trigeminal, and the efferent limb is the vagus. This reflex has a higher incidence in children. Various maneuvers to abolish or obtund the oculocardiac reflex have been promulgated. None of these have been consistently effective, safe, and reliable. Complete vagolytic blockade in the adult mandates 2 to 3 mg of atropine (0.03–0.05 mg/kg). Because the peak effect of intramuscular atropine occurs approximately 30 minutes after administration, it is not surprising that studies with the usual, routine dose have shown inconsistent protection against the oculocardiac reflex. If a cardiac dysrhythmia appears, the surgeon should be asked to cease operative manipulation. Next, the patient's anesthetic depth and ventilatory status should be evaluated. Commonly, heart rate and rhythm return to baseline within 20 seconds after institution of these measures. (See page 980: Oculocardiac Reflex.)

8. **B.** Acetylcholine is commonly used intraocularly after lens extraction to produce miosis. The local use of this drug may occasionally result in systemic effects such as bradycardia, increased salivation, bronchial secretions, and bronchospasm. Echothiophate is a long-acting anticholinesterase miotic that lowers IOP and may prolong the action of succinylcholine. In addition, a delay in metabolism of ester local anesthetics should be expected. It has been shown that cocaine used alone, without topical epinephrine, to shrink the nasal mucosa in conjunction with halothane or enflurane does not sensitize the heart to endogenous epinephrine during halothane or enflurane anesthesia. Cyclopentolate is a mydriatic, with side effects that include central nervous system toxicity, manifested by dysarthria, disorientation, and frank psychotic reactions. Intraocular sulfur hexafluoride has been used for retinal detachment

surgery to facilitate reattachment mechanically. Nitrous oxide should be terminated 15 minutes before gas injection to prevent expansion of intravitreous gas bubble. If the patient requires general anesthesia after this procedure, nitrous oxide should be avoided for 10 days. (See page 980: Anesthetic Ramifications of Ophthalmic Drugs.)

9. **A.** When working with argon laser, orange-tinted goggles should be used. Hibiclens, a 4% chlorhexidine gluconate solution, has been reported to result in serious corneal damage from eye contact. The most common ocular complication of general anesthesia is corneal abrasion; these lesions usually heal in 24 hours. Retinal ischemia or infarction may result from direct ocular pressure; this is particularly true in a hypotensive setting. (See page 991: Postoperative Ocular Complications.)

10. **B.** Although topical epinephrine has been associated with systemic effects, Smith et al. reported that administration of epinephrine into the anterior chamber of patients undergoing cataract surgery in doses up to 68 μg/kg does not lead to much systemic absorption even though the iris, with its rich network of adrenergic receptors, is able to capture most of the agent. Pupillary dilation and capillary decongestion are reliably produced by topical phenylephrine. In patients with coronary artery disease, severe myocardial ischemia, cardiac dysrhythmias, and even myocardial infarction may develop after topical 10% eye drops. Timolol, a nonselective beta-adrenergic agent, should be administered with caution to patients with known obstructive airway disease, congestive heart failure, or greater than first-degree heart block. Life-threatening asthmatic crises have been reported after the administration of timolol drops to some patients with chronic, stable asthma. A newer antiglaucoma drug, betaxolol, a beta$_1$-blocker, is said to be more oculospecific and to have minimal systemic effects. However, patients receiving an oral beta-blocker and betaxolol should be observed for potential additive side effects. (See page 980: Anesthetic Ramifications of Ophthalmic Drugs.)

11. **C.** Since the late 1980s, peribulbar block has become increasingly popular. The advantages of this technique include its safety and the fact that a lid block usually is superfluous because the relatively large volume of injected local anesthetic usually diffuses into the eyelids. Two injections are required, one placed inferotemporally and one between the supraorbital notch and trochlea. Onset is usually slower than with retrobulbar blockade and may be delayed for as long as 15 to 20 minutes. Another disadvantage of peribulbar blockade is that pressure on the eyeball is required to distribute the local anesthetic. However, no cases of either retrobulbar hemorrhage or brainstem anesthesia have been documented associated with peribulbar block. Both retrobulbar and peribulbar blocks are associated with

the oculocardiac reflex. (See page 982: Preoperative Evaluation: Retrobulbar and Peribulbar Blocks.)

12. **A.**   The anesthesiologist involved in caring for a patient with a penetrating eye injury and a full stomach confronts special challenges. He or she must weigh the risk of aspiration against the risk of blindness in the injured eye that could result from elevated IOP and extrusion of ocular contents. As in all cases of trauma, attention should be given to the exclusion of other injuries, such as skull and orbital fractures, intracranial trauma associated with subdural hematoma formation, and the possibility of thoracic or abdominal bleeding. Although regional anesthesia is an often valuable alternative for the management of trauma patients who have recently eaten, such an option is not available for patients with penetrating eye injuries. Retrobulbar blockade is ill advised because extrusion of intraocular contents may ensue. Even though it is conceivable that a well-conducted, extremely smooth awake intubation after topical anesthesia may not increase IOP, it seems much more probable that the coughing and straining that will occur will result in increased IOP.

Succinylcholine offers the distinct advantages of swift onset, superb intubating conditions, and brief duration of action. If administered after careful pretreatment with a nondepolarizing drug and an induction agent, succinylcholine typically produces only a modest increase in IOP. (See page 988: "Open-Eye, Full Stomach" Encounters.)

13. **A.**   Infantile strabismus occurs within the first 6 months of life and is often observed in the neonatal period. Although most patients with strabismus are healthy, the incidence of strabismus is increased in those with central nervous system dysfunction. The use of atropine affords some protection against elicitation of the oculocardiac reflex. For this reason, many anesthesiologists administer intravenous atropine routinely to children scheduled for strabismus surgery. The laryngeal mask airway is gaining popularity for strabismus surgery. To decrease the risk of vomiting, combination therapy with a 5-HT antagonist, metoclopramide, and a glucocorticoid is gaining popularity. Strabismus can be acquired secondary to oculomotor nerve trauma or to sensory abnormalities such as cataracts or refractive aberrations. (See page 989: Strabismus Surgery.)

CHAPTER 34 ■ ANESTHESIA FOR OTOLARYNGOLOGIC SURGERY

For questions 1 through 8, choose the best answer.

1. The most serious complication of tonsillectomy is postoperative hemorrhage. Approximately 75% of postoperative tonsillar hemorrhages occur within how many hours of surgery?

    A. 1
    B. 6
    C. 12
    D. 24
    E. 48

2. All of the following statements regarding emesis after tonsillectomy are true EXCEPT:

    A. It occurs in about 30 to 65% of patients.
    B. It may result from central stimulation of the chemoreceptor trigger zone.
    C. It is sometimes responsive to meperidine.
    D. It may be avoided by decompressing the stomach before extubation.
    E. It may be treated with intravenous ondansetron 0.10 to 0.15 mg/kg.

3. All of the following statements regarding negative pressure pulmonary edema are true EXCEPT:

    A. It is associated with a decrease in pulmonary hydrostatic pressure.
    B. It is caused by the sudden relief of a previously obstructed airway.
    C. Intrapleural pressure in an obstructed airway may reach −30 cm H_2O.
    D. It may be prevented by the application of continuous positive airway pressure during induction of anesthesia.
    E. It is associated with diffuse bilateral infiltrates on chest radiographs.

4. The most common cause of stridor in infants is:

    A. peritonsillar abscess
    B. foreign body obstruction
    C. laryngomalacia
    D. croup
    E. epiglottitis

5. Regarding the pain associated with tonsillectomy, which of the following statements is TRUE?

    A. It is usually less severe when intraoperative hemostasis is achieved with laser and electrocautery rather than with sharp surgical dissection and ligation of blood vessels.
    B. It is usually less severe than after adenoidectomy.
    C. Its severity is often reduced when the peritonsillar space is infiltrated with local anesthetic.
    D. Its occurrence may be reduced with the intraoperative use of corticosteroids.
    E. It is usually related to underlying infection or hematoma formation.

6. A Le Fort III fracture:

    A. passes above the floor of the nose but involves the lower third of the nasal septum
    B. crosses the medial wall of the orbit, including the lacrimal bone
    C. passes through the base of the nose and the orbital plates
    D. is a horizontal fracture of the maxilla
    E. always involves a fracture of the cribiform plate of the ethmoid bone

7. A rigid bronchoscope with an internal diameter of 3.0 mm would have an external diameter of approximately:

    A. 3.5 mm
    B. 4.0 mm

C. 5.0 mm
D. 6.0 mm
E. 7.0 mm

8. The most common site of cervical spine injury in patients presenting with facial fracture sustained in high-velocity trauma is:

A. C1–C2
B. C2–C3
C. C3–C4
D. C4–C5
E. C6–C7

For questions 9 through 17, choose A if 1, 2, and 3 are correct; B if 1 and 3; C if 2 and 4; D if 4; and E if all.

9. Relative contraindications to a superior laryngeal nerve block include:

1. tumor at the site of the block
2. pregnancy
3. infection at the site of the block
4. partially obtunded patient

10. TRUE statements about airway anatomy include:

1. The cricothyroid muscle is innervated by the external branch of the superior laryngeal nerve.
2. The mandible is capable of both translational and rotational motion.
3. The internal branch of the superior laryngeal nerve provides sensory innervation to the vocal cords.
4. Trismus involves spasm of the masseter muscles.

11. TRUE statements about peritonsillar abscesses include:

1. They are located below the laryngeal inlet.
2. They usually interfere with ventilation by mask.
3. They usually impair vocal cord visualization.
4. They often require surgical intervention.

12. According to most guidelines, which of the following patients undergoing adenotonsillectomy should be admitted for inpatient management?

1. A 10-year-old child with Down syndrome
2. A healthy 1-year-old child
3. A 7-year-old child with a peritonsillar abscess
4. A 15-year-old patient with a mild upper respiratory infection

13. Which of the following statements about middle ear surgery is/are TRUE?

1. Patient positioning carries the risk of C1–C2 subluxation in the pediatric population as a result of laxity of the cervical spine ligaments.
2. Maintenance of relative hypotension may be requested to reduce intraoperative bleeding.
3. Nitrous oxide should be avoided during procedures involving tympanic grafts.
4. Dissection carries the potential for injury to the third cranial nerve.

14. TRUE statements about epiglottitis are:

1. Symptoms include sudden onset of fever, dysphagia, and muffled voice.
2. It is associated with a characteristic "steeple sign" appearance on radiological examination.
3. It is caused by *Haemophilus influenzae* type B.
4. It often responds to nebulized racemic epinephrine.

15. TRUE statements about laryngotracheobronchitis include:

1. Symptoms include sudden onset of fever, dysphagia, and muffled voice.
2. It is associated with a characteristic "steeple sign" appearance on radiological examination.
3. It is caused by *Haemophilus influenzae* type B.
4. It often responds to nebulized racemic epinephrine.

16. TRUE statements about laser surgery of the airway include:

1. The energy emitted by the CO_2 laser is absorbed by water in tissue and blood.
2. The neodymium:ytrrium-aluminum-garnet (Nd:YAG) laser has more limited penetrance than the CO_2 laser.
3. Stand polyvinyl chloride (PVC) endotracheal tubes are flammable.
4. The CO_2 laser may cause retinal injury.

17. Findings in a patient with foreign body aspiration may include:

1. refractory wheezing
2. stridor
3. tachypnea
4. fever

ANSWERS

1. **B.**   Approximately 75% of postoperative tonsillar hemorrhages occur within 6 hours of surgery. Most of the remaining 25% occur within the first 24 hours of surgery, although bleeding may not be noted until the

sixth postoperative day. About two-thirds of postoperative bleeding originates from the tonsillar fossa, whereas 27% occurs in the nasopharynx, and 7% involves both regions. (See page 999: Complications.)

2. **C.** The incidence of postoperative emesis after tonsillectomy is approximately 30 to 65%. The exact cause is unclear but is probably multifactorial. Potential causative factors include irritant blood in the stomach, impaired gag reflex resulting from inflammation and edema, and central nervous stimulation of the chemoreceptor trigger zone as a result of gastric distention. Management of postoperative nausea and vomiting commonly includes administration of ondansetron and/or dexamethasone. The use of meperidine for postoperative pain control has been shown to exacerbate symptoms, especially in children. (See page 999: Complications.)

3. **A.** Negative-pressure pulmonary edema is a rare but serious condition caused by the sudden relief of a previously obstructed airway. Under normal circumstances, intrapleural pressures range from −2.5 to −10.0 cm H_2O during inspiration. In the presence of airway obstruction, the intrapleural pressure may reach −30.0 cm H_2O. Rapid relief of airway obstruction results in a decrease in airway pressure, an increase in venous return, and an increase in pulmonary hydrostatic pressure. The net result is the development of pulmonary edema. Mild cases may be asymptomatic. However, in serious cases, the condition is marked by the appearance of frothy pink fluid in the endotracheal tube, decreased O_2 saturation, wheezing, dyspnea, and tachypnea. A chest radiograph illustrating diffuse, usually bilateral, interstitial pulmonary infiltrates, combined with an appropriate clinical history, supports the diagnosis. (See page 999: Complications.)

4. **C.** Laryngomalacia is the most common cause of stridor in infants. Laryngomalacia is most often secondary to a long epiglottis that prolapses posteriorly as well as prominent arytenoid cartilages with redundant aryepiglottic folds that obstruct the glottic opening during inspiration. Symptoms usually present shortly after birth. Peritonsillar abscess, foreign body obstruction, croup, and epiglottitis are also potential but less common causes of stridor in this age group. (See page 1003: Stridor.)

5. **D.** Pain following tonsillectomy is often severe, in contrast to the minimal discomfort usually associated with adenoidectomy. An increase in pain medication requirements has been noted in patients in whom intraoperative hemostasis is achieved using laser or electrocautery as opposed to sharp surgical dissection and ligation of blood vessels. Intraoperative administration of corticosteroids appears to be

somewhat effective at reducing postoperative pain by decreasing edema formation. In contrast, injection of local anesthetic into the peritonsillar space has not been associated with a decrease in postoperative pain. (See page 998: Tonsillectomy and Adenoidectomy.)

6. **C.** In the course of his studies, Le Fort determined the common lines of fracture of the midface. The Le Fort I fracture is a horizontal fracture of the maxilla, passing above the floor of the nose but involving the lower third of the septum, mobilizing the palate, maxillary alveolar process, lower third of the pterygoid plates, and parts of the palatine bones. The Le Fort II fracture crosses the medial wall of the orbit, involving the lacrimal bone, beneath the zygomaticomaxillary suture, crosses the lateral wall of the antrum, and passes through the pterygoid plates. The Le Fort III fracture parallels the base of the skull, passing through the base of the nose and ethmoid as well as the orbital plates. The Le Fort III fracture may, but does not always, involve fracture of the cribiform plate. (See page 1008: Le Fort Classification of Fractures.)

7. **C.** Bronchoscopes are sized based on their internal diameter. Their external diameters are significantly greater than those of endotracheal tubes of similar size. The external diameter of a rigid bronchoscope with an internal diameter of 3.0 mm is 5.0 mm, whereas the external diameter of a comparably sized endotracheal tube would be 4.3 mm. (See page 1003: Bronchoscopy.)

8. **E.** The most common site of cervical spine injury in patients presenting with facial fractures status after high-velocity injury is at the level of C6–C7, accounting for approximately 50% of cases. The second most common site of fracture is at the C2 level. (See page 1009: Patient Evaluation.)

9. **E.** A full stomach, pregnancy, and partially obtunded mental status are relative contraindications to superior laryngeal nerve block because of the possibility of vomiting and aspiration after protective airway reflexes have been blunted. Tumor and infection are considered relative contraindications because of the possibility of dissemination secondary to the manipulation associated with the block. (See page 1010: Awake Intubation.)

10. **E.** Knowledge of airway anatomy is essential to the practicing anesthesiologist, particularly when preparing for an awake intubation. The superior laryngeal nerve has an external branch and an internal branch. The external branch innervates the cricothyroid muscle, a tensor of the vocal cords, whereas the internal branch provides sensory innervation to the vocal cords. The normal mandible has a biphasic motion and anterior-posterior translational movement, as well as rotation

about an axis passing through the condyles. Several conditions cause mechanical dysfunction of the jaw that may complicate tracheal intubation. Trismus is a spasm of the masseter muscles that impairs jaw relaxation. The muscles usually relax in response to anesthetics and muscle relaxants; however, if the jaw has been closed for a prolonged period of time, masseter fibrosis may result in persistent compromise of the jaw's range of motion. (See page 1009: Securing the Airway.)

11. **D.**   Peritonsillar abscess, previously known as quinsy tonsil, is a serious consequence of tonsillar infection that frequently requires surgical drainage. The abscess is usually located in the lateral pharynx above the glottis and laryngeal inlet. It does not typically interfere with mask ventilation or vocal cord visualization. (See page 999: Complications.)

12. **A.**   According to most guidelines, patients who should be admitted to the hospital after adenotonsillectomy include children age 3 years or less, patients with anatomic and medical conditions that could lead to increased risk of bleeding (e.g., abnormal coagulation profile, bleeding diathesis) or airway obstruction (e.g., craniofacial abnormality, achondroplasia, or Treacher Collins, Crouzon, Goldenhar, or Down syndrome.) A patient for whom surgery is being performed because of the presence of an acute peritonsillar abscess would also warrant postoperative inpatient monitoring. However, an otherwise healthy child older than 3 years with a mild upper respiratory infection need not routinely be admitted unless the patient did not meet discharge criteria in the recovery room. (See page 998: Tonsillectomy and Adenoidectomy.)

13. **A.**   Tympanoplasty and mastoidectomy are two of the most common procedures performed on the middle ear and accessory structures, particularly in the pediatric age group. To gain access to the surgical site, the surgeon positions the head on a head rest, which may be lower than the operative table. Extreme degrees of lateral rotation may be requested to facilitate surgical exposure. Extreme tension on the heads of the sternocleidomastoid muscles must be avoided. The laxity of the ligaments of the cervical spine, as well as immaturity of the odontoid process in children, make children especially prone to C1–C2 subluxation. Ear surgery often involves surgical dissection near the facial nerve (cranial nerve VII), thus placing it at risk of being injured if not properly identified and protected. Cranial nerve III, the oculomotor nerve, innervates extrinsic muscles of the eye and is not encountered during typical dissections for middle ear surgery. Bleeding must be kept to a minimum during surgery of the small structures of the middle ear, and maintenance of relative hypotension is often effective at minimizing bleeding. In addition, injection of concentrated epinephrine solution is

performed in the area of the tympanic vessels to produce vasoconstriction. The middle ear and sinuses are air-filled, nondistensible cavities. An increase in the volume of gas contained within these structures results in an increase in pressure. Nitrous oxide diffuses along a concentration gradient into the air-filled middle ear spaces more rapidly than nitrogen moves out. During procedures in which the eardrum is replaced or a perforation is patched, nitrous oxide should therefore be discontinued before the application of the tympanic membrane graft to avoid pressure-related displacement. (See page 1001: Ear Surgery.)

14. **B.**   Acute epiglottitis is most commonly caused by *Haemophilus influenzae* infection. Characteristic signs and symptoms of acute epiglottitis include sudden onset of fever, dysphagia, drooling, thick muffled voice, and preference for the sitting position with the head extended and leaning forward. Retractions, labored breathing, and cyanosis may be observed when obstruction is present. If the clinical situation allows, oxygen should be administered by mask, and lateral radiographs of the soft tissues in the neck may be obtained. Thickening of the aryepiglottic folds as well as swelling of the epiglottis may be noted, producing a classic "thumb sign." In contrast, narrowing of the airway column produces the "steeple sign" on radiographic examination of patients with larygnotracheobronchitis (croup). Treatment of epiglottitis involves establishing an artificial airway. In anticipation of local swelling, the endotracheal tube chosen should be at least one size (0.5 mm) smaller than would normally be chosen. Racemic epinephrine is not part of the standard management of epiglottitis. (See page 1004: Epiglottitis.)

15. **C.**   Laryngotracheobronchitis, or croup, occurs in children 6 months to 6 years of age but is primarily seen in children younger than 3 years. It is usually viral in origin, and its onset is more insidious than that of epiglottitis. The child presents with low-grade fever, inspiratory stridor, and a "barking" cough. Radiological examination confirms the diagnosis; subglottic narrowing of the airway column secondary to circumferential soft-tissue edema produces a characteristic "steeple sign." Treatment includes cool, humidified mist and oxygen therapy usually administered in a tent for mild to moderate cases. More severe cases are accompanied by tachypnea, tachycardia, and cyanosis, and, in these cases, racemic epinephrine administered by nebulizer is often beneficial. The use of steroids is controversial, but a short course may be helpful. (See page 1005: Laryngotracheobronchitis.)

16. **B.**   The CO_2 laser is the most widely used in medical practice, having particular application in the treatment of laryngeal or vocal cord papillomas, laryngeal webs, resection of redundant subglottic

tissue, and coagulation of hemangiomas. The energy emitted by a CO_2 laser is absorbed by water contained in blood and tissues. Human tissue is approximately 80% water, and laser energy absorbed by tissue water rapidly increases the temperature, thus denaturing protein and causing vaporization of the target tissue. The CO_2 laser does not penetrate deeply (0.01 mm); it may cause injury to the cornea, but its energy does not reach the retina. This is in contrast to the Nd:YAG laser, which has a deeper penetration and may therefore cause retinal injury. All standard PVC endotracheal tubes are flammable and can ignite and vaporize when in contact with the laser beam. Endotracheal tubes have been specifically designed for use during laser surgery. Another option is the use of a red rubber tube wrapped with reflective metallic tape. However, the cuff of this tube remains unwrapped and therefore does not completely exclude the potential for laser damage. (See page 1006: Laser Surgery of the Airway.)

17. **E.**   The patient with foreign body aspiration may have coughing, choking, refractory wheezing, stridor, tachypnea, and fever. (See page 1005: Foreign Body Aspiration.)

CHAPTER 35 ■ THE RENAL SYSTEM AND ANESTHESIA FOR UROLOGIC SURGERY

1. Which of the following is believed responsible for blindness following transurethral resection of the prostate (TURP)?

   A. Sorbitol
   B. Glycine
   C. Mannitol
   D. Urea
   E. Glycogen

2. Which of the following tests best predicts the development of acute renal failure (ARF) in critically ill patients?

   A. Serum creatinine (Cr) and blood urea nitrogen (BUN)
   B. Urine sodium concentration (U_{Na})
   C. Creatinine clearance (Ccr)
   D. Fractional excretion of sodium (FENA)
   E. Free water clearance (CH_2O)

For questions 3 to 14, choose A if 1, 2, and 3 are correct; B if 1 and 3; C if 2 and 4; D if 4; and E if all.

3. Which of the following medications have altered pharmacodynamics significant enough to warrant alterations in dosing in patients with end-stage renal disease (ESRD)?

   1. Thiopental
   2. Dexmedetomidine
   3. Midazolam
   4. Isoflurane

4. Causes for increased release of antidiuretic hormone include which of the following?

   1. Increased extracellular sodium
   2. Increased extracellular osmolality
   3. Reduced atrial filling pressures
   4. Arterial baroreceptor stimulation by hypertension

5. Which of the following statements regarding anesthesia and renal function is/are TRUE?

   1. Methoxyflurane is consistently the only agent that produces clinically relevant renal damage.
   2. Anesthesia does not directly affect renal hormonal control.
   3. Most renal injuries during anesthesia are caused by physiologic perturbations.
   4. Spinal anesthesia is the safest anesthetic for the kidney.

6. Alterations in drug administration in patients with chronic renal failure are required because of which of the following alterations in homeostasis?

   1. Alterations in volume of distribution
   2. Alterations in protein binding
   3. Alterations in elimination half-life for various compounds
   4. Alteration in the rise of F_A/F_I for inhaled agents

7. Which of the following intravenous agents have their clinical effects altered in the presence of ESRD?

   1. Thiopental
   2. Etomidate
   3. Valium
   4. Propofol

8. Preoperative factors associated with an increased risk of postoperative renal dysfunction include which of the following?

   1. Pre-existing renal disease
   2. Preoperative hypovolemia
   3. Congestive heart failure
   4. Cirrhosis

9. During aortic surgery, proven techniques to prevent renal injury include which of the following?

   1. Dopamine
   2. Mannitol

   3. Furosemide

   4. Avoidance of hypovolemia and hypotension

10. Qualities of the ideal irrigation solution for TURP include which of the following?

   1. Isotonic

   2. Transparent

   3. Nonhemolytic

   4. Nonelectrolytic

11. Which of the following statements regarding regional anesthesia and TURP is/are TRUE?

   1. A T10 sensory level is required to prevent sensation of bladder distention.

   2. Epidural anesthesia is the regional technique of choice for TURP.

   3. Regional anesthesia may improve detection of TURP syndrome symptoms.

   4. Regional anesthetics have been shown to reduce mortality compared with general anesthesia.

12. Which of the following statements regarding lithotripsy is/are TRUE?

   1. Minimal immersion techniques are devoid of cardiovascular and pulmonary side effects.

   2. Pregnancy is an absolute contraindication.

   3. Small patients are at risk of pulmonary contusion from the shock wave.

   4. Pacemakers are a contraindication to lithotripsy.

13. Risk of pulmonary toxicity secondary to bleomycin exposure is linked to which of the following?

   1. Pre-existing pulmonary disease

   2. Limited duration between bleomycin exposure and high oxygen exposure

   3. Dose of bleomycin of >450 mg

   4. Metastatic disease

14. Endovascular repair of an abdominal aortic aneurysm is gaining in popularity compared with the open approach. Which of the following statements regarding the endovascular approach is/are TRUE?

   1. Typically, hemodynamic alterations are reduced.

   2. Long-term incidences of renal failure or insufficiency are similar.

   3. Patients typically experience less postoperative pain.

   4. It cannot be performed in patients with severe chronic obstructive pulmonary disease.

ANSWERS

1. **B.** All of the above substances (except for glycogen) are used as osmotic agents in TURP procedures. Glycine is the only agent that directly produces transient blindness. It is believed that the blindness is a result of glycine action as an inhibitory neurotransmitter. (See page 1026: Irrigating Solutions for TURP.)

2. **C.** Of all the tests listed, only Ccr is a predictor of imminent ARF, as well as acting as a diagnostic test to assess the kidney's response to treatment. Ccr is a direct measurement of glomerular filtration rate (GFR). Alterations of GFR seen in ARF result in rapid alteration of Ccr. Normally, the test requires a 24-hour collection of urine, but a shorter 2-hour collection correlates well with the 24-hour collection in patients in the intensive care unit. BUN and Cr are good screens for pre-existing renal dysfunction and trend up and down to reflect alterations in kidney function; however, the changes are slow and are affected by numerous other factors. $U_{Na}{}^+$ reflects resuscitative fluids being used. FENA does not serve as an early indicator of ARF. It can differentiate prerenal from renal causes of ARF after the condition is established. (See page 1023: Perioperative Assessment of Renal Function.)

3. **A.** Thiopental, midazolam, and dexmedetomidine all undergo significant protein binding. This binding is reduced in ESRD, resulting in a larger free fraction of the drug. This requires an altered dosing scheme for these medications. Isoflurane pharmacodynamics are not affected by renal failure. (See page 1020: Induction Agents and Sedatives.)

4. **A.** Antidiuretic hormone is released by the posterior pituitary gland in response to increased extracellular sodium or increased osmolality. It is also released during times of hypotension through receptors in the atria and the arterial tree. Antidiuretic hormone release results in increased free water absorption at the distal and the collecting tubules. By increasing the quantity of free water absorbed, the elevated sodium and osmolality levels are diluted, and hypovolemia is abated. (See page 1016: Tubular Resorption of Sodium and Water: Understanding Standards of Care.)

5. **A.** In general, an anesthetic is not injurious to the renal system; an exception is methoxyflurane. During the metabolism of this drug, free fluoride is released, which causes renal injury. Enflurane and sevoflurane also generate free fluoride; however, the quantity released is substantially less than with methoxyflurane, and enflurane and sevoflurane have

not consistently caused clinically relevant renal injury. Regional anesthesia has not been shown to be superior to general anesthesia in preserving renal function. Most renal injury occurs secondary to physiologic perturbations as a result of surgery, as well as complications such as hypoxia, hypovolemia, and hypotension. Anesthetics do not directly alter renal hormonal regulation. (See page 1017: Renal Dysfunction and Anesthesia.)

6. **A.** The pharmacokinetics of most enteral and parenteral medications are altered in patients with chronic renal failure (with the exclusion of inhaled anesthetic agents). There is an increase in the volume of distribution for water-soluble drugs; this results in lower concentration of a drug given as a single bolus. Reduced excretion of the parent drug and any of its active metabolites results in prolonged duration of action for a number of agents. Protein binding is typically reduced in chronic renal failure; this results in a larger free fraction (which produces the effects). There is no alteration in alveolar uptake in patients with chronic renal failure (as long as they are not in congestive heart failure). (See page 1020: Anesthetic Agents in Renal Failure.)

7. **B.** Drug pharmacokinetics are altered in the presence of renal failure. This arises because of the changes in protein binding, increases in volume of distribution, decreased clearance of the parent compound, and any metabolic products with pharmacologic activity. Thiopental, because of its level of protein binding, has a significantly greater free fraction in patients with ESRD; a reduced dose should thus be administered. Etomidate shows little difference in its activity when administered in the standard dose because of its limited side effect profile. Propofol administration can be given at normal doses because of its primary hepatic metabolism. Valium, however, has exaggerated effects if administered in a standard dose; this occurs because of its extensive protein binding and reduced excretion of its active metabolites. (See page 1020: Anesthetic Agents in Renal Failure.)

8. **E.** The single most reliable predictor of postoperative renal dysfunction is preoperative renal dysfunction. Other risk factors include cardiac dysfunction, sepsis, volume depletion, and hepatic failure. Advanced age, by itself, is not predictive of postoperative renal dysfunction. (See page 1022: Patient-Based Risk Factors for Acute Renal Failure.)

9. **D.** No medication (including dopamine, mannitol, or furosemide) has been shown consistently to improve postoperative renal function in aortic surgery. In general, maintenance of adequate intravascular volume and maintenance of blood pressure are the only preventive measures one can

take to preserve renal function. (See page 1024: High-Risk Surgical Procedures.)

10. **E.** TURP involves the use of a fiber-optic scope and an electrocautery loop to resect the prostate from inside the lumen of the urethra. To clear the resected material and blood, an irrigating solution is infused. This irrigating solution must be optically clear and nonconductive toward electricity (because the cautery unit will be in direct contact with fluid). During resection, the fluid used during irrigation is absorbed by the open veins within the prostate, and thus the fluid must be isotonic and nonhemolytic. (See page 1026: Irrigating Solution for TURP.)

11. **B.** Regional anesthesia is used extensively for TURP procedures. There is no difference in mortality between patients receiving general anesthesia and those receiving regional anesthetics. Spinal anesthesia is the technique of choice if a regional technique is selected; this is because spinals provide a more reliable block than epidurals. If a patient selects a regional block for a TURP, one must anesthetize to the T10 level to block sensation from an overdistended bladder. Because patients are awake during regional anesthesia, there is an increased likelihood that the TURP syndrome symptoms would be detected earlier. (See page 1028: Anesthetic Technique for TURP.)

12. **A.** Lithotripsy involves crushing renal calculi with an externally generated shock wave. Early lithotripsy machines transferred the shock wave to the patient by immersing the patient in a water bath. The water transferred the shock wave effectively because tissue and water have similar acoustical properties. Immersion in the water bath can lead to significant physiologic changes including increased central venous pressure, vasodilation, decreased vital capacity, and decreased functional residual capacity. The new minimal immersion techniques are devoid of physiologic derangements. Small patients are at risk of pulmonary contusions, because their lungs lie within the path of the shock wave. Pacemakers were once believed to be a contraindication for lithotripsy, but studies have failed to validate this as a contraindication. Pregnancy is a contraindication to lithotripsy. (See page 1030: Physiologic Effects of Immersion Lithotripsy; see page 1030: Patient Selection for Shock Wave Lithotripsy Procedures.)

13. **A.** Bleomycin is a chemotherapeutic agent commonly used against germ cell tumors. It causes pulmonary damage, which appears to be accelerated with exposure to high concentrations of oxygen. The risk factors for postoperative respiratory failure following bleomycin exposure include a dose of >450 mg, pre-existing pulmonary disease, recent exposure to bleomycin, evidence of renal insufficiency, and exposure to high concentrations of oxygen. There is no link between metastatic disease and pulmonary

toxicity. (See page 1035: Radical Surgery for Testicular Cancer.)

14. **A.** Endovascular procedures to repair abdominal aortic aneurysms typically produce less hemodynamic alterations and, because of the smaller incisions, produce less postoperative pain. Endovascular procedures do not have a lower incidence of long-term renal complications. This is probably because of the similar risk of atheroembolism and because of the significant quantity of radiographic contrast dye used during the procedure. There is no link between metastatic disease and pulmonary toxicity. (See page 1024: High-Risk Surgical Procedures.)

CHAPTER 36 ■ ANESTHESIA AND OBESITY

1. Ideal body weight is defined by which of the following?

   A. Weight in pounds divided by height in inches
   B. Weight in kilograms divided by height in squared centimeters
   C. Weight in pounds divided by height in square inches
   D. Weight in kilograms divided by height in squared meters
   E. Weight in pounds divided by height in squared centimeters

2. Which of the following statements regarding obesity is FALSE?

   A. Angina rarely presents in morbidly obese patients.
   B. Modest obesity is associated with increased risk for complications in the perioperative period.
   C. Risks associated with obesity are related to the distribution of fat.
   D. The effects of obesity are almost exclusively related to the cardiovascular system.
   E. Android distribution is associated with increased oxygen consumption and increased incidence of cardiovascular disease.

3. Which of the following respiratory system changes or parameters does not occur with obesity?

   A. Normal basal metabolic rate
   B. Decreased expiratory reserve volume and functional residual capacity in the upright position
   C. Normal closing capacity in the upright position, but abnormal in supine
   D. Reduced chest-wall and lung compliance
   E. Normal forced vital capacity

4. Cardiovascular system changes that may occur with obesity include all of the following EXCEPT:

   A. arterial hypertension
   B. increased cardiac output in response to exercise or stress

   C. cardiomegaly with an elevated circulating blood volume
   D. impairment of diastolic function with elevated left ventricular end-diastolic pressure
   E. absence of accelerated atherosclerosis

For question 5 to 7, choose A if 1, 2, and 3 are correct; B if 1 and 3; C if 2 and 4; D if 4; and E if all are correct.

5. Which of the following statements is/are pertinent regarding preoperative assessment of the obese patient?

   1. Thorough evaluation of airway with consideration for fiber-optic intubation is indicated.
   2. Serum evaluation of liver function studies for evidence of fatty liver infiltration is recommended.
   3. Aspiration prophylaxis is indicated.
   4. Body mass index (BMI) correlates with the degree of difficulty of intubation.

6. Which statement(s) best describe(s) anesthetic considerations for abdominal surgery in the morbidly obese patient?

   1. Increased BMI is a risk factor for ulnar nerve neuropathy.
   2. Supine positioning may cause ventilatory impairment and compression of the inferior vena cava and aorta.
   3. Lateral decubitus positioning allows for better diaphragmatic movement than the prone position.
   4. Adequate preoxygenation is vital to preventing hypoxemia after loss of consciousness resulting from increased oxygen consumption.

7. Which of the following may apply to the intraoperative anesthetic management of the obese patient?

1. Consideration of an awake fiber-optic intubation should be given in all patients who meet criteria for potential difficult intubation.
2. Stacking is a useful positioning maneuver used to facilitate intubation.
3. Use of intra-arterial monitoring may be necessary in some patients in whom noninvasive blood pressure monitoring may be difficult.
4. Larger induction doses of medications are not necessary in morbidly obese patients.

ANSWERS

---

1. **D.** Ideal body weight is defined by weight in kilograms divided by height in squared meters. This is called the body mass index (BMI). Patients with a BMI >28 are considered obese. Patients with a BMI >35 are considered morbidly obese. (See page 1040: Obesity.)

2. **D.** Even modest obesity is associated with an increased risk of premature death or complications during the perioperative period. Angina or exertional dyspnea rarely presents in morbidly obese patients because of their limited mobility. They may be asymptomatic despite the presence of cardiovascular disease. Truncal distribution of fat, also called android distribution, is associated with increased oxygen consumption and an increased incidence of cardiovascular disease. Multiple physiologic systems are affected by obesity, such as the respiratory, cardiovascular, endocrine and metabolic, and gastrointestinal systems. (See page 1040: Obesity.)

3. **C.** In obesity, oxygen consumption and carbon dioxide production are increased, but the basal metabolic rate is normal because it is related to body surface area. A decreased expiratory reserve volume and a decrease in functional residual capacity occur in the upright position such that tidal volume may encroach upon the range of the closing capacity. This effect is exaggerated in the supine position. The results of this are ventilation–perfusion abnormalities, left-to-right shunting, and hypoxemia. Chest wall compliance is reduced in obesity, although lung compliance is unchanged. Respiratory functions, such as forced vital capacity, forced expiratory volume, and peak expiratory flows, are unchanged in obesity. As obesity increases, hypoventilation syndrome may occur. This is characterized by loss of hypercapnic drive, sleep apnea, hypersomnolence, and airway difficulties. This may progress to pickwickian syndrome (hypercarbia, hypoxia, polycythemia, hypersomnolence, pulmonary hypertension, and biventricular failure). (See page 1041: Respiratory System.)

4. **E.** Arterial hypertension is associated with obesity. Cardiac output increases with exercise and stress. Cardiomegaly may occur, associated with an elevated circulating blood volume and cardiac output and hypertension. Left ventricular wall stress leads to hypertrophy, reduced compliance, and impaired left ventricular filling (diastolic dysfunction) with elevated left ventricular end-diastolic pressure and pulmonary edema. Obesity accelerates atherosclerosis. (See page 1042: Cardiovascular System.)

5. **B.** Evaluation of the airway is critical because of the numerous anatomic changes that could potentially result in difficulty in intubating the obese patient. For example, flexion of the neck could result in difficulty, because of excessive soft tissue. Submental fat may limit mouth opening. A large tongue, fleshy cheeks, redundant palate, and pharyngeal tissue may narrow the airway. Liver function studies are not necessary, because they may not necessarily be indicative of fatty infiltration of the liver. Fatty infiltration of the liver reflects the duration rather than the degree of obesity. Despite histologic and enzymatic changes, no clear correlation exists between routine liver function tests and the capacity of the liver to metabolize drugs. All obese patients should receive aspiration prophylaxis. BMI does not seem to have much influence on difficulty of laryngoscopy. Neck circumference has been identified as the single best predictor of problematic intubation in morbidly obese patients. (See page 1041: Pathophysiology of Obesity.)

6. **E.** There is a documented association between ulnar neuropathy and increasing BMI. It is approximately 30% in patients with a BMI ≥ 38 kg/m^2. Supine positioning causes ventilatory impairment and occlusion of the inferior vena cava and aorta. This may compromise venous return to the heart, with resultant hypotension. Prone positioning in obese patients requires freedom of abdominal movement to prevent detrimental effects on lung compliance, ventilation, and arterial oxygenation. Lateral decubitus positioning is favored over prone positioning whenever possible. Prone positioning decreases functional residual capacity. Adequate preoxygenation is vital to prevent hypoxemia after loss of consciousness resulting from increased oxygen consumption. (See page 1048: Positioning.)

7. **A.** An awake fiber-optic intubation should be considered in all patients who are 75% over ideal body weight because of the greater incidence of difficulty with intubation. Neck circumference is the greatest predictor of problematic intubation. Intra-arterial

blood pressure monitoring may be necessary if proper fit of the blood pressure cuff is not possible. Stacking is a useful maneuver used to facilitate intubation so the chin is at a higher level than the chest. The head-elevated laryngoscopy position (HELP) is a step beyond "stacking." The HELP position elevates the obese patient's head, upper body, and shoulders above the chest to the extent that an imaginary horizontal line connects the sternal notch to the external auditory meatus; this improves the laryngoscopy view. Larger induction doses may be required because obese patients have a larger blood volume, muscle mass, and cardiac output.

(See page 1048: Induction, Intubation, Maintenance.)

CHAPTER 37 ■ ANESTHESIA AND GASTROINTESTINAL DISORDERS

1. Which statement best describes anesthetic considerations for abdominal surgery?

   A. With a 50:50 mixture of nitrous oxide (N_2O), the maximum increase in bowel gas is twofold.
   B. N_2O is 10 times more soluble than nitrogen.
   C. Neostigmine administration results in decreased bowel peristalsis.
   D. Abdominal wall distention occurs with administration of N_2O; however, it cannot result in bowel ischemia.
   E. N_2O should be avoided in all abdominal surgery.

For questions 2 to 7, choose A if 1, 2, and 3 are correct; B if 1 and 3; C if 2 and 4; D if 4 only; and E if all are correct.

2. TRUE statement(s) concerning the gastrointestinal tract include(s):

   1. The esophagus is innervated by intrinsic and extrinsic nerves.
   2. Dopamine and glucagon increase lower esophageal sphincter (LES) tone.
   3. Gastroesophageal reflux is more dependent on barrier pressure than on tone of the LES.
   4. LES tone is not affected by thiopental or propofol.

3. Which of the following statements regarding gastric aspiration is/are TRUE?

   1. Aspiration is most likely to occur during induction of general anesthesia.
   2. Breast milk is cleared more rapidly than other milk products; however, it predisposes to an increased severity of aspiration pneumonitis.
   3. There is a dose-response relationship in the severity of aspiration pneumonitis for both gastric volume and acidity that reaches the lung.
   4. Obesity, pregnancy, and trauma are states that are associated with high gastric volume.

4. The risk of regurgitation and pulmonary aspiration may be reduced by:

   1. use of histamine (H_2)-receptor antagonists
   2. application of the Sellick maneuver (cricoid pressure)
   3. avoiding airway manipulation while under a light depth of anesthesia
   4. application of 1 Newton force to the cricoid

5. Which of the following is/are TRUE concerning the intestine?

   1. Bowel denervation results in no intestinal activity.
   2. Hyperventilation with subsequent hypocapnia is best avoided during colonic surgery.
   3. There is no reason to avoid prokinetic medications (e.g., metoclopramide) during the early postoperative period after colon surgery.
   4. Mesenteric traction syndrome is manifested by sudden tachycardia, hypotension, and cutaneous hyperemia.

6. Which of the following statements regarding carcinoid tumors is/are TRUE?

   1. The gastrointestinal tract is the most common site of origin for carcinoid tumors.
   2. The hormones secreted by nonmetastatic carcinoid tumors are usually deactivated by the liver.
   3. Typical symptoms manifested by metastatic carcinoid disease are extremely variable.
   4. Bronchospasm is usually secondary to bradykinin release.

7. Which of the following statements regarding carcinoid tumors is/are TRUE?

   1. Medical treatment of carcinoid tumors consists of administration of a somatostatin analog.
   2. Octreotide is a synthetic somatostatin analog with a half-life similar to that of somatostatin.

3. Carcinoid heart disease occurs in approximately 60% of patients with carcinoid syndrome and predominantly affects the right side of the heart.

4. Histamine-releasing drugs are not contra-indicated.

ANSWERS

1. **A.** A 50:50 mixture of N_2O will result in a twofold increase in bowel gas. N_2O is 30 times more soluble than nitrogen. In a severely compromised patient, abdominal distention may be so severe as to cause bowel ischemia. N_2O can be used for abdominal surgery, provided no signs of severe distention are present. Neostigmine increases bowel peristalsis. This effect may be ameliorated by the concurrent administration of glycopyrrolate. (See page 1058: Nitrous Oxide and the Bowel; and page 1057: Splanchnic Blood Flow.)

2. **B.** The esophagus is innervated by both intrinsic and extrinsic nerve supply. The intrinsic nerve supply includes the myenteric plexus of Auerbach and submucosal plexus of Meissner. The extrinsic nerve supply is derived from parasympathetic fibers from the vagus with sympathetic fibers from the superior and inferior cervical fourth and fifth sympathetic ganglia. Dopamine, secretin, glucagon, beta-adrenergic agents, thiopental, propofol, opioids, and anticholinergics all reduce LES pressure. In a patient undergoing general anesthesia, the occurrence of reflux is dependent on barrier pressure, which is the difference between LES pressure and gastric pressure. Barrier pressure is more important than LES tone in the production of gastroesophageal reflux. (See page 1053: Esophagus.)

3. **E.** The incidence of regurgitation of gastric contents is low. Aspiration is most likely to occur during induction of anesthesia. Breast milk predisposes to an increased severity of aspiration pneumonitis in comparison with other milk products. Soy-based formulas cause a less severe form of acute lung injury. Breast milk is cleared more rapidly than other milk products. Milk products are cleared more slowly than clear liquids. Obesity, pregnancy, trauma, shock, and pain are examples of physiologic states associated with high gastric volumes. There is a dose-response relationship in the severity of aspiration pneumonitis for both gastric volume and acidity that reaches the lung. (See page 1054: Stomach.)

4. **A.** Anesthesia risk of regurgitation and aspiration may be reduced by all of the following: reducing volume of gastric contents, nasogastric suctioning, inducing emesis, accelerating gastric emptying, increasing LES tone, avoiding airway instrumentation during light anesthesia, and raising the pH level of gastric contents by use of H_2-receptor antagonist or proton pump inhibitors. Cricoid pressure may be used to decrease risk of pulmonary aspiration. Application of 10 Newton force to the cricoid cartilage is suggested while the patient is awake. This will prevent pain, coughing, and retching. Once the patient is anesthetized, 20 Newton force is required to prevent aspiration. (See page 1055: Control of Gastric Contents.)

5. **C.** Parasympathetic stimulation increases the activity of the small intestines. However, bowel denervation results in minimal change in intestinal activity, lending credence to the possibility that humoral secretions play a major role in intestinal activity. Hypocapnia significantly reduces splanchnic blood flow, whereas hypercapnia does the opposite. Therefore, hyperventilation is best avoided after colon resection, to maintain adequate blood flow. Use of prokinetics such as metoclopramide has been associated with colonic anastomotic dehiscence in the early perioperative period. Mesenteric traction syndrome consists of sudden tachycardia, hypotension, and cutaneous hyperemia during mesenteric traction. (See page 1057: Mesenteric Traction Syndrome.)

6. **E.** The gastrointestinal tract is the most common site for carcinoid tumors. Most tumors are small and occur at multiple sites. Twenty percent of carcinoid tumors may be located in the lung. The portal circulation may be a site of inactivation of the hormones secreted by these tumors. The presentation and manifestation of metastatic carcinoid disease are variable. Cutaneous flushing, abdominal pain, vomiting, diarrhea, bronchospasm, hypotension, hypertension, and hyperglycemia are all symptoms of a carcinoid tumor, which are related to secretion of bradykinin and serotonin. Bradykinin produces cutaneous flushing, bronchospasm, and hypotension, whereas serotonin causes hypertension or hypotension. Other substances secreted include histamine, substance P, bradykinin, tachykinin, motilin, corticotrophin, prostaglandins, kallikrein, and neurotensin. (See page 1058: Carcinoid Tumors.)

7. **B.** Complete surgical excision is the most effective treatment for carcinoid tumor. Medical treatment consists of administration of the somatostatin analog octreotide. Octreotide is a somatostatin analog with approximately 50 times the half-life of somatostatin. It has a half-life of approximately 2.5 hours. It may be administered either subcutaneously or intravenously. Therapy may be given prophylactically as well as

intraoperatively to control symptoms. However, octreotide should not be abruptly discontinued in the postoperative period; it should be continued at least 24 hours after surgery. Metastatic carcinoid-secreting tumors will affect the heart and result in lesions on the valves of the right side of the heart (tricuspid and pulmonic valves). Histamine-releasing drugs are contraindicated because they may evoke a carcinoid episode. Other factors that may cause a carcinoid episode include perioperative anxiety, hypothermia, hypercapnia, hypotension, and hypertension.
(See page 1058: Carcinoid Tumors.)

CHAPTER 38 ■ ANESTHESIA FOR MINIMALLY INVASIVE PROCEDURES

For questions 1 to 12, choose A if 1, 2, and 3 are correct; B if 1 and 3; C if 2 and 4; D if 4; and E if all.

1. Potential advantages of video-assisted thoracic surgery (VATS) include which of the following?

   1. Decreased postoperative pain
   2. Improved postoperative pulmonary function
   3. Shorter hospitalization
   4. Earlier return to work

2. Regarding anesthesia for VATS, which of the following is/are TRUE?

   1. It usually is performed with the patient under general anesthesia with one-lung ventilation via a double-lumen tube.
   2. Paravertebral catheters can be placed intraoperatively for pain management.
   3. The anesthetic technique most commonly employed is balanced intravenous and inhalational anesthesia.
   4. VATS can be used in the management of disk herniation.

3. Which of the following statements regarding complications of laparoscopic cholecystectomies is/are TRUE?

   1. Bile duct injuries are more common after laparoscopic than after open cholecystectomies.
   2. Injuries of the bile duct during laporoscopic procedures are typically more extensive and higher in the ductal system.
   3. Most bile duct injuries require a surgical drainage procedure.
   4. Postoperatively, pain and jaundice are the typical presenting features of bile duct injury.

4. Which of the following are potential complications associated with insertion of the trocar for laparoscopic procedures?

   1. Gastrointestinal tract perforation
   2. Hepatic and splenic tears
   3. Major vascular trauma
   4. Bleeding from abdominal wall vessels

5. Which of the following statements regarding positioning for laparoscopic procedures is/are TRUE?

   1. Positioning is required to produce gravitational displacement of abdominal viscera.
   2. The Trendelenburg position of 10 to 20 degrees results in an increase in central blood volume and a decrease in intercostal and diaphragmatic excursion.
   3. The extent of physiologic changes is related to patient age and volume status.
   4. Induction of anesthesia and the reverse Trendelenburg position cause an increase in cardiac index.

6. Potential complications of excessively high intra-abdominal pressure during CO_2 insufflation include:

   1. pneumomediastinum
   2. pneumopericardium
   3. subcutaneous emphysema
   4. ocular emphysema

7. Effects of pneumoperitoneum include:

   1. subcutaneous and retroperitoneal emphysema
   2. pneumothorax
   3. decreased cardiac index, increased systemic vascular resistance, and increased mean arterial pressure
   4. no change in plasma concentration of vasopressin, epinephrine, and norepinephrine

8. Which of the following findings about gas insufflation is/are TRUE?

1. CO_2 is rapidly excreted via the lungs.
2. Helium is insoluble in blood and is difficult to extract should gas embolization occur.
3. Nitrous oxide is potentially dangerous in the presence of electrocautery.
4. Extraperitoneal insufflation of CO_2 may cause a sudden rise in end-tidal CO_2 readings.

9. Possible causes of acute hypotension and/or hypoxemia during laparoscopy include:

    1. reflex increase in vagal tone
    2. pneumothorax
    3. venous gas embolism
    4. hypocarbia

10. Which of the following statements concerning intraoperative hypoxemia during laparoscopy is/are TRUE?

    1. It is uncommon in healthy patients.
    2. It may result from decreased lung compliance, decreased functional residual capacity (FRC), and ventilation–perfusion mismatch.

3. It may result from regurgitation and aspiration.
4. FRC increases.

11. Pulmonary changes during pneumoperitoneum include:

    1. increased peak inspiratory pressure
    2. decreased Pa_{CO_2}
    3. decreased vital capacity
    4. increased FRC

12. Which of the following statements concerning care of the laparoscopy patient is/are TRUE?

    1. Placement of the trocar is via a minilaparotomy approach in selected patients.
    2. Pneumatic compressive devices are recommended to offset the venous stasis associated with an increase in intra-abdominal pressure.
    3. Cuffed endotracheal tubes are usually recommended to decrease the risk of aspiration.
    4. Controlled ventilation is preferred to aid in control of CO_2.

ANSWERS

1. **E.** VATS is associated with decreased postoperative pain, improved postoperative pulmonary function, shorter hospitalizations, and an earlier return to work. (See page 1068: Video-Assisted Thoracic Surgery.)

2. **E.** VATS usually is performed with one-lung ventilation via a double-lumen tube. VATS-assisted placement of paravertebral catheters during thoracoscopic procedures has been reported in the management of postoperative pain. VATS has been reported in the management of multiple diseases of the thoracic spine, including disk herniation. (See page 1068: Video-Assisted Thoracic Surgery.)

3. **E.** Laparoscopic bile duct injuries tend to be more proximal in the ductal system, more common, and more extensive than those after open procedures. They also are associated with less likelihood of a successful repair. Pain and jaundice associated with bile collections are typical features in the postoperative period. When the common bile duct or common hepatic duct is injured, a surgical drainage procedure is usually required. (See page 1067: Postoperative Considerations.)

4. **E.** Trocar insertion is associated with numerous potential complications including perforation of the gastrointestinal tract, hepatic tears, splenic tears, major vascular trauma, and bleeding from abdominal wall vessels. (See page 1066: Specific Intraoperative Complications.)

5. **A.** During laparoscopic surgery, the patient is positioned to produce gravitational displacement of the abdominal viscera away from the surgical site. Gravity has profound effects on the cardiovascular and pulmonary systems. The head-down tilt of 10 to 20 degrees commonly used both in gynecologic procedures and for the initial trocar insertion in laparoscopic cholecystectomy is accompanied by an increase in central blood volume and a decrease in vital capacity and diaphragmatic excursion. The reverse Trendelenburg position favors improved pulmonary dynamics but reduces venous return. The changes associated with positioning may be influenced by the extent of the tilt, the patient's age, intravascular volume status, associated cardiac disease, anesthetic drugs, and ventilation techniques. Induction of anesthesia and the reverse Trendelenburg position cause a significant reduction (35–40%) in cardiac index. (See page 1063: Effects of Patient Position.)

6. **E.** Extravasation of CO_2 during laparoscopic cholecystectomy may result in subcutaneous emphysema associated with pneumomediastinum, pneumopericardium, pneumothorax, and ocular emphysema. Excessively high intra-abdominal pressures during CO_2 insufflation contribute to these complications, which resolve uneventfully

within 24 hours. (See page 1067: Pneumothorax, Pneumopericardium, and Pneumomediastinum.)

7. **A.**   Circulating plasma levels of renin, aldosterone, vasopressin, epinephrine, and norepinephrine increase on creation of pneumoperitoneum. These changes are accompanied by increased systemic vascular resistance, increased central venous pressure, increased blood pressure, and decreased cardiac index. Pneumothorax is a rare but potentially life-threatening complication of pneumoperitoneum. This complication occurs primarily on the right side. Insufflated gas may track around the aortic and esophageal hiatuses of the diaphragm into the mediastinum and may then rupture into the pleural space. (See page 1063: Cardiovascular Effects and Neurohumoral Response.)

8. **E.** CO_2 is the insufflation gas of choice because it is excreted rapidly via the lungs and is stable in vivo. Helium is insoluble in the bloodstream and thus is difficult to extract; this can cause problems if gas embolization occurs. Nitrous oxide supports combustion, which may be dangerous in the presence of electrocautery. Extraperitoneal insufflation has been associated with higher levels of CO_2 absorption than intraperitoneal insufflation and may be the cause of a sudden rise in end-tidal CO_2 during the procedure. (See page 1064: Gas Exchange Effects Carbon Dioxide Absorption.)

9. **A.**   Postulated causes of acute hypotension and/or hypoxemia associated with laparoscopy include the following: (1) hypercarbia, which may induce dysrhythmias; (2) reflex increase in vagal tone from excessive stretching of the peritoneum; (3) pneumothorax, which may present as an increase in airway pressure, hypoxemia, or severe cardiovascular compromise; (4) hemorrhage; and (5) venous gas embolism. (See page 1067: Pneumothorax, Pneumopericardium, and Pneumomediastinum.)

10. **A.**   Intraoperative hypoxemia is uncommon in the healthy patient. Because of both positioning and an increase in intra-abdominal pressures, patients undergoing laparoscopy are at an increased risk of gastric aspiration. If aspiration occurs, hypoxemia will parallel the severity of the aspiration. The reduction in FRC and lung compliance associated with the supine position is further reduced by CO_2 insufflation and cephalad shift of the diaphragm. (See page 1064: Respiratory Effects.)

11. **B.**   Pulmonary changes during pneumoperitoneum include increased peak inspiratory pressure, intrathoracic pressure, and $PaCO_2$ and decreased vital capacity, FRC, and compliance. (See page 1064: Respiratory Effects.)

12. **E.**   Techniques that decrease the risk of complication during laparoscopy include prophylaxis against deep vein thrombosis, use of cuffed endotracheal tubes (to decrease the risk of aspiration syndromes), and controlled ventilation (to offset the effect of abdominal distention). In selected patients, placement of the trocar via a minilaparotomy approach is indicated. (See page 1066: Specific Intraoperative Complications.)

CHAPTER 39 ■ ANESTHESIA AND THE LIVER

For questions 1 to 9, choose the best answer.

1. All of the following statements regarding liver physiology are true EXCEPT:

   A. Hepatic blood flow equals approximately 100 mL/100 g per minute.
   B. Twenty-five percent of total hepatic flow is supplied by the hepatic artery and nearly 50% of hepatic oxygen delivery.
   C. The liver is the largest gland in the human body and weighs approximately 1.5 kg.
   D. The liver receives 40% of the cardiac output.
   E. The portal vein provides 75% of total hepatic blood flow and 50% of its oxygen delivery.

2. All of the following are functions of the liver EXCEPT:

   A. excretion of glycogen after excess carbohydrate ingestion
   B. erythrocyte breakdown and bilirubin excretion
   C. several endocrine functions, which include synthesis of insulin-like growth factor, angiotensinogen, and thrombopoietin
   D. hormone biotransformation and catabolism.
   E. a critical role in glucose buffering and maintenance of euglycemia

3. Choose the FALSE statement regarding pharmacokinetic and liver function.

   A. The liver influences the plasma concentration and availability of most orally and parenterally administered drugs.
   B. Plasma proteins such as albumin and alpha$_1$-acid glycoprotein increase free drug concentrations.
   C. Hepatic clearance is the process by which the liver biotransforms drugs and changes them to inactive water-soluble substances that can be excreted into bile or urine.

   D. Phase 1 and phase 2 reactions are a series of biotransformations.
   E. Phase 1 reactions are much more susceptible to inhibition by advanced age or hepatic disease than phase 2 reactions.

4. All of the following are true regarding laboratory evaluation of liver function EXCEPT:

   A. Aspartate aminotransferase (AST) is detected in increased levels when there is hepatocellular injury and necrosis.
   B. Mild elevations in alanine aminotransferase (ALT) and AST may be seen with fatty liver infiltration, nonalcoholic steatohepatitis, and drug toxicity.
   C. Lactate dehydrogenase (LDH) has poor diagnostic specificity for liver disease and limited clinical usefulness.
   D. Elevation of alkaline phosphatase disproportionate to ALT and AST is indicative of intrahepatic or extrahepatic obstruction.
   E. Prothrombin time (PT) and international normalized ratio (INR) are insensitive indicators of hepatic dysfunction.

5. All of the following statements regarding cirrhosis are true EXCEPT:

   A. The most common causes of hepatic cirrhosis are chronic hepatitic C infection and alcoholism.
   B. Clinical signs are hepatosplenomegaly, ascites, jaundice, spider nevi, and metabolic encephalopathy.
   C. Hyperdynamic circulation exists with high cardiac output, low peripheral vascular resistance, and low to normal blood pressure.
   D. Gastroesophageal varices are the most dreadful complication of portal hypertension.
   E. Portal hypertension is the hallmark of all chronic liver diseases.

6. Which of the following statements regarding hepatorenal syndrome (HRS) is TRUE?

   A. Fifty percent of patients with advanced cirrhosis and ascites develop HRS.
   B. HRS is characterized by intense vasoconstriction of renal circulation, low glomerular filtration, preserved renal tubular function, and normal renal histology.
   C. Patients showing improvement in renal function after vasoconstrictor therapy for HRS do not survive any longer than patients who do not respond to therapy.
   D. Perioperative renal failure does not change the outcome of liver transplantation.
   E. HRS is typed into two categories based upon histologic findings.

7. All of the following are true regarding hepatic encephalopathy (HE) EXCEPT:

   A. HE is a complex, irreversible metabolic encephalopathy presenting with a wide variety of neuropsychiatric abnormalities.
   B. Clinical manifestations are highly variable and range from minimal changes in personality or altered sleep pattern to confusion, lethargy, and coma.
   C. Large dietary protein load, gastrointestinal bleeding, constipation, hypokalemia, diuretics, and azotemia can precipitate HE.
   D. It is believed that HE is caused by substances that under normal circumstances are efficiently metabolized by the liver.
   E. Clinical and neurophysiologic manifestations of HE seem to reflect a global depression of central nervous system function caused by an increase in inhibitory neurotransmitters.

8. All of the following statements regarding uncommon causes of cirrhosis are true EXCEPT:

   A. Wilson disease is a hereditary disease characterized by decreased hepatocellular excretion of copper into bile.
   B. Wilson disease has an autosomal recessive pattern of transmission.
   C. Hematochromatosis is a hereditary disease characterized by excessive iron absorption.
   D. Progression of hematochromatosis may be slowed by repeat phlebotomy.
   E. Primary biliary cirrhosis is a common cause of cirrhosis with an inherited recessive pattern.

9. Which of the following statements regarding the anesthetic management of the patient with advanced liver disease is TRUE?

   A. Physical examination of the patient with chronic liver disease is not valuable because patients do not appear ill before laboratory evidence of hepatic dysfunction.

   B. Increased magnitude of liver dysfunction does not correlate with higher morbidity and mortality.
   C. Drugs administered to patients with advanced hepatic disease require careful titration against effect.
   D. Plasma clearance of fentanyl is not significantly altered.
   E. Decreased doses of vasoconstrictors are needed in these patients.

For questions 10 to 13, choose A if 1, 2, and 3 are correct; B if 1 and 2; C if 2 and 4; D if 4; and E if all.

10. Which of the following is/are TRUE regarding halothane?

    1. In children, halothane hepatitis is extremely rare even with repeated exposure.
    2. In adults, halothane hepatitis is rare with a single exposure, but repeat exposure to halothane in obese middle-aged women substantially increases the risk.
    3. Halothane can markedly reduce hepatic blood flow and oxygen supply and often causes mild transient liver injury.
    4. No reliable test exists for detecting halothane hepatitis or susceptibility to the disease.

11. Which of the following statements regarding maintenance of anesthesia in patients with liver disease is/are TRUE?

    1. The initial dose requirement to achieve relaxation with a nondepolarizing muscle relaxant may be higher.
    2. It is prudent to avoid halothane and enflurane in a patient with liver disease.
    3. Dose requirements for a variety of medications can be unpredictable.
    4. Patients with liver disease have a reduced sensitivity to vasopressor drugs.

12. Which of the following statements regarding postoperative liver disease is/are TRUE?

    1. Postoperative liver dysfunction is common but rarely severe.
    2. It is usually symptomatic and may progress to overt liver failure on rare occasions.
    3. Subclinical hepatocellular injury may occur in 20% of patients who have received enflurane anesthesia.
    4. Jaundice is a late sign of serious hepatic or hepatobiliary dysfunction.

13. Which of the following statements regarding prevention of postoperative liver dysfunction is/are TRUE?

    1. Identification of patients at high risk of developing liver dysfunction or exacerbation of pre-existing liver disease should influence the anesthetic plan.

2. Elective surgery should be postponed when pre-existing liver abnormalities are recognized.
3. Preservation of cardiac output and adequate splanchnic, hepatic, and renal perfusion are

critically important in patients with liver dysfunction who are undergoing a major surgical procedure.
4. Epidural analgesia is contraindicated in patients with severe liver dysfunction.

ANSWERS

1. **D.** The liver is supplied by two large vessels, the hepatic artery and the portal vein. The liver receives approximately 25% of the cardiac output. Hepatic blood flow equals about 100 mL/100 g per minute. The hepatic artery supplies 25% of total hepatic blood flow but 50% of oxygen supply. The portal vein supplies 50% of the oxygen supply and 75% of total hepatic blood flow. The liver weighs approximately 1.4 to 1.8 kg, representing about 2% of the total body weight in the adult. In the neonate, the liver accounts for approximately 5% of body weight. (See page 1073: Hepatic Anatomy.)

2. **A.** The liver has many physiologic functions, including regulation of blood coagulation, synthesis of hormones, erythrocyte breakdown, carbohydrate metabolism, lipid metabolism, amino acid metabolism, synthesis of proteins, and immunologic function. The liver stores glycogen after hyperglycemia following a carbohydrate meal. Endocrine function includes synthesis of insulin-like growth factor, angiotensinogen, and thrombopoietin. The liver is the primary site of thyroxine conversion to triiodothyronine. It also synthesizes thyroid-binding globulin. Corticosteroids, aldosterone, estrogen, androgens, insulin, and antidiuretic hormone are inactivated by the liver. (See page 1077: Major Physiologic Functions of the Liver.)

3. **B.** Drug metabolism is a primary hepatic event. The liver influences plasma concentrations and systemic availability of most orally and parenterally administered drugs. Synthesis of drug binding proteins such as albumin and alpha-acid glycoprotein partitions drugs into various compartments of the body (volume of distribution). These proteins decrease free drug concentration. Hepatic clearance is the sum of all processes by which the liver eliminates drugs from the body. Biotransformation is the metabolism of drugs by the hepatocytes to water-soluble inactive substances that are excreted into the bile or urine. Phase 1 and phase 2 comprise a series of reactions in this biotransformation process. Phase 1 reactions (oxidation, reduction, N-dealkylation) are more susceptible to inhibition by advanced age or hepatic disease than phase 2 reactions. (See page 1079: Immunologic Function.)

4. **E.** Laboratory evaluation of liver function involves measurement of indices of hepatocellular damage and hepatic synthetic function. AST (formally called serum glutamic oxaloacetic transaminase) and ALT (formally called serum glutamic pyruvic transaminase) are detected in increased levels when there is hepatocellular injury and necrosis. Mild elevations in AST and ALT may be seen with fatty infiltration of the liver, nonalcoholic steatohepatitis, and drug toxicity. LDH has poor diagnostic specificity for liver disease and limited clinical usefulness. Elevation of alkaline phosphatase disproportionate to AST and ALT is indicative of intrahepatic or extrahepatic bile obstruction. PT and INR are sensitive indicators of hepatic dysfunction because of the short half-life of factor VII. Mild to moderate hepatic disease may not be detected by PT and INR because coagulation factors are present in quantities that far exceed requirements for normal coagulation. (See page 1091: Cirrhosis: A Paradigm for End-Stage Parenchymal Liver Disease.)

5. **E.** Cirrhosis affects more than 3 million persons in the United States. The most common causes of hepatic cirrhosis are chronic hepatitis and alcoholism. Most common clinical symptoms are anorexia, weakness, nausea, vomiting, and abdominal pain. Clinical signs include hepatosplenomegaly, ascites, jaundice, spider nevi, and metabolic encephalopathy. Patients with cirrhosis and portal hypertension have a hyperdynamic circulation with high cardiac output, low peripheral vascular resistance, low to normal arterial blood pressure, normal to increased stroke volume, normal filling pressures, and mildly elevated heart rate. Portal hypertension can complicate the course of chronic liver disease but is the hallmark of end-stage cirrhosis. Gastroesophageal varices are the most dreadful complication of portal hypertension. They are present in 40 to 60% of patients with cirrhosis. (See page 1091: Cirrhosis: A Paradigm for End-Stage Parenchymal Liver Disease.)

6. **B.** HRS is functional prerenal failure that occurs only in approximately 10% of patients with advanced cirrhosis and ascites. It is characterized by intense vasoconstriction of renal circulation, low glomerular filtration, preserved renal tubular function, and normal renal histology. HRS is diagnosed after all

other causes of renal failure are excluded. There are two major types of HRS, based upon intensity and presentation. Intense renal vasoconstriction results from extreme vasodilation of splanchnic arterial circulation. The resultant abnormal distribution of arterial volume is associated with reduced blood flow to extrasplanchnic areas including the kidneys. Because HRS develops as a result of splanchnic vasodilation, drugs that reduce vasodilation have been used to treat HRS. Patients responding to vasoconstriction therapy survive longer than nonresponders. Transplant survival is reduced in cirrhotic patients with preoperative renal failure. (See page 1095: Hepatorenal Syndrome.)

7. **A.**   HE is a complex, reversible metabolic encephalopathy presenting as a wide spectrum of neuropsychiatric abnormalities. Clinical manifestations are highly variable and range from minimal changes in personality or altered sleep pattern to confusion, lethargy, and coma. Several well-recognized factors can precipitate HE. Large protein load, gastrointestinal hemorrhage, constipation, hypokalemia, diuretics, and azotemia can precipitate HE. It is believed that HE is caused by substances that under normal circumstances are efficiently metabolized by the liver rather than by insufficient synthesis of substances essential for normal neurologic function. Clinical and neurologic manifestations of HE seem to reflect a global depression of central nervous system function caused by an increase in inhibitory neurotransmitters. Treatment with flumazenil in some patients has been effective. (See page 1080: Assessment of Hepatic Function.)

8. **E.**   Wilson disease is a hereditary disease characterized by decreased hepatocellular excretion of copper into bile and decreased binding of copper to ceruloplasm. This results in hepatic copper accumulation and hepatic injury. Wilson disease has an autosomal recessive pattern of inheritance. Hereditary hemachromatosis is a disease characterized by excessive iron absorption from the duodenum, with tissue deposition producing organ damage. Progression of the disease can be slowed by repeat phlebotomy. Established end-organ damage cannot be reversed. Primary biliary cirrhosis is an uncommon disease of the liver of unknown etiology. Genetic factors play a role in development but it is not in a simple dominant or recessive pattern. (See page 1098: Uncommon Causes of Cirrhosis.)

9. **C.**   Physical examination of the patient is particularly valuable because patients may appear ill before there is laboratory evidence of hepatic dysfunction. If no suspicion of liver dysfunction arises, then routine laboratory testing for liver function is not necessary. Regardless of cause, increased magnitude of liver dysfunction correlates with a higher morbidity and

mortality. Drugs administered to patients with advanced liver disease require careful titration. Encephalopathic changes are associated with clinically important alterations in pharmacodynamics and pharmacokinetics of various medications. Plasma clearance of fentanyl is significantly lower in cirrhotic patients. An increase in plasma concentrations of vasodilatory substances in cirrhotic patients results in reduced responses to catecholamines and other vasoconstrictors. (See page 1105: Induction of General Anesthesia and Maintenance of Anesthesia.)

10. **E.**   Clinical use of halothane should take into account the following concerns: Children rarely develop halothane hepatitis even after repeat exposure to the anesthetic. Adults rarely develop the disorder after a single exposure; a risk factor is repeated exposures to halothane over a brief period of time (<6 weeks), especially in middle-aged obese women. There is no reliable test for detecting halothane hepatitis or susceptibility to the disease. Halothane decreases hepatic blood flow and oxygen supply and often causes mild transient liver injury. (See page 1085: Toxic Acute Hepatitis and Volatile Anesthetics.)

11. **E.**   Dose requirements for a variety of medications can be unpredictable because of substantial alterations in pharmacokinetics. Volume of distribution of most nondepolarizing muscle relaxants is increased. Subsequent doses should be decreased owing to decreases in hepatic blood flow, hepatic clearance, and possible concurrent renal disease. It is prudent to avoid halothane and enflurane because they cause the most prominent decreases in hepatic blood and oxygen supply and are associated with the highest incidences of postoperative hepatic dysfunction. Patients with liver disease have a reduced sensitivity to vasopressor drugs. (See page 1073: Hepatic Anatomy.)

12. **B.**   Postoperative liver dysfunction is common but rarely severe. Although it is usually asymptomatic, it may progress to overt liver failure on rare occasions. Mild transient increases in hepatic enzymes can be detected after surgery but rarely persist after 2 days. Subclinical hepatocellular injury may occur in 20% of patients after enflurane anesthesia and in up to 50% of those receiving halothane. Jaundice rarely occurs in healthy patients after minor procedures, but it may occur in 20% of patients after major surgical procedures. Jaundice is typically the earliest sign of serious hepatic or hepatobiliary dysfunction. (See page 1091: Cirrhosis: A Paradigm for End-Stage Parenchymal Liver Disease.)

13. **A.**   Identifying patients at high risk of developing liver dysfunction or of having an exacerbation of liver disease is important for minimizing the morbidity and mortality of patients with liver disease. Patient outcome is optimized by understanding the

interactions of liver disease, surgical procedure, physiologic stress, and anesthetic intervention. This is particularly important in the patient undergoing a major surgical procedure. Any liver abnormalities detected preoperatively should necessitate delaying an elective surgical procedure. The addition of epidural analgesia to general anesthesia may decrease circulating catecholamine levels and mitigate the surgical stress response. The general anesthetic plan should include agents that preserve cardiac output and do not affect the oxygen supply-demand relationship of the liver. Splanchnic, hepatic, and renal perfusion should be preserved. (See page 1101: Hepatic Evaluation and Preparation.)

CHAPTER 40 ■ ANESTHESIA FOR ORTHOPAEDIC SURGERY

For questions 1 to 5, choose the best answer.

1. Which of the following statements regarding peripheral nerve block for the foot is TRUE?

   A. The saphenous, sural, and peroneal nerves are branches of the femoral nerve, which may be blocked at the knee level.
   B. Surgery using tourniquets must be limited to 90 minutes.
   C. Induction or "setup" time may be reduced compared with an intrathecal injection.
   D. Clonidine may be used to prolong surgical anesthesia.
   E. Prolonged block may delay postanesthesia care unit and hospital discharge times.

2. All of the following apply to microvascular surgery EXCEPT:

   A. Phenylephrine should be avoided when correcting the perfusion pressure of a severed limb.
   B. Maintenance of blood flow through anastomoses can be achieved with vasodilators and increasing the perfusion pressure.
   C. Dextran and papaverine can be used to preserve the blood flow.
   D. An epidural catheter placement can improve the perfusion.
   E. Hypothermia can have a deleterious effect.

3. Which of the following statements regarding patients with scoliosis is TRUE?

   A. Scoliosis that requires surgery is usually the result of a neuromuscular disorder.
   B. Resting hypercapnia is the best indicator of the need for postoperative ventilatory support.
   C. They can have associated cyanotic heart disease.
   D. They should be managed with hemodilution or controlled hypotension, but never both.

   E. Moderate, controlled, hypotension is complicated by thrombosis and therefore is not usually beneficial.

4. Which of the following statements regarding neurophysiologic monitoring is TRUE?

   A. Motor-evoked potentials are commonly monitored during spine surgery.
   B. The anesthetic technique of choice when motor-evoked potentials are being monitored is a nitrous-narcotic-relaxant technique.
   C. Somatosensory-evoked potentials (SSEPs) monitor motor function only in those areas of the spinal cord supplied by the anterior spinal artery.
   D. A number of variables can alter SSEP waveforms including acute nerve injury, hypercarbia, hypoxia, and hypotension.
   E. Volatile anesthetics commonly produce a dose-related increase in SSEP amplitude.

5. Risk factors for fat embolism syndrome include all of the following EXCEPT:

   A. generally 20 to 40 years of age
   B. male gender
   C. disorders of lipid metabolism
   D. rheumatoid arthritis
   E. intramedullary instrumentation

For questions 6 to 15, choose A if 1, 2, and 3 are correct; B if 1 and 3; C if 2 and 4; D if 4; and E if all.

6. In conducting an anesthesia technique for orthopaedic hip surgery, the following should be taken into consideration:

   1. The traction table offers the advantages of easy hip manipulation and radiographic images.
   2. An epidural or intrathecal technique can be employed.

3. Using a regional technique can decrease the blood loss during surgery.
4. Calcium channel blockers as well as beta-blockers can be used for deliberate hypotension.

7. Which of the following statements regarding procedures for the upper extremity is/are TRUE?

   1. Regional anesthesia may reduce blood loss as well as lower the incidence of thromboembolism.
   2. Prolonged regional block often delays hospital discharge.
   3. Venous air embolism is uncommon.
   4. Neurapraxia is rare and occurs most commonly after axillary block.

8. Which of the following statements regarding infraclavicular block for surgery at the elbow is/are TRUE?

   1. It should be avoided in outpatients because of the risk of pneumothorax.
   2. Patients must have a postoperative chest radiograph to identify pneumothorax.
   3. It is most reliable for surgery about the proximal humerus.
   4. A pneumothorax of 10% should be treated with a chest tube.

9. Which of the following statements regarding continuous brachial plexus anesthesia using an indwelling catheter is/are TRUE?

   1. It may reduce postoperative vasospasm after limb replantation.
   2. It may be performed using interscalene, infraclavicular, or axillary techniques.
   3. It usually produces profound analgesia in four major nerve distributions.
   4. It reliably provides excellent surgical anesthesia when increased concentrations of local anesthetics are used.

10. Peripheral nerve blocks for surgery on the knee in which a tourniquet will be used must include:

    1. the femoral nerve
    2. the lateral femoral cutaneous nerve
    3. the sciatic nerve
    4. the obturator nerve

11. Which of the following statements regarding the use of regional anesthesia for orthopaedic surgery in children is/are TRUE?

    1. It carries the same advantages as for adults such as decreased nausea and vomiting and decreased time to discharge.

2. Regional techniques are readily adaptable and often underused.
3. Brachial plexus block can be facilitated with a nerve stimulator.
4. Regional techniques are often technically difficult to perform in the pediatric population.

12. Which of the following statements regarding patients with spinal shock is/are TRUE?

    1. They should never receive succinylcholine because of the potential for hyperkalemia.
    2. Hyperventilation and resultant hypocarbia can improve blood flow and "protect" an ischemic spinal cord tissue.
    3. Spinal shock is short-lived and usually improves in 24 to 48 hours.
    4. Spinal shock can mask ongoing hypovolemic shock.

13. Which of the following statements regarding a "wake-up test" is/are TRUE?

    1. Up to 20% of patients will have recall of the test.
    2. Patients who do experience recall frequently describe it as intensely painful.
    3. It is an accurate test with very few false-negative results.
    4. It can be safely and easily performed.

14. Which of the following statements regarding the use of limb tourniquets is/are TRUE?

    1. The tourniquet overlap should always be placed directly over the neurovascular bundle to reduce the likelihood of nerve injury.
    2. When selecting a tourniquet, the width of an inflated cuff should be greater than one-half of the limb diameter.
    3. Cuff pressure must be maintained at no less than 200 mm Hg more than the patient's systolic blood pressure.
    4. Tumor is a relative contraindication to the use of a limb tourniquet.

15. Which of the following statements is/are TRUE?

    1. The optimal treatment of a patient with suspected fat embolism syndrome includes stabilization of long bone fractures.
    2. Autonomic hyperreflexia occurs in approximately 20% of patients with high spinal cord injury.
    3. Nitrous oxide should be discontinued before the use of methyl methacrylate.
    4. Reduction of intraoperative blood pressure during total hip arthroplasty resulting from central neuraxial blockade probably does not reduce blood loss during total hip arthroplasty.

ANSWERS

1. **D.** Innervation of the foot is provided by the femoral nerve (via the saphenous nerve) and by the sciatic nerve (via the posterior tibial, sural, deep, and superficial peroneal nerves). Therefore, central neuraxial blockade and peripheral nerve blocks at the upper leg, knee, or ankle are appropriate regional anesthetic techniques for foot surgery. The selection of the regional technique is based on the surgical site, the use of a calf or thigh tourniquet, the degree of weight bearing or ambulation, and the need for postoperative analgesia. For example, inflation of a thigh tourniquet for >15 to 20 minutes necessitates a general or neuraxial anesthetic, regardless of surgical site. Often patients undergoing lower extremity peripheral techniques may be discharged directly from the operating room to the outpatient nursing station, thus reducing recovery time and charges. The use of long-acting local anesthetics and the addition of epinephrine or clonidine allow prolongation of postoperative analgesia. However, additional onset time is required with bupivacaine and ropivacaine. (See page 1121: Surgery to the Ankle and Foot.)

2. **A.** Microvascular surgery includes both replantation, the reattachment of a completely severed body part, and revascularization, the re-establishment of blood flow through a severed body part. Most replantation surgery involves the upper extremity. Blood flow may be improved by increasing the perfusion pressure, preventing hypothermia, and using vasodilators and sympathetic blockade. Microvascular perfusion pressure depends on both adequate intravascular volume and oncotic pressure. Evidence suggests that use of phenylephrine to support blood pressure does not jeopardize blood flow to the tissue being replanted. Body temperature is also a determinant of blood flow. Hypothermia not only results in peripheral vasoconstriction, but also causes sympathetic activation, shivering, increased oxygen demand, a leftward shift of the oxygen-hemoglobin dissociation curve, and altered coagulation. Therefore, hypothermia must be prevented in microvascular surgical patients. Regional anesthetic techniques provide sympathectomy and vasodilation to the proximal (innervated) segment of an extremity, but they have no effect on vasospasm in the replanted (denervated) tissue. Antithrombotics (heparin), fibrinolytics (streptokinase, urokinase, low-molecular-weight dextran), and smooth muscle relaxants (papaverine, local anesthetics) are also used to preserve blood flow in microvascular anastomoses. A combination of general and continuous regional anesthesia allows prolonged intraoperative anesthesia and postoperative analgesia, reduces the amount of inhalational agent, and increases the patient's acceptance of lengthy surgical procedures. However, regardless of anesthetic technique, conditions that stimulate vasospasm or vasoconstriction, such as pain, hypotension, and hypovolemia, should be avoided. (See page 1122: Microvascular Surgery.)

3. **C.** Idiopathic scoliosis represents 75 to 90% of scoliosis cases. The remaining 10 to 25% of cases are associated with neuromuscular diseases and congenital abnormalities including congenital heart disease, trauma, and mesenchymal disorders. Vital capacity appears to be a reliable prognostic indicator of perioperative respiratory reserve. Postoperative ventilation will most likely be required for patients with a vital capacity of <40% of predicted vital capacity. Scoliosis is also associated with congenital heart conditions, including mitral valve prolapse, coarctation, and cyanotic heart disease, suggesting a common embryonic insult or collagen defect. Normovolemic hemodilution combined with induced hypotension and autotransfusion can decrease or eliminate the need for homologous transfusion. Moderate induced hypotension (reduction of systolic pressure 20 mm Hg from baseline or lowering mean arterial pressure to 65 mm Hg in the normotensive patient) has been shown to decrease blood loss, reduce transfusion requirements by 50%, and shorten operating times. (See page 1114: Scoliosis.)

4. **D.** Although the use of motor-evoked potentials remains limited, SSEP monitoring is widely accepted. However, somatosensory stimulation follows the dorsal column pathways of proprioception and vibration, pathways supplied by the posterior spinal artery. The motor pathway, which is supplied by the anterior spinal artery, is not monitored. Motor-evoked potentials, conversely, monitor motor pathways but are technically more difficult to employ. Muscle relaxants cannot be used in patients having maximum expiratory pressure monitoring. It is critical to note that postoperative paraplegia has occurred in at least one patient with preserved SSEP monitoring intraoperatively.

   Numerous variables are known to alter SSEP waveforms. In addition to neural injury, SSEPs are altered by hypercarbia, hypoxia, hypotension, and hypothermia. All the volatile anesthetics produce a dose-related decrease in the amplitude and an increase in the latency of SSEPs. (See page 1116: Spinal Cord Monitoring.)

5. **C.** Fat embolism syndrome is associated with multiple traumatic injuries and surgery involving long bone fractures. Risk factors include male gender and age (20–30 years), hypovolemic shock, intramedullary instrumentation, rheumatoid arthritis, cemented total hip arthroplasty, and bilateral total knee surgery. The incidence of fat embolism syndrome in isolated long bone fractures is 3 to 4%, and mortality associated

with this condition is significant, 10 to 20%.
(See page 1124: Fat Embolus Syndrome.)

6. **E.**   The lateral decubitus position is frequently used
to facilitate surgical exposure for total hip
replacement, whereas the fracture table is often used
for repair of femur fractures. In transferring the
patient from the supine to lateral decubitus position,
care must be taken to maintain the patient's head and
shoulders in a neutral position. The fracture table
affords two advantages: maintenance of traction on
the fractured extremity, allowing manipulation for
closed reduction and fixation; and access to the
fracture site for radiography in several planes. The
patient must be carefully monitored for hemodynamic
changes during positioning, whether under regional or
general anesthesia. Regional anesthetic techniques are
well suited to procedures involving the hip. Central
neuraxial blockade, including spinal and epidural
blockade, is commonly used. Both hypobaric and
isobaric spinal anesthetic solutions are effective.
Epidural blockade also provides excellent surgical
anesthesia; it allows for prolonged anesthesia as well
as postoperative analgesia. Regional anesthetic
techniques reduce blood loss in patients undergoing
hip surgery. Deliberate hypotension can also be used
with general anesthesia as a means of reducing
surgical blood loss. Diltiazem, nitroprusside with and
without captopril, beta-blockers, and nitroglycerin
have also been used to induce hypotension. (See page
1119: Surgery to the Hip.)

7. **B.**   Regional anesthetics offer several advantages over
general anesthetics in patients undergoing orthopaedic
procedures including improved postoperative
analgesia, decreased incidence of nausea and
vomiting, less respiratory and cardiac depression,
improved perfusion via sympathetic block, reduced
blood loss, and decreased risk of thromboembolism.
Although prolonged blockade of the lower extremities
will interfere with ambulation and therefore delay
outpatient discharge, persistent upper extremity block
is not a contraindication to hospital discharge.
Theoretically, venous air embolism may occur during
surgical procedures to the shoulder because the
operative site is higher than the heart; however, this
complication has not been reported in the literature.
Four percent of patients undergoing total shoulder
arthroplasty have a documented postoperative
neurologic deficit, including 3% of patients with
injury to the brachial plexus. The level of injury is at
the level of the nerve trunks, which is the level at
which an interscalene block is performed, making it
impossible to determine the origin of the nerve injury
(surgical versus anesthetic). Most of these nerve
injuries represent a neurapraxia; 90% will resolve in
3 to 4 months. (See page 1118: Surgery to the Upper
Extremities.)

8. **B.**   Surgical procedures to the distal humerus, elbow,
and forearm are commonly performed using regional

anesthetic techniques. Infraclavicular and
supraclavicular approaches to the brachial plexus are
the most reliable and provide consistent anesthesia to
the four major nerves of the brachial plexus: median,
ulnar, radial, and musculocutaneous. However, the
small but definite risk of pneumothorax associated
with supraclavicular and infraclavicular blocks makes
this approach unsuitable for outpatient procedures.
Typically, the pneumothorax becomes evident 6 to
12 hours after hospital discharge. Therefore, a
postoperative chest radiograph is not helpful.
Although chest tube placement is advised for
pneumothorax >20% of lung volume, the lung may
also be re-expanded with a small Teflon catheter under
fluoroscopic guidance, thus eliminating the need for
hospital admission. The axillary approach to the
brachial plexus eliminates the risk of pneumothorax
and reliably provides adequate anesthesia for surgery
near the elbow. (See page 1119: Surgery to the
Elbow.)

9. **A.**   A continuous infusion of local anesthetic
solution, such as bupivacaine 0.125%, prevents
vasospasm and increases circulation after limb
replantation or vascular repair. More concentrated
solutions of bupivacaine result in complete sensory
block and allow early joint mobilization after painful
surgical procedures to the elbow. Brachial plexus
catheters may be inserted using interscalene,
infraclavicular, and axillary approaches. However, the
axillary approach is most common. Although
analgesia is produced in all nerve distributions, the
block may not provide satisfactory surgical
anesthesia, even with administration of more potent
local anesthetic solutions. Therefore, for surgical
procedures, the continuous brachial plexus block is
often supplemented with a general anesthetic.
(See page 1119: Continuous Brachial Plexus
Anesthesia.)

10. **E.**   Surgical anesthesia for operative procedures on
the knee where a tourniquet will be used requires
blockade of all four nerves (femoral, lateral femoral
cutaneous, obturator, and sciatic) that innervate the
leg. (See page 1120: Total Knee Arthroplasty.)

11. **A.**   Pediatric patients present with a variety of
orthopaedic conditions, including congenital
deformities, traumatic injuries, infections, and
malignancies. Anesthetic management of the pediatric
orthopaedic patient involves not only the usual
pediatric patient considerations, such as airway
management, fluid replacement, and maintenance of
body temperature, but also the unique concerns
associated with orthopaedic surgery. Often regional
anesthetic procedures are technically easier to perform
on children because the relative lack of subcutaneous
tissue facilitates both identification of bony and
vascular landmarks and spread of local anesthetic.
The advantages of regional anesthesia in children
are similar to those in adults and include earlier

ambulation and hospital discharge, decreased incidence of nausea and vomiting, and prolonged postoperative analgesia. However, pediatric patients are often not considered candidates for regional techniques. Neural blockade may be initiated after induction of general anesthesia and before surgical incision, to provide possible pre-emptive analgesia, or on completion of the surgical procedure, to extend the duration of postoperative analgesia. Blockade of the brachial plexus is usually accomplished with perivascular, sheath, or nerve stimulator techniques in children <7 years of age because elicitation of paresthesias is regarded as uncomfortable (and therefore unacceptable) by the younger pediatric patients. (See page 1122: Pediatric Orthopaedic Surgery.)

12. **D.**   In spinal shock, hyperventilation should be avoided because hypocarbia decreases spinal cord blood flow. Spinal shock may persist from a few days to 3 months. It is usually safe to administer succinylcholine for the first 48 hours. Spinal shock can mask underlying hypovolemic shock. (See page 1114: Maintaining Spinal Cord Integrity.)

13. **B.**   If there is satisfactory movement of the hands, but not the feet, the distraction on the rod is released one notch, and the "wake-up test" is repeated. Increasing the blood pressure and blood volume may be attempted to increase spinal cord perfusion. Recall of the event occurs in 0 to 20% of patients and is rarely viewed as unpleasant. It is important to describe what will transpire to the patient preoperatively so anxiety will be minimized should the patient be fully aware. The "wake-up test" is associated with few false-negative results; that is, it is extremely rare for a patient who was neurologically intact when awakened intraoperatively to have a neurologic deficit upon completion of the procedure. However, certain hazards of the "wake-up test" do exist and include recall, pain, air embolism, dislocation of spinal instrumentation, and accidental tracheal extubation or removal of intravenous and arterial lines. In addition, the "wake-up test" requires patient cooperation and may be difficult to perform on young children or mentally deficient patients. (See page 1116: Spinal Cord Monitoring.)

14. **C.**   The cuff should be large enough to circle the limb comfortably to ensure uniform pressure. The point of overlap should be placed 180 degrees from the neurovascular bundle, because there is some area of decreased compression at the overlap point. The width of the inflated cuff should be greater than one-half of the limb diameter. Pressure is usually maintained by compressed gas (air or oxygen) and must be monitored continually while the tourniquet is in use. Before tourniquet inflation, the limb should be elevated for about 1 minute and tightly wrapped with an elastic bandage distally to proximally to ensure exsanguination. Limb tourniquets are relatively contraindicated when there is infection or tumor. Opinions differ as to the pressure required in tourniquets to prevent bleeding. Leg tourniquets are often pressurized more than arm tourniquets, on the theory that larger limbs require more pressure than smaller limbs. In general, a cuff pressure of 100 mm Hg above a patient's measured systolic pressure is adequate for the thigh, and 50 mm Hg above systolic pressure is adequate for the arm, with the understanding that if hypertensive episodes occur, the cuff pressure should be increased. (See page 1123: Tourniquets.)

15. **B.**   Appropriate treatment of fat embolism syndrome requires early surgical stabilization of fracture sites, aggressive respiratory support, and reversal of possible aggravating factors (e.g., hypovolemia). After recovery from spinal shock, 85% of patients will exhibit autonomic hyperreflexia when there has been complete cord transection above T5. The syndrome is characterized by severe paroxysmal hypertension with bradycardia, arrhythmias, and cutaneous vasoconstriction below and vasodilation above the level of the injury. Methyl methacrylate is often injected under pressure, and it is theorized that air embolism may be one of the causes of hypotension that can accompany injection of cement. Nitrous oxide thus should be discontinued several minutes before this point. Multiple studies have demonstrated reduced intraoperative blood loss during total hip arthroplasty completed under central neuraxial blockade as compared with general anesthesia. (See page 1119: Surgery to the Lower Extremities; page 1114: Autonomic Hyperreflexia; page 1124: Fat Embolus Syndrome; and Methyl Methacrylate.)

CHAPTER 41 ■ ANESTHESIA AND THE ENDOCRINE SYSTEM

For questions 1 to 9, choose the best answer.

1. Which of the following patients would not be hyperthyroid?

   A. A patient with elevated thyroxine (T_4) and elevated T_4-binding globulin levels
   B. A patient with elevated T_4 and elevated triiodothyronine (T_3)
   C. A patient with elevated T_4 and normal T_3
   D. A patient with elevated T_4 and low T_4-binding globulin
   E. A patient with normal T_4-binding globulin and elevated T_3

2. Which of the following statements regarding the uptake of radioactive iodine by the thyroid gland is FALSE?

   A. Radioactive iodine uptake (RAIU) is elevated in hyperthyroidism.
   B. RAIU is decreased in cases of hyperthyroidism caused by thyroiditis.
   C. RAIU is increased by dietary deficiency of iodine.
   D. RAIU will increase with corticosteroid use.
   E. No uptake of radioactive iodine may indicate thyroid malignancy.

3. Patients with mild to moderate hypothyroidism:

   A. are at significant risk of perioperative congestive heart failure
   B. can be anesthetized safely without preoperative thyroid supplementation
   C. should have urgent thyroid replacement before surgery if there is a history of coronary artery disease
   D. are very sensitive to the effects of anesthetic drugs
   E. are at significant risk of postoperative ventilatory failure

4. Which of the following will increase ionized serum calcium?

   A. Elevated serum albumin
   B. Alkalosis
   C. Acute hypomagnesemia
   D. Hypoparathyroidism
   E. Acute hyperphosphatemia

5. TRUE statements about perioperative steroid replacement in patients who have received steroids include:

   A. Steroid replacement is not necessary with subarachnoid block or deep general anesthesia.
   B. Steroid replacement always should be given in supraphysiologic doses.
   C. Steroid replacement is not necessary if patients already are steroid dependent.
   D. Steroid replacement in a low-dose regimen has been shown to be ineffective for most patients.
   E. There is no proven optimal regimen for steroid replacement in the perioperative period.

6. Which of the following statements regarding pheochromocytoma is TRUE?

   A. Pheochromocytoma is a common adrenal cortical malignancy.
   B. Pheochromocytoma is a common cause of primary hypertension.
   C. Cardiovascular effects from pheochromocytoma are treated easily with deep anesthesia.
   D. Pheochromocytomas are not directly innervated, and catecholamine release is random.
   E. Pheochromocytoma is diagnosed easily and reliably by measurement of free catecholamines in the urine.

7. Which of the following statements regarding the perioperative anesthetic management of the patient with pheochromocytoma is TRUE?

A. Patients who present with normotension will not require preoperative alpha-adrenergic blocking agents.
B. Patients who present with normotension may be easily managed on an outpatient basis until the time of surgery.
C. If alpha-adrenergic blocking agents have not been instituted before surgery, no special anesthetic induction technique is necessary.
D. Although there is no clear advantage to one anesthetic technique over another, halothane should be avoided.
E. Invasive monitoring is not required for patients whose blood pressure has been well controlled preoperatively.

8. Which of the following statements regarding type 1 diabetes mellitus is TRUE?

A. Patients usually have normal insulin levels and significant insulin resistance in peripheral tissues.
B. Patients often are treated with diet alone.
C. Patients frequently are obese.
D. Patients are prone to ketoacidosis.
E. End-organ damage is rare.

9. Which of the following statements regarding insulin is TRUE?

A. The normal adult pancreas produces 200 to 300 U of insulin/day.
B. The half-life of human insulin is 90 minutes.
C. Hepatic dysfunction will increase circulating insulin levels.
D. Vagal stimulation will decrease circulating insulin levels.
E. alpha-Adrenergic stimulation will increase circulating insulin levels.

For questions 10 to 25, choose A if 1, 2, and 3 are correct; B if 1 and 3; C if 2 and 4; D if 4; and E if all.

10. Which of the following would be appropriate in the preoperative preparation of a patient with Graves disease?

1. Administration of potassium iodide for 7 to 14 days preoperatively
2. A short-term course of T_4 supplementation
3. Administration of propranolol for 1 week preoperatively
4. Administration of propylthiouracil for 3 days preoperatively

11. Which of the following statements regarding hypoparathyroidism is/are TRUE?

1. The cardiovascular manifestations are shortened QT interval and pericardial effusion.
2. Neuronal irritability may cause seizures and muscle tetany.

3. Trousseau sign usually is positive, and Chvostek sign usually is negative.
4. Acute hypoparathyroidism may manifest as stridor and/or apnea.

12. Which of the following statements regarding Cushing syndrome is/are TRUE?

1. Most cases occur secondary to bilateral adrenal hyperplasia.
2. Cushing syndrome usually represents adrenal adenocarcinoma when it occurs in older patients.
3. Twenty-five percent of cases are caused by adrenal neoplasm.
4. Cushing syndrome may occur iatrogenically from steroid treatment of chronic illness.

13. Which of the following statements with respect to patients with Addison disease is/are TRUE?

1. The predominant cause of Addison disease is autoimmune destruction of the adrenal gland.
2. Patients with secondary forms of Addison disease always are hyperpigmented.
3. Treatment includes replacement of mineralocorticoids.
4. Diagnosis is confirmed by an increased adrenal response to adrenocorticotropic hormone (ACTH).

14. Which of the following statements regarding acute adrenal insufficiency is/are TRUE?

1. It rarely, if ever, occurs in the perioperative period.
2. Treatment consists of fluid and electrolyte resuscitation, as well as steroid replacement.
3. Usually it requires continued steroid therapy for 4 to 6 weeks following the acute event.
4. It may require the use of inotropes and invasive monitoring despite aggressive steroid treatment.

15. Hypoaldosteronism:

1. may be defined as failure to increase aldosterone production in response to ACTH
2. commonly occurs in patients with mild renal failure and long-standing diabetes mellitus
3. commonly presents with life-threatening hypokalemia and hypotension
4. may be treated adequately with furosemide alone in the patient with congestive heart failure

16. Which of the following statements regarding the preoperative preparation of the patient with pheochromocytoma is/are TRUE?

1. Preoperative preparation usually is unnecessary if deep opioid anesthesia is planned.
2. Preoperative treatment for 10 to 14 days with phenoxybenzamine is advocated by most clinicians.
3. Preoperative treatment usually is started with beta-adrenergic blocking drugs to avoid reflex tachycardia when alpha-blocking drugs are added.
4. Prazosin is a shorter acting alpha-blocking agent that may be used in place of phenoxybenzamine.

17. Which of the following statements regarding the pharmacologic therapy for pheochromocytoma is/are TRUE?

    1. Acute hypertensive crises are best treated with short-acting drugs, such as sodium nitroprusside, esmolol, and phentolamine.
    2. Labetalol, a combination alpha- and beta-adrenergic antagonist, is an excellent second-line therapy.
    3. alpha-Methyltyrosine is an agent used for reduction of catecholamine biosynthesis in situations in which surgery is contraindicated.
    4. Adrenergic blocking agents should not be given to pregnant patients.

18. Which of the following are potential causes of diabetes mellitus?

    1. Cystic fibrosis
    2. Pancreatic surgery
    3. Pheochromocytoma
    4. Cushing disease

19. Which of the following options may be acceptable in the perioperative management of patients with diabetes mellitus?

    1. Maintain a continuous intravenous infusion of insulin.
    2. Give half the usual insulin dose preoperatively.
    3. Give insulin intraoperatively based on the level of measured glucose level.
    4. Give no insulin.

20. Which of the following statements regarding nonketotic hyperosmolar coma is/are TRUE?

    1. Patients often present with extremely high blood sugar concentrations.
    2. It usually occurs in "brittle" diabetics.
    3. Cerebral edema may result in delayed recovery of mental status.
    4. The mainstay of treatment is high-dose intravenous insulin by continuous infusion.

21. Which of the following statements regarding patients with diabetic ketoacidosis is/are TRUE?

    1. The serum potassium level always will be low.
    2. Total body potassium level always will be low.
    3. With appropriate treatment, the serum potassium level will tend to rise toward the normal range.
    4. All patients with ketoacidosis, except those with acute renal failure, should be given intravenous potassium supplementation.

22. Hypoglycemia in the patient undergoing general anesthesia:

    1. is diagnosed easily by recognition of the usual signs and symptoms
    2. causes effects that are misinterpreted as light anesthesia
    3. rarely occurs in diabetic patients who receive insulin perioperatively
    4. occurs more commonly in diabetic patients with renal insufficiency

23. Which of the following statements regarding the posterior pituitary is/are TRUE?

    1. It is composed of terminal nerve endings that extend from the ventral hypothalamus.
    2. It secretes vasopressin.
    3. It secretes antidiuretic hormone (ADH).
    4. It secretes oxytocin.

24. Which of the following statements regarding vasopressin is/are TRUE?

    1. It promotes the reabsorption of sodium from the thick ascending limb of the loop of Henle.
    2. Serum levels decrease with increasing osmolality.
    3. It functions to relax vascular smooth muscle.
    4. It may be used in the treatment of von Willebrand disease.

25. Which of the following statements regarding diabetes insipidus is/are TRUE?

    1. It can occur following intracranial trauma.
    2. Urine output is highly concentrated.
    3. Symptoms include polydipsia.
    4. There is an excessive secretion of ADH.

ANSWERS

1. **A.** Elevations in T_4-binding globulin concentration are the most common cause of hyperthyroxinemia in the euthyroid patient. Elevations of T_4, T_3, or both in the presence of an elevated thyroid hormone binding rate all indicate hyperthyroidism. (See page 1130: Tests of Thyroid Function.)

2. **D.** Radioactive iodine generally is taken up by normal functioning thyroid tissue. Uptake is under the control of thyroid-stimulating hormone, and factors that decrease thyroid-stimulating hormone, such as corticosteroid use, will decrease RAIU. Hyperfunctioning thyroid tissue will increase RAIU activity, whereas malignant or nonfunctioning tissue

will decrease RAIU. (See page 1131: Radioactive Iodine Uptake.)

3. **B.** Several studies have shown that patients with mild to moderate hypothyroidism may be anesthetized safely without preoperative supplementation and are not at an increased risk of perioperative complications. Patients with a history of coronary artery disease or unstable angina may have symptoms precipitated by supplementation with T_4, and they should have replacement delayed until the postoperative period. (See page 1133: Treatment and Anesthetic Considerations.)

4. **C.** Acute hypomagnesemia causes an increase in parathyroid hormone release and a rise in serum ionized calcium. An increase in serum albumin levels will increase the total serum calcium, as well as calcium binding, and subsequently results in a lowered free or ionized calcium level. Acute hyperphosphatemia and alkalosis lower ionized calcium. (See page 1134: Calcium Physiology.)

5. **E.** Because acute adrenal crisis is life-threatening and because there is relatively little risk in providing steroid coverage for isolated periods of stress, most clinicians empirically administer supplemental steroids to all patients who have received steroid replacement for 1 to 2 weeks during the previous 6 to 12 months. There is no proven optimal regimen for perioperative steroid replacement. A low-dose regimen (125 mg hydrocortisone in 24 hours) has been shown to be equally effective when compared with the more traditional use of supraphysiologic doses. (See page 1140: Steroid Replacement During the Perioperative Period.)

6. **D.** Pheochromocytoma is the only important disease process associated with the adrenal medulla. These tumors, which are not innervated directly, produce, store, and secrete catecholamines. Although pheochromocytomas occur in <1% of hypertensive patients, it is important to evaluate the patient with clinically suspected symptoms aggressively, because surgical excision is curative in >90% of patients. Most deaths in patients with pheochromocytoma are from cardiovascular causes. Malignant spread occurs in approximately 10% of cases. The most common screening tests are measurements of catecholamine metabolites, vanillylmandelic acid, and unconjugated norepinephrine in the urine. However, urinary levels are not always elevated to a significant degree. (See page 1142: Pheochromocytoma.)

7. **D.** Occasionally, a patient with pheochromocytoma may present without hypertension. These patients are noted to be difficult to manage on an outpatient basis because of the fear of clinically significant orthostatic hypotension with alpha-blockade therapy. Because of the unpredictable and potentially lethal nature of the patient's response to the stress of anesthesia and surgery, all patients presenting for pheochromocytoma surgery should receive preoperative alpha-blocking therapy. When this is not possible, sodium nitroprusside infusions often are initiated in anticipation of the marked blood pressure elevations that can occur with laryngoscopy and surgical stimulation. Although there is no clear advantage of any one anesthetic technique, drugs that are known to liberate histamine are avoided. Halothane is also avoided because it sensitizes the myocardium to catecholamines and predisposes to ventricular irritability. Invasive monitors are used in most adult patients. (See page 1144: Perioperative Anesthetic Management.)

8. **D.** Diabetes often is divided into two broad types: type 1, or insulin-dependent diabetes mellitus; and type 2, or non–insulin-dependent diabetes mellitus. Patients with type 1 diabetes typically experience the onset of disease in early life. Consequently, this form also is referred to as juvenile-onset diabetes. Generally, the patient with type 1 diabetes is not obese, has an abrupt onset of the disease, and has very low levels of circulating insulin. Treatment in these patients requires insulin. Patients with type 1 disease are prone to become ketotic and are likely to develop end-organ complications of diabetes. (See page 1144: Diabetes Mellitus.)

9. **C.** Insulin is metabolized in the liver and the kidney. In patients with hepatic dysfunction, the loss of gluconeogenesis and the prolongation of insulin effect increase the risk of hypoglycemia. Normal production of insulin in the adult human is equivalent to 40 to 50 U per day. The half-life of insulin in the circulation is only a few minutes. Insulin release is related to a number of events. First, and most important, is the direct effect of glucose to stimulate insulin release. The mechanism involves interaction with hormones from the gastrointestinal tract released during enteral feeding. An increase in insulin release occurs by vagal stimulation. Insulin release is also caused by beta-adrenergic stimulation blockade. (See page 1145: Physiology.)

10. **B.** The combination of propranolol and potassium iodide every 8 hours for 7 to 14 days can be used to ameliorate cardiovascular symptoms and to reduce the circulating concentration of T_4 and T_3. Although propylthiouracil also is an effective treatment, it would require 6 to 8 weeks to render the patient euthyroid. Patients with Graves disease already have elevated levels of T_4 and should not be given T_4 supplements. (See page 1132: Treatment and Anesthetic Consideration.)

11. **C.** The clinical features of hypoparathyroidism result from hypocalcemia. Neuronal irritability and skeletal muscle spasms, tetany, or seizures reflect a reduced threshold of excitation. Chvostek sign is a contracture of the facial muscle produced by tapping the facial

nerve. Trousseau sign is contraction of the fingers and wrist following application of a blood pressure cuff inflated above the systolic pressure for approximately 3 minutes. Both Chvostek sign and Trousseau sign are indicative of hypocalcemia. The acute onset of hypocalcemia following thyroid or parathyroid surgery may manifest itself as stridor and apnea. (See page 1136: Clinical Features and Treatment.)

12. **E.** Cushing syndrome may be caused either by overproduction of cortisol by the adrenal cortex or by exogenous glucocorticoid therapy. Most cases of Cushing syndrome that occur spontaneously result from bilateral adrenal hyperplasia secondary to ACTH production by an anterior pituitary microadenoma. The primary overproduction of cortisol is caused by an adrenal neoplasm in 20 to 25% of patients. When Cushing syndrome occurs in patients older than 60 years, the most likely causes are adrenal adenocarcinoma or ectopic ACTH produced from a nonendocrine tumor. An increasingly common cause of Cushing syndrome is the prolonged administration of exogenous glucocorticoids used to treat various illnesses. (See page 1137: Glucocorticoid Excess [Cushing Syndrome].)

13. **B.** Addison disease results from a lowered secretion of adrenal cortical hormones. At present, the most frequent cause of Addison disease is autoimmune destruction of the adrenal gland. Primary Addison disease causes hyperpigmentation as ACTH levels rise in response to low cortisol levels. Secondary forms of the disease result from low levels of ACTH, and these patients are never hyperpigmented. The diagnosis of primary adrenal insufficiency is unequivocally confirmed by the failure of the adrenal gland to respond to exogenously administered ACTH. Treatment of the disease involves glucocorticoid (e.g., prednisone or hydrocortisone) and mineralocorticoid (e.g., fludrocortisone) replacement. (See page 1139: Adrenal Insufficiency.)

14. **C.** Acute adrenal insufficiency usually is precipitated by sepsis, trauma, or surgical stress. Immediate therapy is mandatory regardless of cause and consists of fluid and electrolyte resuscitation and steroid replacement. Steroid replacement is continued during the first 24 hours, and if the patient is stable, the steroid dose reduction begins on the second day. If the patient continues to be hemodynamically unstable following adequate fluid resuscitation, inotropic support and invasive monitoring may be necessary. (See page 1139: Treatment and Anesthetic Considerations.)

15. **C.** Mineralocorticoid insufficiency may occur for various reasons and is seen commonly in patients with mild renal failure and long-standing diabetes. It results from a failure to increase aldosterone production in response to salt restriction or volume contraction. Most patients present with hypotension,

hyperkalemia that may be life-threatening, and metabolic acidosis (as a result of impaired sodium and potassium exchange). Patients may be treated with mineralocorticoid replacement. An alternative approach in patients with pre-existing hypertension or congestive heart failure may involve the administration of furosemide alone or in combination with mineralocorticoid. (See page 1141: Mineralocorticoid Insufficiency.)

16. **C.** A dramatic reduction in perioperative mortality has been achieved with the introduction of alpha-antagonists preoperatively. Beta-adrenergic blockade is often added after alpha-blockade has been established. Beta-blockers should not be given until adequate alpha-blockade is achieved to avoid the possibility of unopposed alpha-mediated vasoconstriction. Phenoxybenzamine is a long-acting, noncompetitive, presynaptic alpha$_2$- and postsynaptic alpha$_1$-blocker. Prazosin is a postsynaptic alpha$_1$-blocking agent with a shorter half-life than that of phenoxybenzamine. Both drugs have been used successfully in the preoperative preparation of pheochromocytoma patients. (See page 1143: Anesthetic Considerations.)

17. **A.** Acute hypertensive crises are best treated with intravenous infusions of short-acting drugs. This would include phentolamine, nitroprusside, and esmolol. Labetalol is a beta-antagonist with alpha-blocking activity; it is an effective second-line medication. alpha-Methyltyrosine is an agent that inhibits the enzyme, tyrosine hydroxylase, which is the rate-limiting step in catecholamine biosynthesis. This medication currently is reserved for patients with metastatic disease or in whom surgery is contraindicated. Unrecognized pheochromocytoma during pregnancy may be life-threatening to the mother and the fetus. Although the safety of adrenergic blocking agents during pregnancy has not been established, these agents probably improve fetal survival. (See page 1143: Anesthetic Considerations.)

18. **E.** Diabetes can be a secondary result of a disease that damages the pancreas. Examples include pancreatic surgery, chronic pancreatitis, cystic fibrosis, and hemochromatosis. Diabetes also can result from one of the endocrine diseases that produce a hormone that opposes the action of insulin. Examples of this include glucagonoma, pheochromocytoma, and acromegaly. An increased effect of glucocorticoids either from Cushing disease or from steroid therapy also may oppose the effect of insulin and may thereby elicit clinical diabetes. (See page 1144: Classification.)

19. **E.** There is no consensus about the optimal way to manage perioperative metabolic changes in diabetic patients. For some diabetic patients, the best method of management is to give no insulin. For short procedures in nonstressed patients, particularly if they are not receiving insulin on a long-term basis, there

may be enough endogenous production of insulin to maintain a reasonable glucose balance in the unfed state. (See page 1147: Management Regimens.)

20. **B.** An occasional elderly patient with minimal or mild diabetes may present with remarkably high blood glucose levels and profound dehydration. Such patients usually have enough endogenous insulin activity to prevent ketosis. Marked hyperosmolarity may lead to coma and seizures with increased plasma viscosity, producing a tendency to intravascular thrombosis. It is characteristic of this syndrome that the metabolic disturbance responds quickly to rehydration and small doses of insulin. With rapid correction of hyperosmolarity, cerebral edema is a risk, and recovery of mental acuity may be delayed after the blood glucose level and circulating volume have been normalized. (See page 1147: Hyperosmolar Nonketotic Coma.)

21. **C.** Potassium replacement is a key concern in patients with diabetic ketoacidosis. Because of the hyperglycemia-induced osmotic diuresis, the total body's potassium stores are reduced. However, acidosis by itself causes a shift of potassium ions out of the cell. Thus, the serum potassium concentration may be normal or even slightly elevated while the patient remains acidotic. As soon as the metabolic acidosis is corrected, the potassium ions shift back into cells. Consequently, the serum potassium concentration can decline acutely. Therefore, early and vigorous potassium replacement is required in these patients. (Patients with renal failure are an exception.) (See page 1147: Diabetic Ketoacidosis.)

22. **C.** Hypoglycemia is the clinical occurrence most feared when dealing with diabetic patients and is almost impossible to diagnose in the unconscious patient. With hypoglycemia, there is a reflex catecholamine release that produces overt sympathetic hyperactivity, causing tachycardia, diaphoresis, and hypertension. In the anesthetized patient, the signs of sympathetic hyperactivity can be misinterpreted as inadequate or light anesthesia. Hypoglycemia is more likely to occur in the diabetic surgical patient with renal insufficiency in whom the action of insulin and oral hypoglycemic agents may be prolonged. An avoidable cause of inadvertent hypoglycemia is the administration of insulin to a patient who is not receiving sufficient caloric input. (See page 1148: Hypoglycemia.)

23. **E.** The posterior pituitary, or neurohypophysis, is composed of terminal nerve endings that extend from the ventral hypothalamus. The two hormones it secretes are vasopressin (also called ADH) and oxytocin. (See page 1149: Posterior Pituitary.)

24. **D.** ADH (also called vasopressin because it constricts vascular smooth muscle) promotes reabsorption of free water by increasing the cell membrane's permeability to water. The target sites for ADH are the collecting tubules of the kidneys. The primary stimulus for ADH release is an increase in serum osmolality. ADH may also promote hemostasis through an increase in the level of circulating von Willebrand factor. (See page 1149: Vasopressin.)

25. **B.** Diabetes insipidus results from inadequate secretion of ADH. Failure to secrete an adequate amount of ADH results in polydipsia, hypernatremia, and a high output of poorly concentrated urine. This disorder usually occurs following destruction of the pituitary gland by intracranial trauma, infiltrating lesions, or surgery. (See page 1149: Diabetes Insipidus.)

CHAPTER 42 ■ OBSTETRIC ANESTHESIA

1. Plasma volume and red cell volume increase by which of the following percentages in pregnancy?

   A. Plasma volume, 60%; red cell volume, 40%
   B. Plasma volume, 40%; red cell volume, 40%
   C. Plasma volume, 40%; red cell volume, 20%
   D. Plasma volume, 60%; red cell volume, 20%
   E. Plasma volume, 60%; red cell volume, 60%

2. Which of the following factors does not influence the placental transfer of drugs?

   A. Fetal osmolality
   B. The placental area
   C. Ionization of the drug
   D. Molecular weight
   E. Concentration in fetal blood

3. Which dermatomes are affected in the first stage of labor?

   A. Thoracic 5 to 10
   B. Sacral 2 to 4
   C. Thoracic 10 to lumbar 1
   D. Thoracic 12 to lumbar 2
   E. Thoracic 6 to lumbar 2

4. The most common side effect of neuraxial anesthesia for obstetrics is:

   A. meningitis
   B. decreased variability of fetal heart rate
   C. nausea and vomiting
   D. hypotension
   E. nerve-group damage

5. Considering regional anesthesia for cesarean section, which of the following is TRUE?

   A. Epidural is the most common regional technique.
   B. Prehydration is not necessary when using epidurals.
   C. Epidural anesthesia eliminates visceral discomfort during exteriorization of the uterus.

   D. Spinal drug doses should be carefully based on a patient's height.
   E. Epidural has the advantage of slower onset and controllability.

6. When considering anesthetic complications relating to cesarean section, which of the following is TRUE?

   A. Fatality with general anesthesia is 30 times greater than with regional anesthesia.
   B. There is no difference in hemodynamic stability between patients who receive epidural and spinal anesthesia.
   C. Phenylephrine should not be used to treat hypotension in the pregnant patient.
   D. The risk of pulmonary aspiration is greater in pregnant women thanty in nonpregnant women.
   E. The risk of hypotension with regional anesthesia is increased in women in labor compared with nonlaboring women.

7. The incidence of postdural puncture headache after dural puncture with a 25- or 26-gauge spinal needle in the pregnant woman is:

   A. 0%
   B. 1%
   C. 3%
   D. 5%
   E. 10%

8. Many of the symptoms associated with pre-eclampsia may result from an imbalance between the placental production of:

   A. renin and angiotensin
   B. endothelin and nitric oxide
   C. prostacyclin and thromboxane
   D. platelets and antithrombin III
   E. progesterone and estrogen

9. The greatest change in cardiac output in the pregnant patient occurs:

    A. during the second trimester
    B. after the delivery of the placenta
    C. during the third trimester
    D. during the first stage of labor
    E. during the second stage of labor

10. When considering fetal heart rate, which of the following is TRUE?

    A. The normal fetal heart rate equals 80 to 120 beats/minute.
    B. Acceleration of fetal heart rate in response to fetal stimulation is ominous.
    C. A fetal heart rate of <170 beats/minute can be caused by intravenous narcotics.
    D. Baseline variability of fetal heart rate can be affected by ephedrine.
    E. No good correlation exists between fetal acid-base status and baseline variability.

11. Normal fetal oxygen saturation is?

    A. 90 to 100%
    B. 50 to 100%
    C. 50 to 80%
    D. 30 to 70%
    E. 10 to 50%

12. The normal fetal scalp pH level is:

    A. >7.45
    B. 7.40 to 7.45
    C. 7.25 to 7.40
    D. 7.20 to 7.25
    E. <7.20

13. The peak pressure of the initial breath during neonatal resuscitation should be ____ cm H_2O?

    A. 10 to 15
    B. 15 to 20
    C. 20 to 30
    D. 30 to 40
    E. 40 to 50

14. The four major studies that relate surgery and anesthesia during pregnancy to fetal outcomes have found that:

    A. Both surgery and anesthesia can be correlated with congenital disorders and increased fetal death.
    B. Both surgery and anesthesia can be correlated with fetal death but not an increase in congenital disorders.
    C. Neither surgery nor anesthesia can be correlated with congenital disorders or an increase in fetal death.
    D. Surgery and anesthesia can be correlated with congenital disorders but not an increase in fetal death.

    E. Surgery and anesthesia are associated with a significant incidence of congenital disorders.

For questions 15 to 23, choose A if 1, 2, and 3 are correct; B if 1 and 3; C if 2 and 4; D if 4; and E if all.

15. Which of the following statements concerning lung volume changes during pregnancy is/are TRUE?

    1. Functional residual capacity decreases by 40%.
    2. Inspiratory reserve volume decreases.
    3. Expiratory reserve volume increases.
    4. Total lung capacity remains unchanged.

16. Considering a pregnant patient's response to anesthetic, which of the following is/are TRUE?

    1. Progesterone levels have no effect on minimum alveolar concentration.
    2. Lower doses of local anesthetics are needed per dermatomal segment for an epidural or spinal block.
    3. A decrease in minimum alveolar concentration is not seen until after 20 weeks' gestation.
    4. Pregnancy leads to increased neurosensitivity to local anesthetics.

17. Which of the following is/are side effects of systemic meperidine analgesia for labor?

    1. Decreased variability of the fetal heart rate
    2. Fetal bradycardia
    3. Neonatal depression
    4. Prolongation of the first stage of labor

18. Considering paracervical block, which of the following statements is/are TRUE?

    1. Paracervical block effectively relieves pain during the first stage of labor.
    2. Bupivacaine is the local anesthetic agent of choice.
    3. Paracervical block may cause uterine artery constriction.
    4. Paracervical block is safe for the fetus.

19. Which of the following would cause pre-eclampsia to be classified as severe?

    1. Intrauterine growth retardation
    2. Oliguria
    3. Systolic blood pressure of 170 mm Hg
    4. Epigastric pain

20. Which of the following statements is/are TRUE?

    1. Magnesium increases the duration of action of depolarizing muscle relaxants.
    2. Magnesium does not affect duration of action of nondepolarizing muscle relaxant.
    3. Magnesium decreases the amount of the acetylcholine liberated from motor nerve endings.
    4. Magnesium makes the end plate more sensitive to acetylcholine.

21. The side effects of terbutaline include which of the following?

    1. Hypertension
    2. Bronchospasm
    3. Hyperkalemia
    4. Pulmonary edema

22. When considering neonatal adaptations at birth, which of the following statements is/are TRUE?

    1. There is a dramatic decrease in pulmonary vascular resistance with increasing pulmonary arterial oxygen tension.

2. Functional closure of the ductus arteriosus occurs within hours to days.
3. Prompt expansion of the lungs is of primary importance.
4. The foramen ovale functionally closes almost immediately.

23. Nitrous oxide may affect DNA synthesis by affecting which of the following?

    1. Methionine synthetase
    2. Conversion of homocysteine to alanine
    3. Vitamin B_{12}
    4. Nitric oxide synthetase

ANSWERS

---

1. **C.** Increased mineralocorticoid activity during pregnancy produces sodium retention and increased body water content. Thus, plasma volume and total blood volume begin to increase in early gestation, resulting in a final increase of 40 to 50% and 25 to 40%, respectively, at term. The relatively smaller increase in red blood cell blood volume (20%) accounts for the reduction in hematocrit during pregnancy. (See page 1153: Hematologic Alterations.)

2. **A.** Drugs cross biological membranes by simple diffusion, the rate of which is determined by the Fick principle. The Fick equation is dependent on the diffusion constant of the drug, which depends on molecular size, lipid solubility, and degree of ionization. Other factors important in the Fick equation include surface area available for exchange or placental area, concentration of free drug in maternal blood, concentration of free drug in fetal blood, and thickness of the diffusion barrier. Most drugs commonly used by anesthesiologists have molecular weights of <500 and are easily transferred through the placenta. (See page 1154: Placental Transfer and Fetal Exposure to Anesthetic Drugs.)

3. **C.** In early labor, only the lower thoracic dermatomes T11 and T12 are affected, but with progressing cervical dilation and the transitional phase, adjacent dermatomes may be involved, and pain is referred from T10–L1. In the second stage of labor, additional pain impulses resulting from distention of the vaginal vault and perineum are carried by the pudendal nerve, which is composed of lower sacral fibers S2–S4. (See page 1158: Anesthesia for Labor and Vaginal Delivery.)

4. **D.** Hypotension resulting from sympathectomy is the most frequent complication that occurs with central neuraxial blockade. Therefore, maternal blood pressure must be monitored at regular intervals, typically 2 to 5 minutes for the first 20 minutes after

initiating the block. Meningitis is a rare complication of neuraxial anesthesia, as is nerve group damage. Nausea and vomiting may result from hypotension. Fetal heart rate variability is much less affected using neuraxial anesthesia when compared with intravenous anesthetics. (See page 1158: Regional Anesthesia.)

5. **E.** Subarachnoid or spinal block is the most commonly administered regional anesthetic technique for cesarean delivery because of its speed and reliability. Despite an adequate dermatomal level with either spinal or epidural anesthesia, women may experience varying degrees of visceral discomfort, particularly during exteriorization of the uterus and traction on abdominal viscera. Studies have shown that it is not necessary to adjust the drug based on the patient's height when using a spinal anesthetic. In contrast to spinal anesthesia, epidural anesthesia is associated with slower onset of action and more controllability. Prehydration is necessary when using either spinal or epidural anesthetics because sympathetic tone will be decreased and hypotension is a common side effect of neuraxial anesthesia. (See page 1160: Spinal Anesthesia.)

6. **D.** Regional anesthesia is commonly associated with hypotension, which is related to the rapidity of local anesthetic-induced sympatholysis. More hemodynamic stability is usually observed with epidural anesthesia. A recent study of anesthesia-related death in the United States (between 1979 and 1990) revealed that the case fatality rate with general anesthesia was 16.7 times greater than that of regional anesthesia. The risk of hypotension after regional anesthesia is lower in women who are in labor compared with nonlaboring women. In the presence of maternal tachycardia, phenylephrine 25 to 50 μg may be substituted for ephedrine (which is the first choice for treating hypotension in the pregnant patient). The risk of inhalation of gastric contents

(i.e., pulmonary aspiration) is increased in pregnant women compared with nonpregnant women. (See page 1163: Anesthetic Complications.)

7. **B.** The frequency of postdural puncture headache development is related to the diameter of the puncture needle, ranging from >70% following the use of a 16-gauge needle to <1% with a smaller 25- or 26-gauge spinal needle. The incidence of the headache is reduced with the use of atraumatic pencil-point needles (e.g., Whitaker or Sprotte needles). (See page 1163: Postdural Puncture Headache.)

8. **C.** Many of the symptoms associated with pre-eclampsia, including placental ischemia, systemic vasoconstriction, and increased platelet aggregation, may result from an imbalance between the placental production of prostacyclin and thromboxane. During normal pregnancy, the placenta produces equivalent quantities of these prostaglandins. During pre-eclamptic pregnancy, seven times more thromboxane than prostacyclin are present. (See page 1164: Pre-eclampsia–Eclampsia.)

9. **B.** During labor, cardiac output increases above antepartum levels. Between contractions, the cardiac output increases approximately 30% during the first stage and 45% during the second stage. The greatest change occurs immediately after delivery of the placenta, when cardiac output increases to an average of 80% above prepartum values. In some cases, it may increase by as much as 150%. (See page 1168: Heart Disease.)

10. **D.** The baseline fetal heart rate is measured between contractions and ranges from 120 to 160 beats/minute. An acceleration of fetal heart rate in response to fetal stimulation (e.g., during vaginal examination or fetal capillary blood sampling) is a reassuring sign that the fetus is not acidotic. Persistently elevated fetal heart rates may be associated with chronic fetal distress, maternal fever, or administration of drugs such as ephedrine and atropine. Fetal hypoxia and acidosis often lead to low fetal heart rates. The baseline fetal heart rate variability, which is normally present, reflects the beat-to-beat adjustments of parasympathetic and sympathetic nervous symptoms to various internal and external stimuli. Fetal central nervous system depression by asphyxia may decrease baseline variability. Therefore, a smooth fetal heart rate may be an ominous finding. Studies comparing beat-to-beat variability with fetal acid-base analysis indicate a good correlation between the two parameters. Ephedrine can increase heart rate variability. Intravenous narcotics can cause a slowing of the fetal heart rate. (See page 1170: Biophysical Monitoring.)

11. **D.** Fetal oxygen saturation between 30% and 70% is considered normal. Saturation readings consistently <30% for a prolonged period of time (i.e., 10–15 minutes) are suggestive of acidemia. Fetal blood scalp sampling and/or prompt obstetric intervention may be indicated. (See page 1171: Fetal Pulse Oximetry.)

12. **C.** Assessment of acid-base status of the fetus became possible in the 1960s with the development of fetal capillary blood sampling techniques. Blood is usually obtained from the scalp but may be sampled from a breech presentation. It is collected into a heparinized glass capillary tube, and pH, P_{CO_2}, P_{O_2}, and base deficit are determined immediately with an appropriate electrode system adapted to small sample size. A fetal capillary blood pH of 7.25 is the lowest limit of normal. A pH <7.20 indicates fetal acidosis. Values between 7.20 and 7.24 are considered preacidotic. (See page 1172: Biochemical Monitoring.)

13. **D.** Initial resuscitative methods include rubbing the back and slapping the neonate's feet. If these maneuvers produce no response and the baby remains apneic, ventilation should be instituted at a rate of 40 breaths/minute. The initial breath may require pressures of 30 to 40 cm H_2O. Subsequently, inflation pressure should be reduced to 15 to 20 cm H_2O in an infant with normal lungs. (See page 1174: Treatment of Moderately Depressed Infants.)

14. **B.** Four major studies attempted to relate surgery and anesthesia during human pregnancy to fetal outcome, as determined by anomalies, premature labor, or intrauterine death. Although they failed to correlate surgery and anesthetic exposure with congenital anomalies, all of them demonstrated an increased incidence of fetal deaths, particularly after operations during the first trimester. No particular anesthetic agent or technique has been implicated, and it seems that the condition that necessitated surgery was the most relevant factor. (See page 1175: Anesthesia for Nonobstetric Surgery in the Pregnant Woman.)

15. **D.** From the fifth month, the expiratory reserve volume, residual volume, and functional residual capacity decrease. The latter decreases by 20% when compared with the nonpregnant state. Concomitantly, there is an increase in inspiratory reserve volume so total lung capacity remains unchanged. (See page 1153: Ventilatory Changes.)

16. **C.** The minimum alveolar concentration for inhaled agents is decreased by 8 to 12 weeks of gestation and may be related to an increase in the progesterone levels. Lower doses of local anesthetics are needed per dermatomal segment for epidural or spinal block; this has been attributed to an increased spread of local anesthetic within the epidural and subarachnoid spaces, which occurs as a result of epidural venous engorgement. In addition, an increased neurosensitivity to local anesthetics has been suggested (which may be mediated by progesterone). (See page 1154: Altered Drug Responses.)

17. **B.** Meperidine is the most commonly used systemic opioid during the first stage of labor. The major side effects are nausea and vomiting, dose-related depression of ventilation, orthostatic hypotension, and potential for neonatal depression. Meperidine may cause transient alterations of fetal heart rate, such as decreased beat-to-beat variability and tachycardia. There have been no studies showing that systemic opioids prolong the first stage of labor. (See page 1158: Opioids.)

18. **B.** Although paracervical block effectively relieves pain during the first stage of labor, the technique has fallen out of favor because it was associated with a high incidence of fetal asphyxia and poor neonatal outcome (particularly with the use of bupivacaine). This may be related to uterine artery constriction or increased uterine tone. The technique is basically simple and involves submucosal injection of local anesthesia at the vaginal fornix. (See page 1160: Paracervical Block.)

19. **E.** Pre-eclampsia is classified as severe if it is associated with any of the following: (1) systolic blood pressure of >160 mm Hg, (2) diastolic blood pressure of 110 mm Hg, (3) proteinuria of 5 g/24 hours, (4) oliguria (400 mL/24 hours), (5) cerebral or visual disturbances, (6) pulmonary edema, (7) epigastric pain, and (8) intrauterine growth retardation. (See page 1164: Pre-Eclampsia–Eclampsia.)

20. **B.** Magnesium potentiates the duration and intensity of action of depolarizing and nondepolarizing muscle relaxants. It seems to do this by decreasing the amount of acetylcholine liberated from the motor nerve terminals and diminishing the sensitivity of the end plate to acetylcholine. It has also been found to depress the excitability of the skeletal muscle. (See page 1166: General Management.)

21. **D.** Obstetricians frequently try to inhibit preterm labor to enhance fetal lung maturity. Various agents have been used to suppress uterine activity including terbutaline, which is a beta-adrenergic drug. beta$_2$-Receptor stimulation results in myometrium inhibition, vasodilation, and bronchodilation. Maternal complications include pulmonary edema and hypotension. Severe reactions including hypokalemia, hyperglycemia, myocardial ischemia, and death have been reported. (See page 1168: Preterm Delivery.)

22. **E.** Many morphologic and functional changes occur in the neonate. The onset of ventilation and expansion of the lungs opens the pulmonary vasculature, resulting in decreased resistance and a significant increase in pulmonary blood flow. Pulmonary vascular resistance decreases as oxygen tension increases and the carbon dioxide level decreases. As soon as the pulmonary perfusion increases, the foramen ovale (which constitutes a communication between the inferior vena cava and the left atrium) undergoes functional closure. Cessation of the umbilical circulation reduces pressure in the inferior vena cava and the right atrium. The increase in pulmonary blood flow increases the pressure in the left atrium. The smooth muscle of the ductus arteriosus constricts in response to increased oxygen tension. Catecholamines also help constrict the ductus arteriosus. However, the ductus does not constrict abruptly or completely after birth; in fact, functional closure may take hours or even days. (See page 1173: Neonatal Adaptations at Birth.)

23. **B.** Although the mechanism of the teratogenic effect of nitrous oxide has not been determined, it may be related to an inhibitory effect of the agent on methionine synthetase activity and vitamin B$_{12}$. It is possible that failure of methionine synthetase to convert homocysteine to the amino acid methionine may lead to abnormalities of myelination of nerve fibers. Furthermore, inhibition of methionine synthesis results in decreased thymidine production, which, in turn, can lead to decreased DNA synthesis and inhibition of cell division. (See page 1177: Direct Effects of Anesthetic Agents on Embryo and Fetus.)

CHAPTER 43 ■ NEONATAL ANESTHESIA

For questions 1 to 6, choose the best answer.

1. The neonatal period is defined as the period that begins with the birth and ends at:

   A. 24 hours
   B. 14 days
   C. 30 days
   D. 6 months
   E. 1 year

2. Which of the following statements regarding the fetal circulation is FALSE?

   A. Fetal pulmonary vascular resistance is relatively high compared with the systemic vascular resistance.
   B. The ductus arteriosus allows 90% of the blood leaving the right ventricle to bypass the lungs and flow through the ascending aorta.
   C. Persistent patency of the foramen ovale is seen in 20 to 30% of adult patients.
   D. Pulmonary vascular resistance drops acutely at the time of birth and reaches neonatal levels within 1 hour.
   E. The ductus arteriosus is dilated secondary to a low Pa_{O_2} level.

3. True statements regarding the transition of the cardiopulmonary system and persistent pulmonary hypertension (PPH) include all of the following EXCEPT:

   A. The goal of therapy is to keep Pa_{O_2} between 80 and 90 mm Hg.
   B. Pulmonary circulation is sensitive to O_2, pH, and nitric oxide.
   C. Hypoxia and acidosis are pivotal etiologic factors in PPH.
   D. The use of extracorporeal membrane oxygenation to treat PPH is associated with increased risk of intracranial hemorrhage.

   E. Patency of the ductus arteriosus beyond 4 days of age is abnormal regardless of the gestational age.

4. Which of the following corresponds with the location of glottis in full-term neonates?

   A. C2
   B. C3
   C. C4
   D. C5
   E. C6

5. Which of the following statements regarding O_2 consumption in adult versus neonate is correct?

   A. 7 cc/kg per minute adult; 3 cc/kg per minute neonate
   B. 6 cc/kg per minute adult; 5 cc/kg per minute neonate
   C. 10 cc/kg per minute adult; 4 cc/kg per minute neonate
   D. 3 cc/kg per minute adult; 7 cc/kg per minute neonate
   E. 5 cc/kg per minute adult; 5 cc/kg per minute neonate

6. The ratio of minute ventilation to functional residual capacity is approximately 1.5:1 in adults and approximately ____ :1 in neonates.

   A. 0.5
   B. 1
   C. 1.5
   D. 2
   E. 5

For questions 7 to 24, choose A if 1, 2, and 3 are correct; B if 1 and 3; C if 2 and 4; D if 4; and E if all.

7. Fetal circulation contains which of the following shunts?

1. Placenta
2. Foramen ovale
3. Ductus arteriosus
4. Foramen secundum

8. Persistent pulmonary hypertension (PPH) may be caused by which of the following?

   1. Sepsis
   2. Respiratory distress
   3. Meconium aspiration
   4. No specific etiology

9. Which of the following statements regarding the neonatal kidney is/are TRUE?

   1. The neonatal kidney is >90% mature by 1 week of age.
   2. The renin-angiotensin-aldosterone system is not present in a neonate.
   3. The neonatal kidney conserves sodium completely in the presence of a severe sodium deficit.
   4. Neonates must receive sodium in their intravenous fluid to maintain a normal serum sodium level.

10. Which of the following statements regarding neonatal airway is/are TRUE?

    1. The head is flexed forward when the patient is supine.
    2. Neonates are obligate nose breathers.
    3. They have a relatively large tongue.
    4. The vocal cords are the narrowest portion.

11. Which of the following statements regarding the neonatal pulmonary system is/are TRUE?

    1. Neonates have a high closing volume.
    2. Neonates have rigid ribs.
    3. Neonates have high O_2 consumption.
    4. Neonates have a low ratio of minute ventilation to functional residual capacity.

12. Which of the following statements regarding the neonatal cardiovascular system is/are TRUE?

    1. Increases in cardiac output are achieved primarily through the increase in heart rate.
    2. Hypoxia is a major cause of perioperative bradycardia.
    3. Cardiac output typically may be increased by no more than 40% in neonates.
    4. Neonates have immature baroreceptors.

13. Which of the following statements about muscle relaxants in pediatrics is/are TRUE?

    1. The duration of action of vecuronium is twice as long in children <1 year of age than it is in older children.
    2. The incremental administration of *d*-tubocurarine and atracurium minimizes the release of histamine.
    3. Epinephrine may be indicated following succinylcholine-induced hyperkalemia.

4. Succinylcholine should be used in male children <8 years of age only for rapid sequence induction, difficult airway, and other emergencies.

14. Which of the following statements regarding neonatal anesthetic requirement is/are TRUE?

    1. Neonates require as much anesthetic as older infants.
    2. In a premature infant, minimum alveolar concentration is decreased by 30%.
    3. Premature infants have decreased endorphins.
    4. Immature infants have immature blood-brain barriers.

15. Which of the following statements regarding regional anesthesia in neonates is/are TRUE?

    1. The requirement for intraoperative opioids may be eliminated.
    2. The dose of muscle relaxants needs to be increased.
    3. The most common response to a high spinal is respiratory insufficiency.
    4. The requirement for inhalation anesthetics is unchanged.

16. Which of the following statements regarding anesthetic uptake in infants versus adults is/are TRUE?

    1. The ratio of alveolar ventilation to functional residual capacity is 1.5:1.
    2. Neonates have a greater cardiac index.
    3. Infants have higher blood gas partition coefficient.
    4. In neonates, the brain and heart receive relatively more of cardiac output.

17. Which of the following statements regarding congenital diaphragmatic hernia is/are TRUE?

    1. The 1-minute Apgar score may be normal.
    2. Most congenital diaphragmatic hernias are left sided.
    3. After diagnosis, the patient requires immediate intubation.
    4. High-frequency ventilation significantly improves survival.

18. Omphalocele is associated with:

    1. a 20% incidence of congenital heart disease
    2. a sac (amnion) that increases the extra-abdominal contents
    3. Beckwith-Wiedemann syndrome
    4. more fluid loss preoperatively than is associated with gastroschisis

19. Which of the following statements regarding tracheoesophageal fistula is/are TRUE?

    1. Eighty-five percent of these connections consist of a fistula between the distal trachea and the esophagus, with a blind proximal esophageal pouch.

2. Fifty percent of these patients have associated congenital anomalies.

3. Primary repair can be done 24 to 48 hours after diagnosis.

4. A major complication is dehydration.

20. Which of the following statements regarding meningomyelocele is/are TRUE?

 1. Fifty to 90% of meningomyeloceles are detected by serum alpha-fetoprotein.
 2. Amniotic fluid alpha-fetoprotein is more reliable than serum alpha-fetoprotein.
 3. Meningocele does not contain the neural elements.
 4. Regional anesthesia is absolutely contraindicated in these patients.

21. Which of the following statements regarding postoperative apnea is/are TRUE?

 1. Premature infants with congenital anomalies are at highest risk.
 2. Spinal anesthesia may decrease the incidence of postoperative apnea.
 3. The etiology is multifactorial.
 4. A 44-week postconceptional infant undergoing a spinal anesthetic does not require prolonged postoperative monitoring.

22. Which of the following metabolic abnormalities is/are classically described in a patient with pyloric stenosis?

 1. Hyponatremia
 2. Metabolic acidosis
 3. Hypochloremia
 4. Hyperkalemia

23. Which of the following statements regarding pyloric stenosis is/are TRUE?

 1. It is a surgical emergency.
 2. Dextrose 5% in water should be used for fluid replacement.
 3. It is usually evident in the first week of life.
 4. Postoperative apnea is a concern in these patients.

24. Which of the following statements regarding retinopathy of prematurity is/are TRUE?

 1. The exact cause is unknown.
 2. Hypoxia may be a cause.
 3. Prolonged bright-light exposure may contribute to the cause.
 4. In premature infants, Pa_{O_2} of 70 mm Hg is appropriate.

ANSWERS

---

1. **C.** The neonatal period is defined as the first 30 days of extrauterine life and includes the newborn period. The newborn period is the first 24 hours of life. (See page 1182: Physiology of the Infant and the Transition Period.)

2. **D.** The pulmonary vascular bed has a high vascular resistance because the alveoli are relatively closed and filled with fluid and the blood vessels are compressed. However, the ductus arteriosus represents a low-resistance system, which is dilated secondary to low Pa_{O_2}. Therefore, the blood that leaves the right ventricle by the pulmonary artery is shunted preferentially (90%) through the ductus arteriosus to the aorta, whereas only 10% of the cardiac output of the right ventricle flows through the pulmonary artery into the pulmonary vascular bed. The transition of alveoli from a fluid-filled to an air-filled state results in a reduced compression of the pulmonary alveolar capillaries and thus a reduction in pulmonary vascular resistance. It takes 3 to 4 days for the pulmonary vascular resistance to decrease to the eventual level that it will achieve during the neonatal period. Autopsy studies of healthy hearts demonstrated a 30% incidence of patent foramen ovale during the first 30 years of life and a 20% incidence for persons 30 years of age and older. (See page 1182: Fetal Circulation.)

3. **A.** Patency of the ductus arteriosus beyond the fourth day of life is abnormal regardless of gestational age. The major transition of circulatory system occurs over the first 24 hours of life. The pulmonary circulation is extremely sensitive to O_2, pH, and nitric oxide. Hypoxia and acidosis, along with inflammatory mediators, may cause the pulmonary artery pressure either to persist at a high level or to increase to pathologic levels; the result is PPH. The goals of therapy are to achieve a Pa_{O_2} of between 50 and 70 mm Hg with a Pa_{CO_2} of between 40 and 60 mm Hg. With the use of extracorporeal membrane oxygenation, heparin must be administered, and this may increase the chance of intracranial bleeding. (See page 1183: Patent Ductus Arteriosus and Persistent Pulmonary Hypertension.)

4. **C.** In the healthy adult, the glottis is at the level of C5. In the full-term infant, the glottis is at the level of C4. In a premature infant, it is at a level of C3. (See page 1185: Anatomic and Maturational Factors of Neonates and Their Clinical Significance.)

5. **D.** The O_2 consumption of the infant is 7 to 9 cc/kg per minute, whereas the adult's is 3 cc/kg per minute. Therefore, varying degrees of early obstruction have more impact on O_2 delivery and reserve in the neonate, infant, and child

than in adults. (See page 1186: The Pulmonary System.)

6. **E.** Tidal ventilation for an adult is the same, in cubic centimeters per kilogram, as for the neonate, but O_2 consumption is three times greater; thus, the respiratory rate must be three times greater (which results in an alveolar ventilation that is three times greater). Consequently, the ratio of minute ventilation to functional residual capacity is approximately 5:1 in neonates, whereas in adults it is 1.5:1. (See page 1186: The Pulmonary System.)

7. **A.** Fetal circulation is characterized by presence of three main shunts: the placenta, foramen ovale, and ductus arteriosus. The relatively low pressure in the left atrium and the high pressure in the right atrium cause the foramen ovale to be open. (See page 1182: Fetal Circulation.)

8. **E.** PPH is a syndrome that may be primary, with no recognized origin, or it may be secondary to meconium aspiration, sepsis, pneumonia, respiratory distress, and congenital diaphragmatic hernia. (See page 1183: Persistent Pulmonary Hypertension.)

9. **D.** By the time the healthy full-term infant is 1 month of age, the kidneys are approximately 70% mature. The renin-angiotensin-aldosterone system is a primary compensatory system for the absorption of sodium and water to compensate for the loss of plasma, blood, gastrointestinal tract fluid, and third-space fluid. Although the neonate has a normal renin-angiotensin-aldosterone system, the neonatal kidney cannot completely conserve sodium; the neonate will continue to excrete sodium in the urine even in the presence of severe sodium deficit. For this reason, the neonate is considered an obligate sodium loser. (See page 1185: Transition and Maturation of Renal System.)

10. **A.** Neonates are obligate nose breathers; therefore, anything that obstructs the nares will compromise a neonate's ability to breathe. The large tongue occupies relatively more space in the infant's airway and makes it difficult to laryngoscope and intubate an infant's trachea. The narrowest portion of a neonate's airway is not the vocal cords but the cricoid ring. The neonate has a large occiput, so the head will flex forward onto the chest when the patient is lying supine and the head is in midline. (See page 1185: Anatomic and Maturational Factors of the Neonate and Their Clinical Significance.)

11. **B.** Anatomically and physiologically, the neonatal pulmonary system differs in at least four respects from that of the adult: high O_2 consumption, high closing volumes, high ratio of minute ventilation to functional residual capacity, and pliable ribs. (See page 1186: The Pulmonary System.)

12. **E.** Any increase in cardiac output must be accomplished by an increase in the heart rate. For this reason, the infant is said to be rate dependent for its cardiac output. Hypoxia is a major cause of bradycardia in neonates. The neonatal heart can increase cardiac output by 30 to 40%. Neonates have immature baroreceptors; the baroreceptors are responsible for the reflex tachycardia that occurs in response to hypotension. (See page 1188: Heart and Sympathetic Nervous System.)

13. **E.** *D*-Tubocurarine causes a dose-related histamine release; however, incremental administration will minimize the effect on the blood pressure. In infants <1 year of age, the duration of action of vecuronium is approximately twice that observed in older children (because of their immature livers). The reports of hyperkalemia with cardiac arrest in male children <age 8 years (unrecognized muscular dystrophy) have caused some clinicians to recommend that succinylcholine should not be used routinely in this age group. However, succinylcholine is still recommended in rapid sequence situations, a potential difficult airway, or if airway emergencies develop with desaturation. If the circulation is unstable with severe bradycardia, hypotension, and/or cardiac arrest, the first drug of choice is epinephrine. (See page 1189: Non-Depolarizing Agents.)

14. **C.** Neonates and premature infants have lower anesthetic requirements than older infants and children. In premature infants, the minimum alveolar concentration value will decrease by 20 to 30%. The reason for the lower minimum alveolar concentration requirements is thought to be multifactorial: an immature nervous system, progesterone from the mother, elevated levels of endorphins, and an immature blood-brain barrier. (See page 1191: Anesthetic Dose Requirements of Neonates.)

15. **B.** Regional anesthetic techniques allow for early extubation in neonates because they can eliminate the need for intraoperative narcotics, reduce the need for muscle relaxants, and reduce the concentration of volatile agents needed. A high spinal presents as respiratory insufficiency rather than hypotension; the reason for this is the lack of sympathetic tone. (See page 1191: Regional Anesthesia.)

16. **C.** Various reasons for the faster uptake of anesthetic in infants have been proposed: the ratio of alveolar ventilation to functional residual capacity is 5:1 in infants and 1.5:1 in adults; in neonates, more of the cardiac output goes to the vessel-rich group of organs, which include the heart and the brain; neonates have a greater cardiac output per kilogram of body mass; and the infant has a lower blood gas partition coefficient for volatile anesthetics. (See page 1191: Uptake and Distribution of Anesthetic in Neonates.)

17. **A.** The left side of the diaphragm closes later than the right side, and this results in a higher incidence (90%) of left-sided congenital diaphragmatic hernias (foramen of Bochdalek). Because the infant's status immediately following birth is determined primarily by the placental oxygenation, the 1-minute Apgar score may be normal. Immediate supportive care includes tracheal intubation and control of the airway, along with decompression of the stomach. High-frequency ventilation has been used in place of conventional ventilation in an attempt to reduce barotrauma, but it has not been shown to improve survival. (See page 1194: Congenital Diaphragmatic Hernia.)

18. **A.** Failure of part or all of the intestinal content to return to the abdominal cavity results in omphalocele that is covered with a membrane called an amnion. The amnion protects the abdominal contents from infection and loss of extracellular fluid. In gastroschisis, the intestines and viscera are not covered by any membrane and are susceptible to infection and loss of extracellular fluid. There is a high instance of associated congenital anomalies with omphalocele, but none with gastroschisis. The Beckwith-Wiedemann syndrome consists of mental retardation, hypoglycemia, congenital heart disease, enlarged tongue, and omphalocele. Congenital heart defects are found in approximately 20% of infants with omphalocele. (See page 1196: Omphalocele and Gastroschisis.)

19. **E.** Approximately 85% of tracheoesophageal fistulae consist of a fistula from the distal trachea to the esophagus and a blind proximal esophageal pouch. Fifty percent of affected infants have associated congenital anomalies, of which approximately 15 to 20% involve the cardiovascular system. The two major complications of esophageal atresia with a distal tracheal fistula are aspiration pneumonia and dehydration. If the infant is in good condition, primary repair can be performed 24 to 48 hours after diagnosis. (See page 1198: Tracheoesophageal Fistula.)

20. **A.** Elevation of maternal serum alpha-fetoprotein will detect 50 to 90% of open neural tube defects, but this test has a false-positive rate of 5%. Amniotic fluid alpha-fetoprotein is more reliable. By definition, the lesion involves both meninges and neural components, as compared with meningocele, which does not contain neural elements. Regional anesthesia has been reported as a safe alternative to general anesthesia in neonates with meningomyelocele. (See page 1199: Meningomyelocele.)

21. **A.** The infants at highest risk for postoperative apnea are those born prematurely, those with multiple congenital anomalies, those with a history of apnea and bradycardia, and those with chronic lung disease. The etiology of apnea is multifactorial. Spinal anesthesia without supplemental sedation decreases the incidence of postoperative apnea and bradycardia in high-risk infants. The most widely accepted guideline at present is to monitor all infants <50 weeks' postconceptional age for at least 12 hours after surgery; this includes infants who have had a spinal regimen as their sole anesthetic. (See page 1193: Postoperative Apnea.)

22. **B.** The classic electrolyte pattern in infants with severe vomiting consists of hyponatremia, hypokalemia, hypochloremia, and metabolic alkalosis with compensatory respiratory acidosis. (See page 1201: Pyloric Stenosis.)

23. **D.** Pyloric stenosis is a medical emergency and not a surgical one. These patients need fluid resuscitation (full strength, balanced salt solution), and after the infant begins to urinate, potassium chloride should be added. Pyloric stenosis can appear as early as the second week of life. The risk of postoperative apnea in these patients is a concern. (See page 1201: Pyloric Stenosis.)

24. **E.** Although the exact cause of retinopathy of prematurity is unknown, variations in arterial oxygenation (hypoxia or hyperoxia) and prolonged exposure to bright light are believed to play significant roles. The guidelines for administration of O_2 in premature infants is a goal of 50 to 80 mm Hg. An O_2 saturation of 90 to 95% represents a PaO_2 of somewhere between 60 and 80 mm Hg. (See page 1193: Retinopathy of Prematurity.)

CHAPTER 44 ■ PEDIATRIC ANESTHESIA

1. Choose the correct statement regarding pediatric anesthesia:

   A. Appropriate fluid management remains the single most important aspect of delivering safe pediatric anesthesia.
   B. Intramuscular succinylcholine is recommended when relaxation is required and intravenous access is not available.
   C. Practice guidelines from the American Society of Anesthesiology state that pediatric patients should be NPO at least 4 hours before surgery.
   D. Chlorohydrate is the most commonly used premedicant in children.
   E. The most commonly used form of regional anesthesia in children is the spinal block.

2. In the younger infant who still feeds frequently, formula should be given up to ____ hours preoperatively.

   A. 2
   B. 4
   C. 6
   D. 8
   E. 10

3. Choose the TRUE statement regarding oral premedications.

   A. The effect of oral midazolam lasts about 2 hours.
   B. The onset of peak effect is faster for ketamine than for midazolam.
   C. Patients receiving midazolam have more oral secretions than those receiving ketamine.
   D. The recommended dose of oral ketamine is 1 mg/kg.
   E. The appropriate dose of midazolam is 0.1 mg/kg.

4. The pediatric airway differs from that of the adult with respect to all of the following EXCEPT:

   A. Larger head size relative to body size
   B. Larger tongue size relative to body size
   C. Larger surface-to-body ratio
   D. Larger functional residual capacity (FRC) relative to total lung capacity
   E. Larger oxygen consumption

5. An otherwise healthy 10-kg, 2-year-old girl presents for 2-hour eye muscle surgery. She has been fasting since 10 PM and enters the operating room at 8 AM. Approximately how much intravenous fluid should she receive during the first hour of anesthesia?

   A. 50 mL
   B. 100 mL
   C. 150 mL
   D. 250 mL
   E. 350 mL

6. The average hourly maintenance fluid requirement for a 22-kg child is approximately ____ mL?

   A. 42
   B. 52
   C. 54
   D. 62
   E. 84

7. All the following statements regarding pediatric patients suffering from an upper respiratory infection (URI) are true EXCEPT:

   A. They are at a higher risk if they live in a household with parents who smoke.
   B. Bronchial hyperreactivity resolves within 4 weeks after a URI.
   C. They have fewer perioperative complications if a mask anesthetic is used rather than an endotracheal tube.
   D. Children <1 year of age with a URI are at a greater risk than are older children undergoing anesthesia.

E. Children with sickle cell disease are at a greater risk.

8. Healthy children undergoing elective minor surgery require the following preoperative tests:

A. Coagulation screening (bleeding time)
B. Hematocrit
C. Chest radiograph
D. Urinalysis
E. None of the above

9. Choose the correct statement regarding the American Society of Anesthesiologists practice guidelines for preoperative fasting:

A. Solids are always prohibited after midnight.
B. Formula is allowed until 8 hours of surgery.
C. Breast milk is allowed until 4 hours of surgery.
D. Flat cola is not allowed within 6 hours of surgery.
E. Apple juice is not allowed within 4 hours of surgery.

10. All the following statements regarding the use of succinylcholine in pediatric patients are true EXCEPT:

A. When given in a dose of 1.5 to 2.0 mg/kg, it consistently produces excellent intubating conditions in 30 seconds.
B. It is absolutely contraindicated in patients with a recent burn injury.
C. Its use in all children is relatively contraindicated.
D. The requirement for succinylcholine has been reduced by the availability of fast-acting nondepolarizing agents such as rocuronium.
E. It is recommended only when ultrarapid onset and short duration of action are required.

11. Choose the correct statement regarding postoperative nausea and vomiting (PONV) in pediatric patients:

A. The effectiveness of ondansetron as the best rescue medication has been proven.
B. Droperidol should be avoided because of prolongation of the P-R interval.
C. PONV is common after orchiopexy, strabismus surgery, and tonsillectomy.
D. The type of anesthetic technique has no effect on PONV.
E. Patients should eat and/or drink before discharge.

12. The hourly maintenance fluid requirement for a pediatric patient weighing 16 kg is:

A. 36 mL/hour
B. 42 mL/hour
C. 46 mL/hour
D. 52 mL/hour
E. 56 mL/hour

13. What is the maximum allowable blood loss (MABL) for a 4-kg term infant with a starting hematocrit of 32% and a target hematocrit of 24%?

A. 70 mL
B. 80 mL
C. 90 mL
D. 100 mL
E. 110 mL

For questions 14 to 19, choose A if 1, 2, and 3 are correct; B if 1 and 3; C if 2 and 4; D if 4; and E if all.

14. A child with a URI or who is recovering from a URI is at increased risk to develop:

1. laryngospasm
2. bronchospasm
3. postoperative atelectasis
4. croup

15. Which of the following patient(s) may be at increased risk for developing postoperative apnea following general anesthesia?

1. A 2-year-old child undergoing strabismus surgery
2. A 4-month-old infant who was delivered at 35 weeks
3. A 1-year-old child undergoing inguinal hernia surgery
4. A 3-month-old infant with a history of apnea and bradycardia

16. Which of the following are appropriate drug/dose amounts for oral preoperative sedation?

1. Midazolam 0.5 to 0.75 mg/kg
2. Ketamine 2 mg/kg
3. Clonidine 4 μg/kg
4. Methohexital 25 mg/kg

17. Choose the correct statement(s) regarding mask induction of general anesthesia in pediatric patients:

1. A right-to left intracardiac shunt slows the rate of mask induction.
2. Desflurane has an unacceptable incidence of laryngospasm when used for mask induction.
3. The incidence of bradycardia, hypotension, and cardiac arrest is highest in patients <1 year of age.
4. The minimum alveolar concentration (MAC) of sevoflurane is approximately 2.5% for young infants compared with 2% for adolescents and adults.

18. Choose the correct statement(s) regarding airway management in pediatric patients:

1. After the endotracheal tube is placed, air should leak out at 20 to 25 cm H_2O.
2. The narrowest portion of the pediatric airway is at the level of the cricoid cartilage.
3. The appropriate-sized endotracheal tube can be determined by comparison with the fifth digit.
4. If a cuffed tube is used, the cuff pressure should not exceed 20 cm H_2O.

19. Which of the following statement(s) regarding regional anesthesia in pediatric patients is/are FALSE:

1. The dural sac is at the S1 level at 1 year of age.
2. The recommended dose of bupivacaine for a caudal anesthetic is 1.5 mL/kg of 0.25% solution.

3. The sitting position facilitates free flow of cerebrospinal fluid when placing a spinal block in neonates.
4. A spinal anesthetic is contraindicated in preterm infants.

ANSWERS

1. B. The American Society of Anesthesiologists has recently issued practice guidelines regarding preoperative fasting. Solids are prohibited within 6 to 8 hours of surgery (generally after midnight), formula within 6 hours, breast milk within 4 hours of surgery, and clear liquids within 2 hours of surgery. Oral midazolam is the most commonly used sedative premedicant. Succinylcholine is recommended when ultrarapid onset and short duration of action are of paramount importance (laryngospasm), when relaxation is required, or when intravenous access is not available and intramuscular administration is required. Appropriate airway management remains the single most important aspect of delivering safe pediatric anesthesia. The most commonly used form of regional anesthesia in children is the caudal block. (See page 1205: Key Points.)

2. C. Solids are prohibited within 6 to 8 hours of surgery, formula within 6 hours, breast milk until 4 hours preoperatively, and clear liquids up to 2 hours preoperatively. (See page 1207: Preoperative Fasting Period.)

3. B. By far the most popular oral premedication at this time is midazolam, in a dose of 0.5 to 0.75 mg/kg. The effect of this medication peaks in about 30 minutes after administration and lasts about 60 minutes. Maximal sedation occurs within 20 minutes after oral ketamine administration; nystagmus occurs in 60% of the patients, and increased oral secretions occur in 33%. Oral ketamine has been used as a sedative at a dose of 5 to 6 mg/kg. (See page 1208: Preoperative Sedatives.)

4. D. Oxygen consumption is two to three times greater in infants that adults, whereas the FRC is half as large as adults. The anesthetic implication of a reduced FRC is rapid oxygen desaturation following apnea. (See page 1205: Key Points; see page 1206: Table 44-1.)

5. D. The hourly maintenance fluid requirement for a child <10 kg is 4 mL/kg. This child would have an hourly requirement of 40 mL (10 kg × 4 mL/kg). The fluid deficit is then calculated by multiplying the hourly fluid requirement by the time since the last oral fluid intake (40 mL × 10 hours = 400 mL). Generally, half of the total deficit (200 mL) is replaced in the first hour of the anesthetic, in addition to the scheduled maintenance under anesthesia. Because the third-space and evaporative losses are minimal during eye surgery, the hourly intraoperative maintenance is approximately 4 mL/kg. Hence, approximately 240 mL should be given in the first hour. (See page 1213: Table 44-4.)

6. D. For the "first" 10 kg, the hourly fluid requirement is 4 mL/kg per hour. For the "next" 10 kg, it is 2 mL/ kg per hour. For the "remaining" kg, it is 1 mL/kg per hour. Hence, the average hourly maintenance fluid requirement is 62 mL (40 + 20 + 2). (See page 1213: Table 44-4.)

7. B. Children with asthma, infants and young children with bronchopulmonary dysplasia, children <1 year of age, children with sickle cell disease, children who live in a household that includes parents who smoke, and children who are to undergo bronchoscopy are at a higher risk to develop perioperative morbidity if they are suffering from an URI. It is unclear how long surgery should be delayed following an URI because bronchial hyperreactivity may exist for up to 7 weeks. (See page 1206: Coexisting Health Conditions.)

8. E. It is currently the standard of care that healthy children undergoing elective minor surgery require no laboratory evaluation. Routine chest radiographs and urinary analysis are also unnecessary. Commonly used coagulation screening tests, such as bleeding time and prothrombin time, do not reliably predict abnormal perioperative bleeding. (See page 1207: Laboratory Evaluation.)

9. C. According to the American Society of Anesthesiologists practice guidelines for preoperative fasting, solids are prohibited within 6 to 8 hours of surgery, formula within 6 hours, breast milk within 4 hours of surgery, and clear liquids within 2 hours of surgery. Indeed, liquids such as apple or grape juice, flat cola, and sugar water may be encouraged up to 2 hours before the induction of anesthesia because their consumption has been shown to decrease the gastric residual volume. (See page 1207: Preoperative Fasting Period.)

10. **A.** When given in a dose of 1.5 to 2.0 mg/kg, succinylcholine produces excellent intubating conditions (reliably) in 60 seconds. Its use is absolutely contraindicated in patients with muscular dystrophy, recent burn injury, spinal cord transection, and/or immobilization, as well as in any child with a family history of malignant hyperthermia. Succinylcholine is currently listed as relatively contraindicated for use in all children by the Food and Drug Administration (FDA). The requirement for succinylcholine has been decreased by the availability of fast-acting nondepolarizing agents such as rocuronium. Succinylcholine can be recommended only when ultrarapid onset and short duration of action are of paramount importance (laryngospasm), when relaxation is required, or when intravenous access is not available and intramuscular administration is required. (See page 1212: Muscle Relaxants.)

11. **C.** PONV is particularly prominent after certain surgical procedures such as orchiopexy, strabismus surgery, and tonsillectomy. The type of anesthetic employed for a particular surgical procedure will also influence the incidence of PONV. For instance, when propofol is used in place of inhaled agents as the primary anesthetic, there is evidence that PONV is less common after high-risk procedures. The FDA issued a report warning of prolonged QT syndrome and possible torsades de pointes with droperidol use. The practice of requiring patients to eat and/or drink before discharge will only increase PONV rates and does not appear to improve outcomes. (See page 1212: Antiemetics.)

12. **D.** The hourly maintenance fluid requirement for pediatric patients is 4 mL/kg for the first 10 kg plus 2 mL/kg for each kilogram between 11 and 20 kg and 1 mL/kg for each kilogram over 20 kg. For the foregoing example with a 16-kg patient, this would be: 40 mL/hour (first 10 kg) + 2 mL/hour × 6 kg = 52 mL/hour. (See page 1213: Fluid and Blood Product Management.)

13. **C.** MABL is estimated as follows:

$$\text{MABL} = \frac{\text{EBV} \times (\text{starting hematocrit} - \text{target hematocrit})}{\text{starting hematocrit}}.$$

In general, estimated blood volume (EBV) is 90 mL/kg for the term infant, so the EBV = 4 kg × 90 mL/kg = 360 cc. Therefore,

$$\text{MABL} = 360 \text{ mL} \times \frac{32-24\%}{32\%} = 90 \text{ mL}.$$

(See page 1213: Fluid and Blood Product Management.)

14. **E.** Multiple investigations have found that a child with a URI or one who is recovering from a URI is at increased risk to develop laryngospasm, bronchospasm, oxygen desaturation, postoperative atelectasis and croup. Although these complications usually do not cause significant morbidity in otherwise healthy children, they may be very significant in children with underlying conditions. (See page 1206: Coexisting Health Conditions.)

15. **C.** Research indicates that former preterm infants are more likely to develop postoperative apnea following general anesthesia. These reports indicate that the risk of postoperative apnea is inversely related to postconceptional age, and those infants with a history of apnea and bradycardia, respiratory distress, and mechanical ventilation may be at increased risk. Infants 52 to 60 weeks postconceptional age should generally be admitted to the hospital and monitored following anesthesia. (See page 1206: Coexisting Health Conditions.)

16. **B.** Midazolam is the most commonly used sedative premedicant used in the United States. It has rapid onset and predictable effect without causing cardiorespiratory depression. In an oral dose of 0.5 to 0.75 mg/kg, midazolam peaks approximately 30 minutes after administration, and its effect lasts approximately 30 minutes. Oral ketamine has been used as a sedation medication in doses of 5 to 6 mg/kg for children 1 to 6 years of age. Orally administered clonidine in a dose of 4 μg/kg has been demonstrated reliably to cause sedation, decrease anesthetic requirements, and decrease the requirement for postoperative analgesics. (See page 1208: Preoperative Sedatives.)

17. **E.** Mask induction of general anesthesia remains the most common induction technique for pediatric anesthesia in the United States. The incidence of bradycardia, hypotension, and cardiac arrest during mask induction is higher in infants <1 year of age than in older children and adults. There is actually a small increase in MAC between birth and 2 to 3 months of age that represents the age of highest MAC requirement. For sevoflurane, the change in MAC is marked, with a value of approximately 2.5% for young infants compared with 2% for adolescents and adults. A right-to-left shunt slows the inhaled induction of anesthesia because the anesthetic concentration in the arterial blood increases more slowly. Desflurane has an unacceptable incidence of laryngospasm when used for inhalational induction. (See page 1209: Anesthetic Agents.)

18. **E.** Because the narrowest portion of the pediatric airway is at the level of the cricoid cartilage, uncuffed tubes can be used and will create a functional seal when appropriately sized. Several formulas have been used for tube selection in children older than 1 year of age, the most common being (16 + age)/4. One may also estimate the size by comparing the

size of the fifth digit or of a nostril. Once the tube is in place, it should be checked to determine at what pressure air can escape around the tube. Air should leak out at no higher than 20 to 25 cm H_2O to minimize the risk of postextubation croup. Cuffed tubes can also be safely used in children by selecting a tube 0.5 mm smaller in internal diameter than the uncuffed choice. Care should be taken to check the pressure in the cuff to ensure that it does not exceed 20 cm H_2O. (See page 1214: Airway Management.)

19. C.   When using bupivacaine for a caudal block, a 0.175% solution in a dose of 1 mL/kg is used, and if larger volumes are needed, the use of 0.125% is recommended. When considering spinal anesthesia, it is important to note that the dural sac migrates cephalad during the first year of life, and in a neonate it is at S3, whereas after the age of 1 year it is at the S1 level. The sitting position may be especially helpful in neonates to maintain midline needle position and free flow of spinal fluid. (See page 1216: Regional Anesthesia.)

CHAPTER 45 ■ ANESTHESIA FOR THE GERIATRIC PATIENT

For questions 1 to 4, choose the best answer.

1. All of the following are associated with age-related changes in the kidney EXCEPT:

   A. decreased serum creatinine concentration
   B. decreased number of glomeruli
   C. renal perfusion shifted to the medulla
   D. decreased glomerular filtration rate
   E. decreased overall renal tissue mass

2. Which of the following is a species-specific fixed biological parameter that quantitates maximum attainable individual age?

   A. Geriatrics
   B. Age
   C. Life expectancy
   D. Life span
   E. Longevity

3. Which of the following statements regarding cardiovascular changes associated with aging is FALSE?

   A. There is a modest decrease in resting cardiac index.
   B. The maximal heart rate is age limited.
   C. There is myocardial muscle atrophy.
   D. There is decreased ventricular compliance.
   E. There is impaired diastolic relaxation.

4. Choose the TRUE statement regarding anesthetic requirements in the elderly:

   A. The median effective dose (ED_{50}) for neuromuscular blocking agents is reduced.
   B. A reduced volume of local anesthetic is required for spinal anesthesia.
   C. Parenteral morphine requirements are directly related to patient age.
   D. Minimum alveolar concentration (MAC) values decline >75% than in young adulthood.

   E. The brain becomes more sensitive to etomidate and less sensitive to narcotics.

For questions 5 to 12, choose A if 1, 2, and 3 are correct; B if 1 and 3; C if 2 and 4; D if 4; and E if all are correct.

5. Which of the following statements regarding the cardiovascular system and aging is/are TRUE?

   1. There is elastic replacement of fibrous tissue within the cardiovascular system.
   2. Vascular impedance increases.
   3. Ventricular wall hypertrophy occurs only as a result of arterial hypertension.
   4. Maximal cardiac output decreases.

6. Which of the following statements regarding the pulmonary system in the geriatric patient is/are TRUE?

   1. Pulmonary shunting increases.
   2. Pulmonary dead space increases.
   3. Vital capacity decreases.
   4. Lung elasticity decreases.

7. Which of the following statements regarding an 80-year-old patient compared with a 20-year-old patient is/are TRUE?

   1. Liver tissue mass decreases by 40%.
   2. Renal blood flow decreases by 50%.
   3. Glomeruli decrease by 30%.
   4. Renal tissue mass decreases by 30%.

8. Which of the following statements regarding central nervous system changes in elderly patients is/are TRUE?

   1. The adult brain weight is 20% less by age 80 years.
   2. The cerebrospinal fluid decreases in the 80-year-old patient.

3. There is a >30% decrease of the neuronal population of the cerebral cortex.
4. Cerebral blood flow in the gray matter is maintained in the elderly patient.

9. Which of the following statements regarding the peripheral nervous system in the elderly patient is/are TRUE?

1. The postjunctional muscle membrane is thicker.
2. The dose requirements for competitive neuromuscular blocking drugs are not significantly reduced.
3. Motor nerve conduction velocity decreases.
4. The total number of acetylcholine receptors increases.

10. Which of the following statements regarding the geriatric patient and neuromuscular blocking agents is/are TRUE?

1. The time to onset of neuromuscular blockade is decreased.
2. The dose requirement decreases in parallel with age-related decline in skeletal muscle mass.

3. Age is the primary determinant of the completeness of antagonism of neuromuscular block.
4. The clinical duration of action of most neuromuscular blocking agents is increased.

11. Which of the following statements regarding the nervous system in the aged is/are TRUE?

1. The contractile properties of peripheral vascular smooth muscle remain intact.
2. Cortisol secretion declines at least 15%.
3. "Endogenous beta-blockade" occurs.
4. Plasma concentrations of norepinephrine are two to four times greater than in younger patients.

12. Which of the following statements regarding the pulmonary system in elderly patients is/are TRUE?

1. Closing capacity typically becomes greater than the volume of the lung at rest.
2. Hypoxic pulmonary vasoconstriction remains intact during general anesthesia.
3. Elderly patients are predisposed to acute postoperative ventilatory failure.
4. The cardiovascular and ventilatory responses to hypoxia are increased in onset.

ANSWERS

1. **A.** Despite compromise of renal functional reserve, serum creatinine concentration usually remains within the normal range in elderly patients because their declining skeletal muscle mass generates a progressively smaller creatinine load. Thirty percent of renal tissue mass is lost by the eighth decade. More than one-third of the glomeruli and their associated nephron tubular structures disappear in the elderly. The renal cortex appears to be particularly sensitive to progressive reduction of tissue vascularity, with relative sparing of the renal medulla. Shifting of renal perfusion from cortex to medulla appears to produce a slight compensatory increase in filtration fraction in the elderly. (See page 1222: Pharmacokinetics, Hepatorenal, and Immune Function.)

2. **D.** Life span is an idealized, species-specific, relatively fixed biological parameter that quantifies maximum attainable individual age under optimal conditions. In contrast, life expectancy describes typical longevity under prevailing conditions in society. (See page 1219: Concepts of Aging and Geriatrics.)

3. **C.** The heart, unlike other major organs, does not atrophy significantly with age, and both heart size and myocardial tissue mass actually increase. The modest decrease in resting cardiac index observed in most healthy elderly persons

is not from a degenerative process, but rather represents an appropriate and integrated response to the reduced requirements for perfusion and metabolism that occur with age-related atrophy of skeletal muscle and the loss of tissue mass in many other major organs. The maximal heart rate is age limited. The ventricle is less compliant with aging. Age-related diastolic dysfunction makes elderly persons significantly more dependent on the synchronous atrial contraction of sinus rhythm for complete ventricular filling at end diastole. (See page 1221: Cardiopulmonary Function.)

4. **B.** Despite the inevitable loss of skeletal muscle mass in elderly persons, the ED_{50} and steady-state plasma concentrations required for half-maximal neuromuscular blocking effect remain virtually unchanged or may actually increase slightly in the elderly patient. When a fixed dose and volume of local anesthetic is used, higher levels of sensory blockade occur in elderly patients than in young patients undergoing spinal anesthesia. Parenteral morphine requirements are inversely related to patient age and are essentially independent of body weight. Between young adulthood and the geriatric age range, relative MAC values for the newer inhalational agents decline by as much as 30%. Most studies suggest that aging increases brain sensitivity to narcotics, with insignificant pharmacodynamic effects for

barbiturates. (See page 1224: Analgesic and Anesthetic Requirement.)

5. **C.** Systolic arterial hypertension results from fibrotic replacement of the elastic tissues within the cardiovascular system. This results in an increase in vascular impedance to cardiac ejection. Thus, left ventricular wall hypertrophy can occur even in the absence of arterial hypertension. There is a lower limit on maximal cardiac output in the elderly patient compared with a younger patient. (See page 1221: Cardiopulmonary Function.)

6. **E.** Elderly patients experience inevitable emphysema-like increases in lung compliance because lung elasticity declines. Vital capacity is compromised significantly as residual volume increases (along with decreasing inspiratory and expiratory reserve volumes). There is an increase in both anatomic and physiologic dead space as well as increased shunting in the elderly patient. (See page 1221: Cardiopulmonary Function.)

7. **E.** Liver tissue mass decreases 40% by the age of 80 years, and splanchnic blood flow and hepatic blood flow are reduced proportionately. Thirty percent of the maximum young adult value for bilateral renal tissue mass is lost by the eighth decade. More than one-third of the glomeruli and their associated nephron tubular structures will disappear by the age of 80 years. Total renal blood flow decreases 50% by age 80; a decline of 10% per decade begins in early adulthood. (See page 1222: Pharmacokinetics, Hepatorenal, and Immune Function.)

8. **B.** Aging reduces brain size; the 80-year-old brain weighs 20% less than the young adult brain. The decrease in brain matter results in the compensatory increase in cerebrospinal fluid. The neuronal population of the cerebral cortex decreases 30 to 50% in the elderly person. Cerebral blood flow in the gray matter declines 20 to 30% from the maximal value seen in the young adult. (See page 1223: Central Nervous System.)

9. **E.** Peripheral motor nerve conduction velocity decreases in the elderly patient. The postjunctional muscle membrane thickens. There is an increase in the total number of acetylcholine receptors both at the end plate and in the surrounding areas of the muscle cell. Despite the loss of skeletal muscle mass, the dose requirements for competitive neuromuscular blocking drugs in elderly patients are not reduced. (See page 1223: Peripheral Nervous System.)

10. **D.** The dosages of nondepolarizing neuromuscular blocking drugs do not decline in parallel with the age-related atrophy of skeletal muscle. The time required for onset of neuromuscular blocking agents appears to be slightly, but consistently, increased relative to that of younger patients. However, the clinical duration of their effects is markedly prolonged if their elimination from the plasma is dependent on organ function. The effectiveness of reversal of neuromuscular blockade is not dependent on the patient's age but on the intensity of neuromuscular block and the dose of the reversal agent. (See page 1224: Analgesic and Anesthetic Requirement.)

11. **E.** Plasma concentrations of norepinephrine are two- to fourfold higher in elderly persons than in younger adults during sleep, at rest, and even in response to exercise-induced physical stress. Aging markedly depresses beta-adrenergic end-organ responsiveness. In effect, aging produces "endogenous beta-blockade." There appears to be little change in alpha-adrenoceptor or muscarinic cholinoceptor activity in older adults and no intrinsic changes in the basic contractile properties of peripheral vascular smooth muscle. Adrenal tissues atrophy and cortisol secretion declines at least 15% by the age of 80 years. (See page 1224: Autonomic Nervous System.)

12. **B.** Small airway patency, normally maintained by elastic recoil, may become compromised with aging, and closing capacity typically becomes greater than the volume of the lung at rest. General anesthesia leads to depression of active pulmonary vasoconstriction. Skeletal calcification and increased airway resistance increase the work of breathing in elderly persons and predispose them to acute postoperative ventilatory failure. The cardiovascular and ventilatory responses to imposed hypoxia or hypercarbia are also delayed in onset. (See page 1221: Cardiopulmonary Function.)

CHAPTER 46 ■ ANESTHESIA FOR AMBULATORY SURGERY

For questions 1 to 4, choose the best answer.

1. Which of the following is not a candidate for outpatient surgery requiring general anesthesia?

   A. A term 3-month-old infant with a sibling who died of sudden infant death syndrome
   B. An asymptomatic ex-premature child who is 62 weeks' postconceptional age
   C. A patient in whom a blood transfusion is anticipated
   D. Any patient in American Society of Anesthesiologists (ASA) class IV
   E. A patient scheduled for surgery lasting >3 hours

2. Which of the following statements concerning inhalation agents is FALSE?

   A. Sevoflurane is less pungent than isoflurane or desflurane.
   B. Desflurane and sevoflurane have relatively low blood gas partition coefficients.
   C. Sevoflurane provides for a smoother inhalation induction than desflurane.
   D. Desflurane is more likely than sevoflurane to produce toxic breakdown products in the presence of CO_2 absorbers.
   E. Rapid induction with desflurane may induce significant sympathetic activity.

3. Which of the following statements regarding spinal anesthesia in premature or former premature infants is TRUE?

   A. Raising the infant's legs after placing the spinal anesthetic is necessary to ensure adequate spread of the local anesthetic.
   B. The lateral position is the preferred position for placing the spinal anesthetic.
   C. Discharge of an infant <50 weeks' postconceptional age <24 hours after surgery with spinal anesthesia is appropriate.

   D. Adding clonidine to the spinal anesthetic has no effect on the duration of block in infants.
   E. Hypotension is uncommon after spinal anesthesia in infants.

4. Which of the following statements regarding children with current or recent upper respiratory tract infections (URI) is TRUE?

   A. The incidence of laryngospasm and/or bronchospasm is no different in children with a current URI compared with children who had a URI within the last 4 weeks.
   B. Children with recent URIs are more likely to desaturate (<90%) than children with current URIs.
   C. The risk of adverse respiratory events is the same whether an endotracheal tube or a laryngeal mask airway is used.
   D. Children of parents who smoke have the same risk of adverse airway reactions compared with children of nonsmoking parents.
   E. Nonproductive cough carries the same risk of adverse airway reactions as does cough accompanied by copious secretions.

For questions 5 to 9, choose A if 1, 2, and 3 are correct; B if 1 and 3; C if 2 and 4; D if 4; and E if all.

5. Which of the following statements reflect(s) the current thinking on preoperative fasting and the risk of pulmonary aspiration of gastric contents in ambulatory adult patients?

   1. The longer the withholding of liquids, the safer the gastric environment will be.
   2. In outpatients, 50 mL of clear fluid given 2 hours preoperatively increases gastric volume.
   3. It is acceptable to allow a patient to have a small solid meal the morning of surgery.

4. Coffee drinkers should be encouraged to drink black coffee the morning of surgery to avoid the risk of withdrawal.

6. Which of the following statements regarding perioperative opioids and nonsteroidal anti-inflammatory drugs is/are TRUE?

   1. Preoperative opioids help control hypertension during tracheal intubation and provide for pre-emptive analgesia.
   2. Meperidine is helpful in controlling shivering.
   3. Preoperative celecoxib is accompanied by a reduced need for supplemental analgesia in the postanesthesia care unit (PACU).
   4. Opioids are particularly effective agents in relieving anxiety in adults in the preoperative period.

7. Which of the following statements regarding postoperative nausea and vomiting (PONV) with ambulatory surgery is/are TRUE?

   1. Granisetron (serotonin [5-HT$_3$] antagonist) at 40 μg/kg is a superior antiemetic compared with metoclopramide 0.25 mg/kg.
   2. Midazolam may possess some antiemetic properties.
   3. The ReliefBand acustimulation device is as effective as ondansetron in treating PONV in patients who are still nauseous after having received metoclopramide and droperidol.
   4. If a dose of ondansetron is given in the operating room and the patient complains of nausea

in the PACU, a repeat dose is often effective.

8. Which of the following statements regarding spinal anesthesia is/are TRUE?

   1. Chloroprocaine carries the same risk of transient neurologic symptoms (TNS) as does lidocaine.
   2. Adding fentanyl to the local anesthetic in the spinal technique improves the tolerance for tourniquet pain.
   3. Nausea after spinal or epidural anesthesia is the same as after general anesthesia.
   4. Early ambulation after spinal anesthesia may decrease the incidence of postdural puncture headache.

9. Which of the following statements regarding depth of anesthesia is/are TRUE?

   1. The use of bispectral index (BIS) monitoring has been shown to reduce the use of intraoperative anesthetics by up to 20%.
   2. The use of sympatholytics to treat hemodynamics is associated with faster recovery and fewer side effects than treating the hemodynamics with inhalational agents.
   3. The use of BIS monitoring can result in quicker awakening from general anesthetics.
   4. The use of BIS monitoring has significantly reduced the length of stay in the hospital and significantly decreased the incidence of PONV.

ANSWERS

1. **A.** Ex-premature infants >50 weeks' postconceptional age without a history of apnea may be suitable candidates for outpatient surgery. However, anemia with a hematocrit of <30 is associated with an increased incidence of apnea in preterm infants <60 conceptional weeks. Ex-premature infants with a recent history (in the last 2–3 months) of lingering symptoms such as wheezing or apnea are not candidates for outpatient surgery. It is also prudent to monitor an infant <6 months old who had a sibling die of sudden infant death syndrome for 18 to 24 hours postoperatively. Patients classified as ASA III and IV are considered for outpatient procedures, provided their systemic disease is medically controlled. Little relationship exists between length of anesthesia and recovery; thus, length of surgery is not a criterion for ambulatory procedures. The need for transfusion also is not a contraindication for ambulatory procedures. (See page 1230: Places, Procedures, and Patient Selection.)

2. **D.** Desflurane and sevoflurane, newer halogenated anesthetics with low blood gas partition coefficients,

may be indicated for patients undergoing ambulatory surgery. Unlike desflurane, sevoflurane allows for smooth inhalation induction of anesthesia. Desflurane can be problematic in patients with hypertension when the concentration of the drug is increased rapidly. Rapid changes in the concentration of isoflurane or desflurane have been associated with sympathetic and renin-angiotensin system activity and with transient increases in arterial blood pressure and heart rate. Sevoflurane may generate toxic breakdown products in the presence of CO_2 absorbers. (See page 1238: General Anesthesia: Maintenance.)

3. **E.** Spinal anesthesia is useful for ambulatory procedures in children born prematurely. The procedure is best performed with the child in the sitting position, head supported and somewhat extended, to prevent occlusion of the airway. Because raising the legs may cause the spinal anesthetic to go higher, the child must be kept flat when, for example, the electrosurgical unit pad is placed. Hypotension is less common after spinal anesthesia in infants than in adults. Spinal

anesthesia with a local anesthetic alone may not last long enough. In one study, when clonidine was added to bupivacaine, the length of spinal block increased from an average of 67 minutes to 111 minutes (after 1 μg/kg clonidine). (See page 1234: Place, Procedure, and Patient Selection: Regional Techniques/Spinal Anesthesia.)

4. **A.** One study of 1,078 children 1 month to 18 years old could find no difference in laryngospasm or bronchospasm when the children had active URIs, a URI within 4 weeks, or no symptoms. However, children with active or recent URIs had more episodes of breath-holding, incidences of desaturation <90%, and more respiratory events compared with children without symptoms. Independent risk factors for adverse respiratory events in children with URIs include use of an endotracheal tube (versus use of a laryngeal mask airway), a history of prematurity, a history of reactive airway disease, a history of parental smoking, surgery involving the airway, presence of copious secretions, and nasal congestion. Generally, if a patient with a URI has a normal appetite, does not have a fever or an elevated respiratory rate, and does not appear toxic, it is probably safe to proceed with the planned procedure. (See page 1231: Upper Respiratory Tract Infection [URI].)

5. **D.** For patients who are not at an increased risk of aspiration, prolonged fasting does not improve the gastric environment when compared with patients who received clear liquids 2 hours preoperatively. The clear liquids promote emptying and probably dilute the endogenous gastric secretions to some extent. At present, because of the risk of particulate pulmonary aspiration, it is still recommended strictly to avoid ingestion of solid foods on the day of surgery. Coffee is free of particulate matter and is accepted as a clear liquid. Coffee drinkers should be encouraged to drink coffee before their procedures, because physical signs of withdrawal (e.g., headache) can easily occur. (See page 1231: Restriction of Food and Liquids Before Ambulatory Surgery.)

6. **A.** Preoperative opioids can be used to sedate patients, to control hypertension with tracheal intubation, and to decrease pain before surgery. However, the effectiveness of these agents in relieving anxiety is controversial, particularly in adults. Meperidine is known to help control postoperative shivering. Preoperative administration of nonsteroidal anti-inflammatory drugs is also useful in the early postoperative period. Celecoxib has been shown to reduce postoperative pain. (See page 1233: Opioids and Nonsteroidal Analgesics.)

7. **A.** The 5-HT$_3$ antagonists seem particularly effective. For example, in one study of children who underwent strabismus surgery and were then nauseous during the first 3 hours after recovery from anesthesia, emesis-free episodes were greater after granisetron 40 μg/kg (88%), compared with droperidol 40 μg/kg (63%) or metoclopramide 0.25 mg/kg (58%). Midazolam and propofol, although more commonly used for sedation, have antiemetic effects that are longer in duration than their effects on sedation. When a ReliefBand acustimulation device was compared with ondansetron for patients who were nauseous in the PACU after receiving metoclopramide or droperidol and who were undergoing laparoscopic surgery, nausea was most effectively treated with both the ReliefBand and ondansetron, although both therapies were equally effective individually in treating PONV. If patients have already received ondansetron prophylaxis in the operating room, and are nauseous in the PACU, another repeat dose is not particularly effective. (See page 1242: Nausea and Vomiting.)

8. **C.** Nausea is much less frequent after epidural or spinal anesthesia than after general anesthesia. Lidocaine use has been problematic because of TNS. When fentanyl was added to spinal local anesthetic, tourniquet tolerance was improved. Bed rest does not reduce the frequency of headache. Indeed, early ambulation may decrease the incidence. Lidocaine is associated with a higher rate of TNS than chloroprocaine. (See page 1234: Spinal Anesthesia.)

9. **A.** BIS monitors are thought to decrease anesthesia used during general anesthesia. Because less anesthesia is used, titration of anesthesia with these monitors results in earlier emergence from anesthesia. In a meta-analysis of BIS monitoring for ambulatory anesthesia, BIS monitoring was shown to reduce anesthetic use by 19%, with more modest decreases in PACU duration (4 minutes) and PONV (6%). Sympatholytic drugs, instead of anesthesia, can be used to control autonomic responses to anesthesia. In fact, recovery is faster and side effects are fewer in ambulatory patients whose blood pressure is controlled by sympatholytics instead of inhalation agents. (See page 1240: Depth of Anesthesia.)

CHAPTER 47 ■ MONITORED ANESTHESIA CARE

1. Sedation/analgesia:

   A. is now replaced by the term "conscious sedation" in the American Society of Anesthesiologists (ASA) practice guidelines
   B. describes a state in which a patient's only response is reflex withdrawal from a painful stimulus
   C. describes a state that allows the patient to respond purposefully to a verbal command or tactile stimulation
   D. is a deeper level of sedation than that provided by monitored anesthesia care (MAC)
   E. was a term first introduced by the American Dental Association

2. The condition in which a patient has no movement in response to a painful stimulus describes:

   A. conscious sedation
   B. intravenous sedation
   C. MAC
   D. sedation/analgesia
   E. general anesthesia

3. All of the following statements regarding MAC are true EXCEPT:

   A. The patient remains able to protect the airway for most of the procedure.
   B. It always involves the administration of sedative drugs.
   C. It requires performance of a preanesthesia examination and evaluation.
   D. It is reimbursed at the same level as general or regional anesthesia.
   E. It may include the administration of bronchodilators.

4. The context-sensitive half-time:

   A. is directly related to the elimination half-time
   B. is independent of the duration of infusion

   C. is the half-time of equilibration between drug concentration in the blood and its effect
   D. depends on both metabolism and distribution phenomena
   E. generally is measured by serum assay of drug concentrations

5. Select the TRUE statement regarding drug interactions.

   A. Coexisting respiratory disease is not related to the frequency of respiratory depression in patients receiving opioid-benzodiazepine combinations.
   B. There is no difference in the incidence of adverse respiratory effects when midazolam is used alone or in combination with fentanyl.
   C. Most of the fatalities reported after the use of midazolam and opioids were related to adverse cardiac events.
   D. Opioids and benzodiazepines are synergistic in producing hypnosis.
   E. When an opioid is used in the analgesic dose range, there is little risk of adverse cardiorespiratory interaction.

6. When used for MAC, propofol:

   A. causes greater respiratory depression than midazolam when combined with an opioid
   B. reliably causes amnesia
   C. possesses antiemetic effects
   D. has excellent analgesic properties
   E. has a context-sensitive half-time that depends markedly on the duration of the infusion

7. Advantages of midazolam over diazepam include all of the following EXCEPT:

   A. It has a lower incidence of resedation.
   B. Clearance is unaffected by cimetidine.
   C. Thrombophlebitis is rare.
   D. It is usually painless on injection.

E. Active metabolites work synergistically with parent drug.

8. Choose the TRUE statement regarding remifentanil.

   A. Compared with other opioids, a bolus of remifentanil is associated with an increased incidence of respiratory depression.
   B. It is predominately metabolized by the P450 hepatic enzyme system.
   C. When used with midazolam, remifentanil causes less respiratory depression than with other opioids.
   D. The initial infusion rate should be 1 μg/kg per minute.
   E. It is supplied in a multidose vial that should be refrigerated.

9. Choose the correct order of symptoms observed with worsening local anesthetic toxicity.

   A. Muscle twitching, metallic taste, vertigo
   B. Tinnitus, numbness of the tongue, seizure
   C. Slurred speech, muscle twitching, restlessness
   D. Sedation, tinnitus, seizure
   E. Blurred vision, circumoral numbness, vertigo

10. Dexmedetomidine:

    A. has the same half-life as clonidine
    B. decreases cardiac vagal activity
    C. is not associated with hypotension
    D. is a selective alpha$_2$-receptor antagonist
    E. is administered as an initial bolus of 0.5 to 1.0 μg/kg

11. Choose the correct answer regarding ketamine:

    A. It has been shown to preserve airway reflexes when used in large doses.
    B. It is a good choice for open globe injuries.
    C. It produces a dissociative state.
    D. Doses of 0.3 mg/kg are frequently associated with significant cardiorespiratory depression.
    E. It is a di-isophenol derivative.

For questions 12 to 23, choose A if 1, 2, and 3 are correct; B if 1 and 3; C if 2 and 4; D if 4; and E if all.

12. MAC:

    1. includes diagnosis and treatment of clinical problems that occur during a procedure
    2. may be provided by intensive care unit nurses
    3. conceptually should allow for a more rapid recovery than general anesthesia
    4. does not include postprocedure anesthesia management

13. MAC resembles general anesthesia in that both:

    1. include preoperative assessment
    2. require continual physical presence of the anesthesiologist or nurse anesthetist
    3. include intraoperative monitoring
    4. involve the administration of sedative drugs

14. The ideal sedation technique for MAC:

    1. should provide rapid and complete recovery at the end of the procedure
    2. should have a low incidence of side effects
    3. may provide deeper sedation than that provided during "sedation/analgesia"
    4. allows the patient to be able to communicate during the procedure

15. Sedation may depress:

    1. protective laryngeal and pharyngeal reflexes
    2. the ventilatory response to hypoxia and hypercapnia
    3. the swallowing reflex
    4. the resting arterial partial pressure of oxygen

16. Agitation during MAC could be caused by:

    1. hypoxia
    2. local anesthetic toxicity
    3. distended bladder
    4. cerebral hypoperfusion

17. Advantages of administration of drugs by continuous infusion rather than by intermittent dosing during MAC include:

    1. reduced total amount of drug administered
    2. facilitation of a more rapid recovery
    3. fewer episodes of excessive sedation
    4. fewer episodes of inadequate sedation

18. Select the TRUE statement(s) regarding the advantages of propofol over benzodiazepines for conscious sedation.

    1. Immediate recovery is faster.
    2. Psychomotor function returns to baseline earlier.
    3. There is less postoperative clumsiness.
    4. The postanesthesia care unit stay is markedly shorter.

19. Flumazenil reversal of benzodiazepine-induced sedation:

    1. is inexpensive and should be routine
    2. is associated with undesirable hemodynamic effects
    3. does not reverse the amnestic effect
    4. may be associated with resedation because of its short elimination half-life

20. Which of the following statements about the use of opioids during MAC is/are TRUE?

    1. They are a good choice for sedation during a working spinal anesthetic.
    2. Alfentanil is a good choice for brief, intense analgesia.
    3. They are associated with reliable amnesia.

4. They are associated with a significant risk of nausea.

21. Oxygen administration during MAC:

    1. can "mask" significant alveolar hypoventilation
    2. must be administered in high concentrations to be effective
    3. may be required in the postoperative period
    4. is required by the ASA standards for basic monitoring

22. Bispectral index monitoring:

    1. may help avoid complications of overdosing medications
    2. is a processed electroencephalogram parameter

3. ideally should be used as an adjunct to clinical evaluation
4. increases upon deepening of sedation

23. The ASA practice guidelines for sedation and analgesia by nonanesthesiologists:

    1. suggest that the individual performing the procedure also monitor the patient's vital signs
    2. suggest the routine administration of supplemental oxygen
    3. emphasize the importance of preprocedure patient evaluations but not fasting
    4. suggest that an individual with advanced life support skills be present during the procedure

---

ANSWERS

---

1. **C.** Sedation/analgesia is the term currently used by the ASA in its practice guidelines for sedation and analgesia by nonanesthesiologists. The current ASA definition of sedation/analgesia is "a state that allows patients to tolerate unpleasant procedures while maintaining adequate cardiorespiratory functions and the ability to respond purposefully to verbal command or tactile stimulation." Thus, sedation/analgesia is intended to be a lighter level of sedation than may be encountered during MAC. The term sedation/analgesia is used most frequently in the context of care provided by nonanesthesiologists and implies a level of vigilance that is less than that required for general anesthesia. The ASA specifically states that those patients whose only response is reflex withdrawal from a painful stimulus are sedated to a greater degree than encompassed by the term sedation/analgesia. (See page 1247: Terminology.)

2. **E.** General anesthesia describes those patients who are medicated to the extent that they have no movement in response to a painful stimulus. (See page 1247: Terminology.)

3. **B.** MAC refers to those clinical situations in which the patient remains able to protect the airway during most of the procedure. Because MAC is a physician service provided to an individual patient and is based on medical necessity, it should be subject to the same level of reimbursement as general or regional anesthesia. The ASA states that MAC must include performance of a preanesthetic examination and evaluation. Also, the ASA states that all institutional regulations pertaining to anesthesia services shall be observed, and all the usual services performed by an anesthesiologist should be provided including administration of sedatives, tranquilizers, antiemetics, narcotics, other analgesics, and beta-blockers,

vasopressors, bronchodilators, antihypertensives, or other pharmacologic therapy as may be required in the judgment of the anesthesiologist. (See page 1247: Terminology.)

4. **D.** The context-sensitive half-time is the time required for the plasma drug concentration to decline by 50% after terminating an infusion of a particular duration. The context-sensitive half-time takes into account both metabolism and distribution effects. It is highly dependent on the duration of infusion, particularly for drugs such as thiopental and fentanyl. It bears no constant relationship to the elimination half-times. Generally, it is calculated by computer simulation of multicompartmental pharmacokinetic models. (See page 1249: Context-Sensitive Half-Time.)

5. **D.** During MAC, the maximum benefit of opioid supplementation in terms of potentiation of other administered sedatives will accrue when the opioid is used in the analgesic dose range. Within this dose range, there is great potential for adverse cardiorespiratory interaction. Opioid-benzodiazepine combinations are frequently used to achieve the components of hypnosis, amnesia, and analgesia. The opioid-benzodiazepine combination displays marked synergism in producing hypnosis. Several fatalities have been reported after the use of midazolam, most of these related to adverse respiratory events. In many of these cases, midazolam was used in combination with an opioid. Studies have shown that midazolam usually does not produce significant respiratory effects when used alone; however, the combination of midazolam and fentanyl has a higher incidence of hypoxemia in study subjects. The respiratory depressive effects of this drug combination are likely to be even more significant in patients with coexisting

respiratory or central nervous system disease or at the extremes of age. (See page 1250: Drug Interactions in Monitored Anesthesia Care.)

6. **C.** Propofol has many ideal properties of drug for use during MAC. The context-sensitive half-time remains short regardless of the length of infusion, and rapid onset allows for easier titration. It appears to have antiemetic properties but no analgesic or amnestic effects. When combined with opioids, propofol appears to result in minimal respiratory depression. This is in contrast to benzodiazepine-opioid combinations, which can cause severe respiratory depression. (See page 1251: Specific Drugs Used for Monitored Anesthesia Care.)

7. **E.** The major advantages of midazolam over diazepam include the following: midazolam is water soluble, it is usually painless upon injection, thrombophlebitis is rare, it has a short elimination half-life of 1 to 4 hours, the clearance is unaffected by histamine (H_2)-antagonists, it has inactive metabolites, and resedation is unlikely. (See page 1251: Specific Drugs Used for Monitored Anesthesia Care.)

8. **A.** Unlike previously available opioids, remifentanil is predominately metabolized by nonspecific esterases generating an extremely rapid clearance and offset of effect. Published data suggest that bolus administration of remifentanil is associated with an increased incidence of respiratory depression and chest wall rigidity. Because these side effects are likely to be related to high peak concentration of drug, it is recommended that remifentanil boluses be administered slowly or by using a pure infusion technique. The most logical method for the administration of remifentanil during MAC is by an adjustable infusion. Most investigators have used infusion rates that start at 0.1 μg/kg per minute approximately 5 minutes before the first painful stimulus. This initial loading infusion is then weaned to approximately 0.05 μg/kg per minute to maintain patient comfort. Remifentanil is supplied as a powder that must be reconstituted before use. (See page 1251: Specific Drugs Used for Monitored Anesthesia Care.)

9. **D.** The clinically recognizable effects of local anesthetic toxicity on the central nervous system are concentration dependent. Initial symptoms are sedation, numbness of the tongue and circumoral tissues, and a metallic taste. As concentrations increase, restlessness, vertigo, tinnitus, and difficulty focusing may occur. Higher concentrations result in slurred speech and skeletal muscle twitching, which often herald the onset of tonic-clonic seizures. (See page 1258: Preparedness to Recognize and Treat Local Anesthetic Toxicity.)

10. **E.** Dexmedetomidine, like clonidine, is a selective alpha$_2$-receptor agonist. Stimulation of alpha$_2$-receptors produces sedation and analgesia, a reduction of sympathetic outflow, and an increase in cardiac vagal activity. The use of clonidine in the perioperative period is limited by its long half-life of 6 to 10 hours. However, dexmedetomidine has a much shorter half-life and greater alpha$_2$-receptor selectivity. Despite its alpha$_2$-selectivity, dexmedetomidine may still cause significant bradycardia and hypotension. Initial bolus doses range from 0.5 to 1.0 μg/kg over 10 to 20 minutes followed by a continuous infusion of 0.2 to 0.7 μg/kg per hour (See page 1251: Specific-Drugs Used for Monitored Anesthesia Care.)

11. **C.** Ketamine is a phencyclidine derivative. When used in small doses (0.25–0.5 mg/kg), its use is associated with minimal respiratory and cardiovascular depression. Ketamine produces a dissociative state in which the eyes remain open with a nystagmic gaze. Ketamine can elevate intraocular pressure and is thus relatively contraindicated in patients with open globe injuries. Increased oral secretions make laryngospasm more likely. Although it has been suggested that airway reflexes are relatively preserved with ketamine, no convincing evidence supports this notion. (See page 1251: Specific Drugs Used for Monitored Anesthesia Care.)

12. **B.** MAC includes all aspects of anesthesia care: a preoperative visit, intraoperative care, and postprocedure anesthesia management. During MAC, the anesthesiologist or a member of the anesthesia care team provides a number of specific services including but not limited to monitoring of vital signs, maintenance of the patient's airway, continual evaluation of vital functions, and diagnosis and treatment of clinical problems that occur during the procedure. (See page 1247: Terminology.)

13. **A.** MAC usually is provided to conscious patients undergoing therapeutic or diagnostic procedures that would otherwise be unacceptably uncomfortable or unsafe without the attention of an anesthesiologist. As with general anesthesia, there must be a preanesthetic examination and evaluation, a prescription of anesthesia care, personal participation in or medical direction of the entire plan of care, and continuous physical presence of the anesthesia care provider. MAC always involves monitoring of a patient but does not necessarily require the administration of sedative drugs. (See page 1247: Preoperative Assessment.)

14. **E.** The ideal sedation technique involves the administration of either individual or combinations of analgesic, amnestic, and hypnotic drugs. There should be a minimal incidence of side effects such as cardiorespiratory depression, nausea and vomiting, delayed emergence, and dysphoria. Recovery after the completion of the procedure should be rapid and complete. (See page 1247: Techniques of Monitored Anesthesia Care.)

15. E. Protective laryngeal and pharyngeal reflexes are depressed by sedation and may render the patient vulnerable to aspiration. The swallowing reflex can be depressed for a long time following the return of consciousness. Opioids depress the normal ventilatory response to hypoxia and hypercapnia. Benzodiazepines appear to have a variable effect on ventilatory response, although they clearly potentiate the respiratory depression of opioids. Hypoventilation will lead to reduced oxygen saturation in the absence of supplemental inspired oxygen. (See page 1256: Sedation and Protective Airway Reflexes.)

16. E. Agitation during MAC may be a result of pain or anxiety, but it is of paramount importance that hypoxia and cerebral hypoperfusion be excluded. Other possible causes of agitation include local anesthetic toxicity, hypothermia, distended bladder, nausea, uncomfortable position or equipment, and prolonged tourniquet inflation. (See page 1247: Techniques of Monitored Anesthesia Care.)

17. E. Continuous infusions of sedative drugs are superior to intermittent bolus dosing because they produce less fluctuation in drug concentration, thus reducing the number of episodes of inadequate or excessive sedation. Also, the total amount of drug will be lower, thereby facilitating a more prompt recovery. (See page 1248: Pharmacologic Basis of Conscious Sedation Techniques—Optimizing Drug Administration.)

18. A. A study by Mackenzie showed that a group of patients receiving propofol had faster immediate recovery than did the group of patients that received midazolam. Furthermore, psychomotor function was comparable to baseline values immediately following propofol sedation but did not return to baseline until 2 hours after midazolam administration. Another study by White et al. showed that propofol produced less postoperative sedation, drowsiness, confusion, and clumsiness than midazolam; however, both had similar discharge times. (See page 1251: Specific Drugs Used for Monitored Anesthesia Care: Propofol.)

19. D. Flumazenil is a specific benzodiazepine antagonist. It reverses the sedative and anesthetic effects without adverse side effects. It has a short elimination half-time, so there is a potential for resedation after the flumazenil has been cleared. The routine use of flumazenil represents a significant cost disadvantage compared with propofol sedation. (See page 1252: Benzodiazepines.)

20. C. Opioids are best used to provide the analgesic component during MAC. They are not appropriate for a sedative or anesthetic component because they cannot reliably produce sedation without significant respiratory depression, and they lack significant amnestic properties. Propofol and midazolam produce more specific sedative effects. Opioids are associated with a significant risk of nausea and vomiting in ambulatory patients. Alfentanil's pharmacokinetic profile makes it well suited for treatment of brief painful periods such as placement of a retrobulbar block. (See page 1252: Opioids.)

21. B. Even in moderate concentrations, oxygen administration is very effective for increasing a low oxygen saturation resulting from hypoventilation. However, when the patient is receiving oxygen, significant hypoventilation and hypercarbia can exist even though the oxygen saturation is normal. Oxygen administration is not required by the ASA standards but should be highly considered whenever sedatives or respiratory depressants are used. Respiratory depression can persist into the recovery period; measurement of oxygen saturation on room air may be useful before discharging a patient from the postanesthesia care unit without supplemental oxygen. (See page 1256: Supplemental Oxygen Administration.)

22. A. The bispectral index is a processed electroencephalogram parameter. Sedation monitoring is attractive because of the potential to titrate drugs more accurately and thus avoid the adverse effects of both overdosing and underdosing. An increased depth of sedation is associated with a predictable decrease in the bispectral index. Although the use of the bispectral index to monitor sedation is appealing, conventional assessment of sedation is an important mechanism whereby continuous patient contact is maintained. Ideally, bispectral index monitoring will be employed in the future as an adjunct to clinical evaluation, rather than as the primary monitor of consciousness. (See page 1258: Bispectral Index Monitoring During Monitored Anesthesia Care.)

23. C. The ASA practice guidelines for sedation and analgesia by nonanesthesiologists emphasize the importance of preprocedure patient evaluation, patient preparation, and appropriate fasting periods. These guidelines also suggest that an individual other than the person performing the procedure be available to monitor the patient's comfort and physiologic status. The routine administration of supplemental oxygen is recommended. At least one person with advanced life support skills should be present during the procedure. (See page 1259: Sedation and Analgesia by Nonanesthesiologists.)

CHAPTER 48 ■ TRAUMA AND BURNS

1. Which of the following statements is FALSE?

   A. Blind passage of a nasopharyngeal airway should be avoided if a basilar skull fracture is suspected.
   B. A cuffed oropharyngeal airway provides good protection against aspiration of gastric contents.
   C. Cricothyrotomy is contraindicated in patients <12 years of age.
   D. The esophageal-tracheal Combitube has been associated with esophageal lacerations leading to subcutaneous emphysema, pneumomediastinum, and pneumoperitoneum.
   E. Cricothyrotomy is contraindicated in patients suspected of having laryngeal trauma.

2. Which of the following statements is FALSE?

   A. The intubating laryngeal mask provides adequate ventilation and higher success with blind intubation, and it can accommodate an endotracheal tube up to 8 mm.
   B. Complications of coughing and bucking at the time of intubation in trauma patients include brain herniation, extrusion of eye contents, or dislodgment of a hemostatic clot.
   C. Cricoid pressure and manual inline stabilization aids in the placement of a laryngeal mask airway (LMA).
   D. Serious airway compromise may develop within a few hours in up to 50% of patients with major penetrating facial injuries.
   E. The presence of cartilaginous fractures or mucosal abnormalities of the airway necessitates awake intubation.

3. Of the following statements, which is FALSE?

   A. Immediate treatment for tension pneumothorax is insertion of a 14-gauge angiocatheter via the second intercostal space on the midclavicular line.
   B. A flail chest results in impaired respiratory mechanics, and therefore, intubation and mechanical ventilation are the primary treatments of choice.
   C. Classic symptoms of tension pneumothorax include cyanosis, tachypnea, hypotension, and neck vein distention.
   D. An underlying pulmonary contusion with increased elastic recoil of the lung and work of breathing is the main cause of respiratory insufficiency in flail chest.
   E. A flail chest can result from sternal and rib fractures.

4. Which of the following statements is TRUE?

   A. The most common cause for hypotension in the hypotensive trauma patient is pericardial tamponade.
   B. Fluid resuscitation with lactated Ringer's solution of 2000 mL over 15 minutes in adults should normalize the vital signs in a patient with moderate hemorrhage (20–40% blood volume).
   C. The base deficit, blood lactate level, and probably sublingual P_{CO_2} (SLP_{CO_2}) are the most useful and practical markers of organ perfusion that can be used to set the goals of resuscitation in trauma patients.
   D. Intraosseous cannulation has many severe side effects.
   E. Intraosseous cannulation should not be used in children <5 years old.

5. Which one of the following statements is FALSE?

   A. Following primary head injury, a leading cause of morbidity is the progression of secondary injury resulting from tissue hypoxia.
   B. A maximally dilated and unresponsive pupil suggests uncal herniation under the falx cerebri.
   C. The most important therapeutic maneuvers in head-injured patients are aimed at maintaining cerebral perfusion pressure and O_2 delivery.

D. A reduction in intracranial pressure with pentobarbital is an effective means of cerebral protection and should be instituted in all instances of head injury.

E. The Glasgow Coma Scale is a valuable tool in the evaluation of head-injured patients.

6. Which of the following statements is FALSE?

A. Traumatic herniation following diaphragmatic injury is more common on the left side than on the right side.

B. A focused approach with sonography for trauma requires one-third of the time the conventional approach requires.

C. Laparoscopy is an excellent screening tool in abdominal trauma patients.

D. Significant intra-abdominal bleeding is typically accompanied by considerable changes in abdominal girth.

E. Isolated intestinal injuries are uncommon after blunt trauma.

7. Of the following methods of intraoperative monitoring for the trauma patient, which single monitor is the most necessary before surgery?

A. Right radial intra-arterial blood pressure monitor
B. Esophageal temperature monitoring
C. Central venous pressure monitoring
D. Transesophageal echocardiography
E. Electrocardiogram

8. Choose the FALSE statement.

A. Patients with a burn of >30% total body surface area develop resistance to most nondepolarizing muscle relaxants.

B. The current recommendation for administration of hydroxyethyl starch is not to exceed 20 mL/kg.

C. Patients with hemorrhagic shock often exhibit bradycardia and respond readily to catecholamine infusions.

D. Hypothermia leads to impaired O_2 release from red blood cells because of a leftward shift of the O_2 dissociation curve.

E. A level of fibrin degradation products >40 mg/dL is diagnostic of disseminated intravascular coagulation.

9. Alcoholic ketoacidosis is managed most appropriately by which of the following?

A. Benzodiazepines
B. O_2 therapy
C. Sodium bicarbonate
D. Insulin
E. Intravenous dextrose

For questions 10 to 18, choose A if 1, 2, and 3 are correct; B if 1 and 3; C if 2 and 4; D if 4; and E if all.

10. Regarding spine and spinal cord injuries, identify the TRUE statement(s).

1. Intact sensory perception over the sacral distribution and voluntary contraction of the anus (sacral sparing) are present in incomplete spinal cord injuries.

2. The best radiological examinations for spine injury are with the patient in an upright position with a radiolucent neck collar.

3. Any intubation technique is safe as long as the patient's neck is held in a neutral position.

4. Cricoid pressure should be forcefully applied when intubating patients with cervical spine injuries.

11. Regarding neck and chest injuries, identify the TRUE statement(s).

1. Signs of airway injury include respiratory distress, subcutaneous crepitus, and laryngeal tenderness.

2. First rib fractures are an indication of severe underlying trauma.

3. The most definitive test for pneumothorax in the supine patient is the computed tomographic (CT) scan.

4. After placement of a thoracostomy tube, drainage of 1,000 mL of blood and collection of >200 mL/hour are indications for thoracotomy.

12. Which of the following statements is/are TRUE?

1. Following pelvic fracture, retroperitoneal hematomas may lead to respiratory difficulty because of pressure on the diaphragm.

2. Angiographic embolization is indicated to treat arterial bleeding following pelvic fracture.

3. Open fractures of the extremities should be repaired within 6 hours to reduce the likelihood of sepsis.

4. Immediate surgery is indicated for compartment syndrome when intracompartmental pressure exceeds 15 cm H_2O.

13. Identify the TRUE statement(s).

1. Fourth-degree burns involve muscle, fascia, and bone, thus necessitating complete excision and leaving the patient with limited function.

2. Full-thickness burns involving >10% of the total body surface area are considered major burns.

3. Sources of airway compromise following burn include upper airway edema from fluid resuscitation and copious thick secretions.

4. Because swelling of the airway following thermal injury is only minimal in children, intubation is often not necessary in pediatric patients.

14. Identify the TRUE statement(s).

1. Methylene blue is the main treatment for cyanide toxicity.

2. The classic cherry red color of the blood occurs only at carboxyhemoglobin (HbCO) concentrations >40%.

3. Patients with an HbCO level of >10% at admission are recommended for hyperbaric O_2 therapy.

4. Immediate O_2 administration and removal from the toxic environment often obviate the need for specific treatment of cyanide toxicity resulting from smoke inhalation.

15. Identify the TRUE statement(s).

1. Fluid flux in burn patients is enhanced by increased intravascular hydrostatic and interstitial osmotic pressures and decreased interstitial hydrostatic pressure.

2. Colloid solutions are preferred for resuscitation during the first day following a burn injury.

3. Fluid resuscitation is essential in the early care of the burned patient with an injury >15% of the total body surface area; smaller burns can be managed with replacement at 150% of the calculated maintenance rate.

4. The hematocrit in burn patients should be kept >30%.

16. Identify the TRUE statement(s).

1. Sublingual P_{CO_2} is an acceptable marker of organ perfusion.

2. An O_2 delivery index of 500 mL/m^2 per minute is an acceptable goal for optimal shock resuscitation.

3. An arterial–end-tidal–arterial CO_2 difference of >10 mmHg predicts mortality after resuscitation in trauma patients.

4. Unrecognized hypoperfusion may allow the passage of luminal microorganisms across the intestinal wall and leads to sepsis and multiple organ failure.

17. Identify the TRUE statement(s).

1. Hemorrhage and hypovolemia following trauma increase the effects of intravenous anesthetic agents on the brain and the heart.

2. The calculated dose for etomidate in patients with shock is approximately one-half of that given to healthy patients.

3. All inhalational anesthetics increase cerebral blood flow and cerebral blood volume and thus increase intracranial pressure.

4. In spontaneously breathing patients, opioids decrease mean arterial pressure and intracranial pressure.

18. Identify the FALSE statement(s).

1. The wake-up time following a midazolam infusion for postoperative sedation can be up to six times longer than the wake-up time following a propofol infusion.

2. A urine output of <0.5 mL/kg is the most sensitive indicator of acute renal failure.

3. Intra-abdominal pressures of >20 to 25 mm Hg indicate the need for immediate abdominal decompression.

4. In trauma patients, deep venous thrombosis (DVT) usually occurs more than 1 week after the injury.

ANSWERS

1. **B.** The cuffed oropharyngeal airways and LMAs provide for an adequate airway, but they do not protect against gastric aspiration. Blind passage of a nasopharyngeal airway in a patient with a basilar skull fracture may actually enter the anterior cranial fossa and therefore is contraindicated with this injury. Cricothyrotomy is contraindicated in patients <12 years old and in patients suspected of having laryngeal trauma. Permanent laryngeal damage may occur in young patients, whereas uncorrectable airway obstruction may occur in patients with laryngeal trauma. The esophageal-tracheal Combitube is an acceptable airway alternative. It is not, however, without complications, such as esophageal laceration and its sequelae. (See page 1263: Airway Obstruction.)

2. **C.** Difficulty may be encountered when inserting an LMA in the presence of cricoid pressure and manual inline stabilization of the cervical spine. The intubating laryngeal mask was developed specifically for blind intubation and can accommodate an 8-mm tube, rather than the 6-mm tube via conventional LMAs. Adequate anesthesia should, if possible, be supplied to trauma patients to prevent hemodynamic changes and coughing to reduce their sequelae such as brain herniation, extrusion of eye contents, and dislodgment of a hemostatic clot. Serious airway compromise may develop within a few hours in up to 50% of patients with major penetrating facial injuries or multiple trauma as a result of progressive inflammation or edema resulting from liberal administration of fluids. The presence of cartilaginous fractures or mucosal abnormalities necessitates awake intubation with a fiber-optic bronchoscope or awake tracheostomy. (See page 1264: Full Stomach; and Head, Open Eye, and Contained Major Vessel Injuries; page 1265: Cervical Spine Injury; and page 1266: Cervical Airway Injuries.)

3. **B.** A flail chest results from comminuted fractures of at least three adjacent ribs or rib fractures with associated costochondral separation or sternal fracture. Without significant gas exchange

abnormalities, chest wall instability alone is not an indication for respiratory support. There is evidence that liberal use of mechanical ventilation in the presence of a flail chest or pulmonary contusion increases the rate of pulmonary complications and mortality and prolongs the hospital stay. Effective pain relief by itself can improve respiratory function and often avoids the need for mechanical ventilation. Tension pneumothorax can be manifested by cyanosis, tachypnea, hypoxia, and neck vein distention. The definitive treatment for this is chest tube placement with suction. The emergency treatment of tension pneumothorax, however, may require insertion of a 14-gauge angiocatheter via the second intercostal space at the midclavicular line on the affected side. (See page 1266: Management of Breathing Abnormalities.)

4. **C.** Some of the proven markers of organ perfusion can be used during early management to set the goals of resuscitation. Of these, the base deficit, blood lactate level, and probably $SLPCO_2$ are the most useful and practical tools during all phases of shock. Hemorrhage is the most common cause of traumatic hypotension and shock. Other sources include abnormal pump function, pericardial tamponade, pre-existing cardiac disease, pneumothorax or hemothorax, and spinal cord injury. Response to fluids aids in the assessment of hypovolemia. Two liters of lactated Ringer's solution over 15 minutes in adults should normalize vital signs if hemorrhage is mild (10–20% blood volume), transiently improve moderate hemorrhage (20–40% blood volume), and have no response in patients with severe hemorrhage (>40% blood volume). Intraosseous cannulation is an acceptable form of vascular access in children younger than 5 years and has a low incidence of complications. (See page 1267: Management of Shock.)

5. **D.** Hypoxia is a major cause of secondary injury and is a major factor in trauma death of head-injured patients. Therefore, rapid diagnosis and treatment of head injury are paramount. The Glasgow Coma Scale is a valuable tool in the evaluation of head-injured patients and provides a standard means of evaluating the patient's neurologic status. Physical signs of brain injury include motor dysfunction, which, in turn, includes ocular motor abnormalities such as unresponsive pupils. Management of head-injured patients should be aimed at maintaining cerebral perfusion and O_2 delivery. Decreasing intracranial pressure is a major step in this process. High-dose barbiturates, (e.g., pentobarbital), however, are of no routine value and are used only for refractory intracranial pressure elevation. A maximally dilated and unresponsive pupil suggests uncal herniation under the falx cerebri. (See page 1269: Early Management of Specific Injuries: Head Injury.)

6. **D.** Laparoscopy is an excellent screening tool in abdominal trauma patients. FAST (focused-approach

abdominal sonography for trauma) requires one-third of the time as the conventional approach. Isolated intestinal injuries are uncommon after blunt trauma. The liver protects the right side of the diaphragm; thus, traumatic herniation is more common on the left side. Absence of abdominal distention does not rule out intra-abdominal bleeding; at least 1 L of blood can accumulate before the smallest change in girth is apparent, and the diaphragm can also move cephalad, allowing further significant blood loss without any change in abdominal circumference. (See page 1277: Diaphragmatic Injury and Abdominal and Pelvic Injuries.)

7. **A.** Intra-arterial pressure monitoring allows beat-to-beat data acquisition and sampling for blood gases. A relatively stable patient may rapidly decompensate when the abdomen or chest is open. Thus, arterial pressure is valuable for therapeutic decisions. Central venous pressure monitoring is often unnecessary in young, healthy patients, although in elderly patients or when myocardial damage is likely, this approach can guide fluid replacement. Because central venous pressure or pulmonary capillary wedge pressure measurements are subject to error in the presence of decreased ventricular compliance or pulmonary contusion, pulmonary artery catheters, with the ability to measure right ventricular output, may be helpful to determine proper organ perfusion. Normothermia is critical in the trauma patient, but devices for temperature monitoring should not delay the start of surgery. Transesophageal echocardiography provides valuable diagnostic information, including right and left ventricular volumes, ejection fraction, and wall motion abnormalities. Visualization of fat and air entry into the right side of the heart and monitoring ventricular volume are added benefits. Despite this, transesophageal echocardiography insertion before surgery is not critical. (See page 1282: Monitoring.)

8. **C.** Burns of >30% total body surface area lead to resistance to all nondepolarizing muscle relaxants except mivacurium beginning at 1 week and peaking around 5 to 6 weeks following injury. Current dosing recommendations for hydroxyethyl starch are to give no more than 20 mL/kg in 24 hours. This is because of potential coagulation abnormalities resulting from reduced platelet function, reduced fibrinogen levels, reduced factor VIII, and reduced von Willebrand factor. Confusion can arise concerning whether a patient is experiencing hemorrhagic shock or neurogenic shock. Indeed, a trauma patient may be experiencing both types of shock simultaneously. However, the hallmark of neurogenic shock is that patients exhibit bradycardia and readily respond to fluids and catecholamine infusions. Hemorrhagic shock manifests as tachycardia and hypotension. Patients with hypothermia have a left shift of their O_2 dissociation curve, which impairs tissue oxygenation. Also, hypothermia may impair platelet and clotting

enzyme function and cause abnormalities in potassium and calcium homeostasis. Disseminated intravascular coagulation can be a devastating complication in the trauma patient. A level of fibrin degradation products >40 mg/dL is diagnostic of disseminated intravascular coagulation. (See page 1285: Anesthetic and Adjunct Drugs: Burns; and page 1288: Management of Intraoperative Complications: Persistent Hypotension, Hypothermia, and Coagulation Abnormalities.)

9. **E.** Alcoholic ketoacidosis is treated with intravenous dextrose, whereas diabetic ketoacidosis is managed with insulin. Symptomatic treatment with sodium bicarbonate has serious disadvantages, including leftward shift of the oxyhemoglobin dissociation curve causing decreased O_2 unloading, a hyperosmolar state secondary to the excessive sodium load, hypokalemia, further hemodynamic depression, overshoot alkalosis a few hours after giving the drug, and intracellular acidosis if adequate ventilation or pulmonary blood flow cannot be provided. (See page 1288: Management of Intraoperative Complications: Electrolyte and Acid-Base Disturbances.)

10. **B.** Depending on the degree of deficit, spinal cord injuries are categorized as complete or incomplete. Sacral sparing is present in incomplete injuries, whereas lack of sacral sparing is present in complete injuries. The possibility of neurologic recovery is slight to none in a complete injury, whereas functional restoration may occur in up to 50% of patients with incomplete injuries. Any radiological examination should be performed with the patient in supine position until a spinal injury is ruled out, so the risk of displacement of the fracture is minimized. If a cervical spine fracture is suspected, immobilization or manual inline stabilization of the neck is necessary before the patient is moved. Any intubation technique is safe as long as the neck is maintained in a neutral position. Cricoid pressure should be applied with great care in the patient with a possible cervical spine injury, because it may produce undue motion of the spine if excessive force is used. (See page 1272: Spine and Spinal Cord Injury: Initial Evaluation, Radiological Evaluation, and Immobilization and Intubation.)

11. **E.** Respiratory distress, cyanosis, and stridor are obvious signs of airway injury. Other signs that strongly suggest airway injury are dysphonia, hoarseness, cough, hemoptysis, air bubbling from the wound, subcutaneous crepitus, laryngeal tenderness, pneumothorax, and hemothorax. First rib fractures, owing to the high amount of injury required for fracture, indicate severe underlying trauma, particularly to the aorta, the subclavian vessels, the heart, the brain, and/or the spinal cord. Likewise, scapula fractures suggest severe thoracic injury, particularly cardiac and lung injuries. Paradoxically, sternal fractures are usually not associated with serious trauma to the thoracic or abdominal viscera. Upright plain radiographs provide the best

opportunity for detection of pleural air. This position, however, may be impossible or contraindicated in some trauma patients. Although a chest radiograph and an ultrasound scan can complement each other, a CT scan is the most definitive radiological test for detecting pneumothorax. Initial drainage of 1,000 mL of blood, or collection of >200 mL/hour for several hours after thoracostomy, is an indication for thoracotomy. Additional indications are a "white lung" appearance on the anteroposterior chest radiograph, a continuous major air leak from the chest tube, and evidence of pericardial tamponade. (See page 1274: Neck Injury, Chest Wall Injury, and Pleural Injury.)

12. **A.** Pelvic fractures can often result in significant bleeding, but the bleeding tends to be venous in nature and will often tamponade itself. Arterial bleeding, in turn, may lead to large retroperitoneal hematomas and can lead to respiratory difficulty. Thus, angiography and embolization are indicated for treatment of arterial bleeding. Delayed fracture repair is associated with an increased risk of sepsis, pneumonia, DVT, and cerebral complications of fat embolism. Therefore, fixation should occur as soon as possible. In particular, open fractures should be repaired within 6 hours to reduce the risk of sepsis. Compartment syndrome, which is characterized by severe pain in the affected extremity, should be recognized early so emergency fasciotomy can be effective in preventing irreversible muscle and nerve damage. The definitive diagnosis is made by measuring compartment pressures. Pressures exceeding 40 cm H_2O are an indication for immediate surgery. (See page 1278: Fractures of the Pelvis and Extremity Injuries.)

13. **A.** Burns are classified as first, second, third, and fourth degree. First- and second-degree burns are partial thickness, whereas third- and fourth-degree burns are full thickness. Fourth-degree burns are the most severe and leave the patient with the highest likelihood of decreased function. Major burns include the following: (1) full-thickness burns of >10% of total body surface area; (2) partial-thickness burns of >25% of total body surface area in adults and >20% of total body surface area at extremes of age; (3) burns involving the face, hands, feet, or perineum; (4) inhalational, chemical, or electrical burns; and (5) burns in patients with severe pre-existing medical conditions. In the upper airway, glottic and periglottic edema as well as copious, thick secretions may produce respiratory obstruction; this may be aggravated by fluid resuscitation even in the absence of significant inhalation injury. The pediatric airway can be greatly compromised by even minimal amounts of swelling, because of its small diameter. Prophylactic intubation may often be required in children who are suspected of having an inhalational injury, even though they are not yet in respiratory distress. (See page 1279: Burns and Airway Complications.)

14. C. Carbon monoxide interferes with mitochondrial function and produces tissue hypoxia by shifting the hemoglobin dissociation curve to the left. The ultimate effect of this is impaired release of O_2 to tissues. This effect can be offset by high concentrations of inspired O_2. The classic cherry red color of blood occurs at an HbCO concentration of >40%, but this may be obscured by coexistent hypoxia and cyanosis. Therefore, HbCO concentration is the most sensitive indicator of carbon monoxide toxicity. The most effective treatment to date for carbon monoxide toxicity is hyperbaric O_2 therapy. An HbCO level of 30% or more is an indication for this therapy. Cyanide toxicity can accompany smoke inhalation in victims of fires within a closed space. Specific treatments for cyanide toxicity include amyl nitrate, sodium nitrite, and thiosulfate. The half-life of cyanide, however, is short, approximately 1 hour, and thus removal from the toxic environment and treatment with O_2 are often all that are necessary to reduce the cyanide levels. (See page 1280: Carbon Monoxide Toxicity and Cyanide Toxicity.)

15. B. Fluid flux in burn patients is enhanced by increased intravascular hydrostatic and interstitial osmotic pressures and decreased interstitial hydrostatic pressure. Intravascular volume can be restored with either crystalloid or colloid solutions. Crystalloid solutions are preferred for resuscitation during the first day following a burn injury; leakage of colloids during this phase may increase edema. Fluid resuscitation is essential in the early care of the burned patient with an injury >15% of the total body surface area; smaller burns can be managed with replacement at 150% of the calculated maintenance rate and careful monitoring of fluid status. Patients often tolerate a decreased hematocrit following burn injury. Transfusion is usually not initiated until the hematocrit is <15 to 20% in healthy patients, ~25% in healthy patients who need extensive procedures, and ≥30% or more when there is a history of pre-existing cardiac disease. (See page 1281: Fluid Replacement.)

16. E. O_2 transport variables, base deficit, blood lactate levels, gastric intramucosal pH, and sublingual P_{CO_2} are considered acceptable markers of organ hypoperfusion in the apparently resuscitated patient and may be used to set the optimal end points of resuscitation. An O_2 delivery index of 500 mL/m^2 per minute has been shown to be an acceptable goal for optimal shock resuscitation. A parameter that has been recently used intraoperatively as a guide to resuscitation during emergency surgery for trauma patients is the end-tidal–arterial CO_2 difference $(Pa\text{-}ET)_{CO_2}$. Values >10 mm Hg after resuscitation predict mortality. It may also be useful in the decision about when to perform damage control surgery, and intraoperatively, in guiding resuscitation with fluids, inotropes, and vasopressors. Unrecognized hypoperfusion may lead to splanchnic ischemia with resulting acidosis in the intestinal wall, thus permitting the passage of luminal microorganisms into the circulation and release of inflammatory mediators causing sepsis and multiple organ failure. (See page 1284: Organ Perfusion and Oxygen Utilization.)

17. B. Hemorrhage and hypovolemia lead to a higher blood concentration following a given dose of an intravenous agent. Increased sensitivity of the brain to anesthetics, preferential distribution of the cardiac output to the brain and heart, cerebral hypoxia, dilutional hypoproteinemia, and acidosis all increase the effects of drugs on the brain and the heart. The etomidate dose does not require adjustment for shock. All inhalation anesthetics increase cerebral blood flow, cerebral blood volume, and thus intracranial pressure. In spontaneously breathing patients, opioids may produce hypoventilation with an associated increase in cerebral blood flow and intracranial pressure. (See page 1285: Anesthetic and Adjunct Drugs: Hypovolemia, Head and Open Eye Injuries.)

18. C. Postoperative sedation with midazolam for mechanically ventilated patients can result in mean wake-up times of 660 ± 440 minutes, whereas the wake-up time for the same group of patients sedated with propofol was 110 ± 50 minutes. Although both drugs are safe and effective, propofol clearly results in a faster wake-up time and earlier ability to examine a patient's neurologic status extensively. Urine output is a relatively insensitive test for diagnosing acute renal failure. More objective data are obtained by calculating free-water clearance and/or creatinine clearance. A creatinine clearance of <25 mL/minute or free-water clearance of >15 mL/hour suggests the likelihood of acute renal failure. Abdominal compartment syndrome results from increased intra-abdominal pressure and associated decreased organ perfusion pressure; this leads to multiple organ failure and death. A normal intra-abdominal pressure is 3 to 10 mm Hg, whereas values of >20 to 25 mm Hg indicate the need for immediate decompression. Trauma patients are at extreme risk of DVT. The overall incidence of DVT is approximately 18% in trauma patients. Almost half of all cases of pulmonary embolus occur within the first week, suggesting that DVT develops shortly after trauma. (See page 1291: Early Postoperative Considerations: Sedation and Analgesia, Acute Renal Failure, Abdominal Compartment Syndrome, and Thromboembolism.)

CHAPTER 49 ■ THE ALLERGIC RESPONSE

For questions 1 to 8, choose the best answer.

1. The humoral defense system includes all the following EXCEPT:

   A. antibodies
   B. cytokines
   C. complement
   D. lymphocytes
   E. circulating proteins

2. Which type of T cell does not require specific antigen stimulation to initiate its function?

   A. Cytotoxic
   B. Lymphotrophic
   C. Suppressor
   D. Helper
   E. Killer

3. Which of the following statements regarding antibodies is TRUE?

   A. Each antibody has two heavy chains and one light chain.
   B. The Fab segment binds the antigen.
   C. The light chain is responsible for the unique biological properties of the different classes of immunoglobulins.
   D. There are six major classes of antibodies in humans.
   E. The light chain determines the structure and function of each molecule.

4. The attachment of an antibody or complement fragment to the surface of foreign cells is called:

   A. immunogenicity
   B. haptogenicity
   C. opsonization

   D. lymphotrophism
   E. lymphokinesis

5. Which are the cells that regulate immune responses by presenting antigens to result in microbicidal function?

   A. Eosinophils
   B. Basophils
   C. Neutrophils
   D. Mast cells
   E. Macrophages

6. Complement can be activated by all of the following EXCEPT:

   A. immunoglobulin G (IgG)
   B. plasmin
   C. killer T cells
   D. endotoxin
   E. the alternate pathway

7. True statements concerning the secondary treatment of anaphylaxis include all of the following EXCEPT:

   A. Bicarbonate should be given to treat severe acidemia.
   B. Corticosteroids require 12 to 24 hours to work.
   C. Corticosteroids are recommended for IgE-mediated reactions
   D. Antihistamines inhibit histamine release.
   E. Aminophylline decreases histamine release from mast cells.

8. The purpose of _____ is to determine basophil activation.

   A. skin testing
   B. the leukocyte histamine release test
   C. the enzyme-linked immunosorbent assay test
   D. the radioallergosorbent test
   E. the protamine test

For questions 9 to 13, choose A if 1, 2, and 3 are correct; B if 1 and 3; C if 2 and 4; D if 4; and E if all.

9. Type II reactions include which of the following EXCEPT:

   1. ABO incompatibility reactions
   2. heparin-induced thrombocytopenia
   3. drug-induced immune hemolytic anemia
   4. classic serum sickness

10. Which of the following statements regarding intraoperative allergic reactions is/are TRUE?

    1. They occur once every 5,000 to 25,000 anesthetics.
    2. The mortality is approximately 3.4%.
    3. In the anesthetized patient, the most common life-threatening manifestation of an allergic reaction is circulatory collapse.
    4. Most reactions occur >10 minutes following an intravenous drug injection.

11. Which of the following statements regarding chemical mediators of inflammation is/are TRUE?

    1. Leukotrienes are derived from arachidonic acid metabolism of phospholipid membranes.

    2. Prostaglandins are potent mast cell mediators.
    3. Prostaglandin D_2 produces bronchospasm.
    4. Kinins are synthesized in mast cells.

12. Which of the following statements regarding anaphylactic reactions is/are TRUE?

    1. There is a >40% loss of intracellular fluid during anaphylactic reactions.
    2. Inhalation anesthetics are the bronchodilators of choice following anaphylaxis.
    3. Corticosteroids are important in attenuating the late-phase reactions that occur 1 to 2 hours after anaphylaxis.
    4. Aminophylline increases right and left ventricular contractility.

13. Which of the following statements regarding latex reactions is/are TRUE?

    1. There is a 24% incidence of contact dermatitis among anesthesiologists.
    2. Patients with an allergy to bananas have antibodies that can cross-react to latex.
    3. A history of atopy is a risk factor for latex sensitization.
    4. Pretreatment always prevents anaphylaxis.

ANSWERS

---

1. **D.** The host defense systems can be divided into cellular and humoral elements. The humoral system includes complement, cytokines, antibodies, and other circulating proteins. The cellular system defense is mediated by specific lymphocytes of the T-cell series. (See page 1299: Basic Immunologic Principles.)

2. **E.** The thymus of the fetus differentiates immature lymphocytes into thymus-derived cells (T cells). The two types of regulator T cells are helper cells and suppressor cells. Helper cells are important for effective cell responses. Suppressor cells inhibit immune function. Killer cells do not require specific antigen stimulation to initiate their function. Cytotoxic T cells destroy mycobacteria, fungi, and viruses. (See page 1299: Thymus-Derived Lymphocytes [T-Cell Lymphocytes] and Bursa-Derived Lymphocytes [B-cell Lymphocytes].)

3. **B.** Each antibody has two heavy chains and two light chains that are bound together by disulfide bonds. The Fab fragment has the ability to bind antigen, whereas the Fc (crystallizable) is responsible for the unique biological properties of the different classes of immunoglobulins. There are five major classes of antibodies in humans: IgG, IgA, IgM, IgD, and IgE. The heavy chain determines the structure and function of each molecule. (See page 1299: Antibodies.)

4. **C.** The attachment of an antibody or complement fragment on the surface of foreign cells is called opsonization, a process that facilitates effector cell killing of foreign cells. Haptens are small molecules that form a bond with either host proteins or cell membranes to form a complete antigen. The ability to act as an antigen is referred to as immunogenicity. (See page 1300: Effector Cells and Proteins of the Immune Response Cells.)

5. **E.** Neutrophils are the first cells to appear in acute inflammatory reaction. Eosinophils accumulate at sites of parasitic infection, tumor, and allergic reactions. Mast cells are tissue fixed and located in the perivascular spaces of the skin and intestine; once activated, they release a broad spectrum of physiologically active mediators. Basophils possess IgE receptors on their surface and function similarly to mast cells. Macrophages regulate immune responses by presenting antigens to result in microbicidal function. (See page 1300: Effector Cells and Proteins of the Immune Response Cells.)

6. **C.** Complement activation can be initiated by IgG or IgM, by plasmin through the classic pathway, by endotoxin, or by drugs through the alternate pathway. The major function of the complement system is to recognize bacteria both directly and indirectly by the attraction of phagocytes. The primary humoral

response to antigen and antibody binding is activation of the complement system. T cells are a component of the cellular immune response system. (See page 1300: Complement.)

7. **D.**   Administration of a histamine (H_1) antagonist may be useful in treating acute anaphylaxis; it does not inhibit histamine release but competes with histamine at the receptor sites. Aminophylline is a phosphodiesterase inhibitor that works by increasing intracellular cyclic adenosine monophosphate. Steroids should be considered a secondary treatment in the management of anaphylactic bronchospasm. They require 12 to 24 hours to exert their peak clinical effect. Although the exact corticosteroid dose and preparation are unclear, investigators have recommended 0.25 to 1 g intravenously of hydrocortisone in IgE-mediated reactions. Acidosis frequently accompanies persistent hypotension. Acidemia decreases the effectiveness of administered epinephrine on the myocardium. Therefore, with refractory hypotension and acidemia, sodium bicarbonate should be given as indicated by arterial blood gas evaluation. (See page 1304: Nonimmunologic Release of Histamine and Treatment Plan and Secondary Treatment.)

8. **B.**   The leukocyte histamine release test is performed by incubating the patient's leukocytes with the offending drug and measuring the histamine release as a marker for basophil activation. The radioallergosorbent test allows in vitro detection of specific IgE directed toward particular antigens by linking them to insoluble material to make them immunoabsorbent. The enzyme-linked immunoabsorbent assay measures antigens and specific antibodies. (See page 1309: Testing for Allergy.)

9. **D.**   Type II reactions also are known as antibody-dependent cytotoxic hypersensitivity reactions. These reactions are mediated by IgG or IgM antibodies directed against antigens on the surface of foreign cells. Examples of type II reactions in humans are ABO-incompatible transfusion reactions, drug-induced immune hemolytic anemia, and heparin-induced thrombocytopenia. Classic serum sickness is an example of a type III reaction. (See page 1301: Type II Reactions.)

10. **A.**   Intraoperative allergic reactions occur once every 5,000 to 25,000 anesthetics, with a reported mortality of 3.4%. More than 90% of the allergic reactions evoked by intravenous drugs occur within 5 minutes of their administration. In the anesthetized patient, the most common life-threatening manifestation of an allergic reaction is circulatory collapse. (See page 1302: Intraoperative Allergic Reactions.)

11. **E.**   Various leukotrienes are synthesized following mast cell activation from arachidonic acid metabolism of phospholipid cell membranes via the lipoxygenase pathway. Prostaglandins are potent mast cell mediators that produce vasodilation, bronchospasm, pulmonary hypertension, and increased capillary permeability. Prostaglandin D_2, the major metabolite of mast cells, produces bronchospasm and vasodilation. Kinins are synthesized in mast cells and basophils and produce vasodilation, increased capillary permeability, and bronchoconstriction. (See page 1302: Anaphylactic Reactions.)

12. **D.**   Aminophylline, a phosphodiesterase inhibitor, causes bronchodilation and decreases histamine release from mast cells. In addition, it increases right and left ventricular contractility and decreases pulmonary vascular resistance. Inhalation anesthetics are not the bronchodilators of choice for treating bronchospasm following anaphylaxis. These anesthetics interfere with the body's compensatory response to the cardiovascular collapse associated with anaphylaxis. Up to a 40% loss of intravascular fluid into the interstitial space during reactions has been reported. Corticosteroids may be important in attenuating the late-phase reactions reported to occur 12 to 24 hours after anaphylaxis. (See page 1305: Initial Therapy.)

13. **A.**   There is a 24% incidence of contact dermatitis among anesthesiologists. Patients with an allergy to bananas have antibodies that can cross-react to latex. A history of atopy is a risk factor for latex sensitization. Pretreatment can help to prevent anaphylaxis. (See page 1309: Latex Allergy.)

CHAPTER 50 ■ DRUG INTERACTIONS

1. Pronounced drug interactions are not commonly seen by anesthesiologists because of all of the following EXCEPT:

   A. Interactions may occur, but they usually do not present a problem.
   B. Variability in response to anesthetic drugs is commonly seen.
   C. The qualitative nature of most anesthetic interactions is predictable even though the magnitude of the responses may not be known with certainty.
   D. Many intravenous anesthetic drugs have small safety margins, particularly when respiration is supported.
   E. It is likely that many instances of anesthetic drug interactions go unrecognized.

2. Pharmacokinetic interaction is defined as one drug altering what property of another drug?

   A. Absorption
   B. Distribution
   C. Metabolism
   D. Elimination
   E. All of the above

3. Monoamine oxidase (MAO) inhibitors:

   A. can increase the effect of indirect-acting sympathomimetics
   B. can interact with morphine to increase brain concentration of serotonin
   C. can interfere with beta-blockers
   D. can be safely given with meperidine
   E. should be discontinued for 24 hours before elective surgery to return enzyme levels to baseline.

4. Choose the FALSE statement concerning hepatic biotransformation.

   A. Drugs undergo oxidative metabolism by cytochrome P450.
   B. Cytochrome P450 has low substrate specificity.
   C. Removal of drug from blood by hepatic clearance is a function of hepatic blood flow and intrinsic clearance.
   D. With low-extraction-ratio drugs, hepatic blood flow is the major rate-limiting factor in overall hepatic clearance.
   E. With low-extraction-ratio drugs, hepatic enzyme activity is a rate-limiting factor.

5. Choose the FALSE statement.

   A. A pharmacodynamic interaction occurs when one drug alters the sensitivity of a target receptor or tissue to the effects of a second drug.
   B. Additive interactions are most likely to occur when drugs with identical mechanisms are combined.
   C. There usually is an additive effect between succinylcholine and the nondepolarizing relaxants.
   D. Synergistic interactions are characterized by small doses of two or more drugs that produce very large effects.
   E. Isobolographic analysis is used for quantitatively assessing the effects of drug combinations to see whether synergism occurs.

For questions 6 to 8, choose A if 1, 2, and 3 are correct, B if 1 and 3; C if 2 and 4; D if 4; and E if all are correct.

6. Which of the following statements is/are examples of a pharmaceutical reaction?

   1. Bicarbonate added to bupivacaine causes a precipitation reaction.
   2. Halogenated anesthetics have been shown to interact with dry soda lyme or baralyme to produce carbon monoxide.
   3. Nitric oxide reacts with oxygen to form nitrogen dioxide.

247

4. Orally administered tetracycline can be inactivated by chelation when given with antacids containing magnesium, calcium, or aluminum.

7. Distribution changes resulting from drug-drug interactions can occur secondary to:
   1. alterations in hemodynamics
   2. changes in drug ionization
   3. changes in binding to plasma and tissue proteins
   4. changes in drug metabolism

8. Which of the following is/are TRUE?
   1. Enzyme induction is an explanation for increased intrinsic clearance.
   2. A single inducer can affect the products of several gene families.
   3. Phenobarbital can increase the amount of P450 enzyme and can therefore increase the clearance of many drugs.
   4. Cimetidine forms an inactive complex with cytochrome P450 and therefore inhibits the metabolism of many drugs, including warfarin and diazepam.

ANSWERS

1. **D.** Drug interactions are not commonly seen in the operating rooms, even though patients routinely take antihypertensives, antidepressants, or gastrointestinal drugs in the preoperative period, and most of them receive five to 10 drugs during general anesthesia. One does not normally hear about significant complications attributable to drug interaction, and numerous explanations for this are possible. First, interactions may occur, but they usually do not present a problem. Anesthesia practitioners are always prepared to titrate drugs and deal with the possibility of significant respiratory, central nervous system, or cardiovascular depression. Toxicity from a drug interaction is likely to become a source of morbidity primarily when it occurs in a setting where it is not rapidly recognized and treated. An example of this is when opioid-midazolam combination agents were first used by nonanesthesia personnel for endoscopic and radiological procedures. The unexpectedly large sedative and ventilatory effects led to numerous deaths. A second explanation is variability in response to anesthetic drugs. As a rule, different patients may have a three- to fivefold difference in the therapeutic and toxic effects of a given dose even when a drug is given alone. Third, the qualitative nature of most anesthetic interactions is predictable, although the magnitude of the response may not be known with certainty. For example, two cardiovascular depressants will almost always produce more hypotension. Similarly, combinations of central nervous system depressants will produce more, not less, depression. Drug interactions that produce a totally unexpected or dangerous effect stand out because of their rarity. Fourth, many intravenous anesthetic drugs have large safety margins, particularly when respiration is supported, so small changes in drug concentration are not extremely important. The mere fact that a measurable interaction exists does not mean that it will cause a difference in outcome or the need for intervention. It is noteworthy that clinically meaningful interactions most often involve drugs such as warfarin, digoxin, and theophylline (drugs with only small differences between therapeutic and toxic concentrations). Finally, it is likely that many instances of anesthetic drug interactions go unrecognized (the clinician must consider the possibility to make the diagnosis). Excessive drug effects are often attributed to some ill-defined "patient sensitivity." When a drug fails to produce an effect, it is because a patient is "tolerant" or "resistant." It is almost never considered a drug reaction or interaction. (See page 1314: Problems Created by Drug–Drug Interaction.)

2. **E.** A pharmacokinetic interaction occurs when one drug alters the absorption, distribution, metabolism, or elimination of another. A pharmacodynamic interaction occurs when one drug alters the sensitivity of a target receptor to the effects of a second drug. This means that the dose-response or concentration-response curve is shifted by another medication. An example of a drug-delayed absorption by a change in the physiologic environment is morphine decreasing gastrointestinal motility so absorption of orally administered acetaminophen is slowed. Another example of a drug's influencing the absorption of another is the common addition of epinephrine to a local anesthetic solution to retard uptake of the local anesthetic from the site of action. This effect also influences the distribution of the local anesthetic. Distribution of a drug can also be influenced by coadministering a second drug that changes the pH of the environment. Also, administering two drugs that compete for protein binding sites results in an increase of the free (active) fraction of each drug. Metabolism of one drug can be either increased or decreased by the presence of another; an example is neostigmine's inhibiting both motor end plate acetylcholinesterase and plasma pseudocholinesterase, which can prolong the effect of succinylcholine (and potentially ester-type local anesthetics in the bloodstream). (See page 1315: Pharmacokinetic Interactions and Pharmacodynamic Interactions.)

3. A. MAO is found in tissues throughout the body, but the largest amounts are found in the liver, kidney, and brain. MAO acts to regulate the presynaptic pool of norepinephrine, dopamine, epinephrine, and serotonin available for synaptic transmission. MAO exists in two isoforms: MAO-A preferentially metabolizes serotonin, dopamine, and norepinephrine, whereas MAO-B preferentially metabolizes phenylethylamine and tyramine. MAO inhibitors are used mainly for the treatment of refractory depression and certain other mood disorders. Interaction with indirect-acting sympathomimetic drugs (ephedrine, amphetamine, metaraminol) occurs because MAO inhibitor treatment increases the amount of presynaptic transmitters that can be released by these drugs. Normal doses of ephedrine can produce exaggerated sympathetic responses including a severe hypertensive crisis. Deaths have been attributed to severe hyperpyrexia and cerebral hemorrhage. The "wine and cheese reaction" is essentially the same interaction. Many foods, such as aged cheese, contain tyramine, a phenylethylamine that has ephedrine-like actions at sympathetic nerve endings. Normal exogenous tyramine is degraded by MAO in the gut wall and liver, but patients taking MAO inhibitors may achieve high systemic concentrations and consequently have a hypertensive crisis. Because MAO plays little role in the metabolism of compounds in the synaptic cleft, the response to sympathomimetics, which act directly on postsynaptic receptor sites (phenylephrine, norepinephrine, epinephrine), should be less affected by such interactions. Beta-blockers can be safely used in these patients. The most important interaction of MAO inhibitors is unquestionably with meperidine. When meperidine is given to a patient on an MAO inhibitor, a life-threatening reaction may occur accompanied by excitation, hyperpyrexia, hypertension, profuse sweating, and rigidity. This may progress to seizures, coma, and death. This reaction does not occur in every instance. The mechanism of meperidine-MAO inhibitor interaction is unknown, but animal modes suggest that it involves elevation in the brain concentration of serotonin. Current clinical opinion probably favors continuing MAO inhibitor therapy up to the time of therapy. Most patients are receiving these drugs for moderate to severe psychiatric disorders that have not responded to other treatments. It is unpleasant and possibly risky for a patient with refractory depression to endure 2 to 3 weeks without effective therapy. If a general anesthetic is planned, it seems prudent to use as few drugs as possible. Avoiding drugs with substantial sympathetic effects probably makes sense. Because opioids, such as fentanyl, appear safe and there are no major interactions with local anesthetics or nonsteroidal anti-inflammatory analgesics, providing anesthesia without meperidine should not be a hardship. (See page 1317: Monoamine Oxidase [MAO] Interaction.)

4. D. Many anesthetic drugs undergo oxidative metabolism by one of the isoforms of the cytochrome P450 found in liver microsomes. The P450 isoforms have low substrate specificity, which means that drugs of diverse structures can be biotransformed by a single group of enzymes. The removal of drug from the blood by hepatic biotransformation (hepatic clearance) is a function of two independent variables, the hepatic blood flow and the intrinsic clearance (the maximal ability of the liver to metabolize that drug). The intrinsic clearance is often expressed as the extraction ratio, defined as the fraction of drug that can be metabolized in a single pass through the liver. Drugs may be classed broadly as high extraction and low extraction, a distinction with important implications for drug interactions. For drugs with a high extraction ratio (e.g., lidocaine, propranolol), hepatic blood flow is a rate-limiting factor in overall hepatic clearance (i.e., the delivery of drug to the liver determines the amount cleared). Clearance is decreased by drugs or maneuvers that lower hepatic blood flow. Clearance of these rapidly metabolized drugs is much less sensitive to changes in enzyme activity. Plasma-protein binding does not have a large effect, either. Low-extraction drugs (e.g., diazepam, mepivacaine) behave quite differently because hepatic enzyme activity is rate limiting (hepatic clearance is limited by intrinsic clearance). Stimulation or inhibition of enzyme activity can have a large effect on overall pharmacokinetics. Protein binding is also more likely to affect clearance because the bound forms of these drugs are protected from hepatic metabolism. (See page 1318: Hepatic Biotransformation.)

5. C. A pharmacodynamic interaction occurs when one drug alters the sensitivity of a target receptor or tissue to the effects of a second drug. This means that the dose-response or concentration-response curve for one drug is shifted by another. Additive interactions are most likely to occur when drugs with identical mechanisms are combined. There is an antagonistic interaction between succinylcholine and the nondepolarizing relaxants. Antagonistic drug interactions are those involving deliberate reversal with drugs that compete at the same receptor site. Synergistic drug interactions, in which small doses of two or more drugs can produce very large effects, are most likely to occur when drugs of different classes, or even those with slightly different mechanisms, are used to produce the same effects. Two of the most common techniques used by experimental pharmacologists to study the effects of drug combinations are algebraic (fractional) analysis and isobolographic analysis. (See page 1320: Pharmacodynamic Interactions.)

6. A. A pharmaceutical interaction is a chemical or physical interaction that occurs before a drug is administered or absorbed systemically. The most obvious pharmaceutical drug interactions are the incompatibilities that can occur between intravenous drugs and solution. In addition, two drugs may interact chemically to form a toxic compound. An example of the former is precipitation of barbiturate when thiopental is injected together with succinylcholine into an intravenous line. An example of the latter occurs when halogenated anesthetics produce carbon monoxide when interacting with dry soda lyme or nitric oxide–forming nitrogen dioxide when it contacts oxygen. Tetracycline inactivation by antacids is an example of a pharmacokinetic reaction. (See page 1315: Pharmaceutical Interactions.)

7. **A.**   Many drug-drug interactions occur when one drug alters the distribution of a second. This may result from alterations in hemodynamics, drug ionization, or binding to plasma or tissue proteins. Drug-induced hemodynamic compromise can affect pharmacokinetics. Drugs such as beta-blockers, calcium channel blockers, and vasodilators can decrease cardiac output by a variety of mechanisms and can produce significant changes in drug distribution. For a given rate of drug administration, a decrease of cardiac output will increase the arterial drug concentration to highly perfused tissues such as the brain and myocardium. Drug-induced changes in pH in a particular body region or fluid compartment can alter the distribution of other drugs by so-called "ion trapping." A drug that is protein bound will not be filtered by a normal glomerulus and (for some drugs) will not be acted upon by drug-metabolizing enzymes. A drug that is highly bound to plasma protein effectively exists as a depot,

similar to a deep intramuscular injection. The potential therefore exists that one drug can alter the disposition, clearance, or biological effect of another by altering its binding. An example of this is illustrated by a highly bound potentially toxic drug such as warfarin, which is more than 98% bound to albumin. When another drug is given (e.g., phenylbutazone) that competes for the same binding sites, it displaces warfarin and increases the free fraction and therefore increases the anticoagulant effect. (See page 1315: Distribution.)

8. **E.**   The most common reason for increased intrinsic clearance is enzyme induction. Many drugs of importance in anesthesiology are metabolized by the cytochrome P450 enzymes. Hundreds of drugs and environmental toxins can stimulate (or induce) microsomal enzymes. Typically, a single inducer can affect the products of several gene families. Phenobarbital increases the amount of many P450 enzymes. The increase in the quantity of enzyme protein can therefore increase the clearance of many drugs simultaneously. Cimetidine has an imidazole group that binds to the heme iron of cytochrome P450 and forms an inactive complex. Cimetidine inhibits the metabolism of many drugs including warfarin, diazepam, phenytoin, and morphine. (See page 1318: Hepatic Biotransformation.)

CHAPTER 51 ■ ANESTHESIA PROVIDED AT ALTERNATE SITES

For the following questions, choose: A if 1, 2, and 3 are correct; B if 1 and 3; C if 2 and 4; D if 4; and E if all.

1. Anesthesia equipment required in alternate sites includes which of the following:

   1. Central oxygen supply
   2. Wall suction
   3. Spare oxygen cylinder
   4. Gas scavenger system

2. Which of the following statements regarding conscious sedation is/are TRUE?

   1. The patient is relaxed.
   2. The patient should be able to respond to verbal stimulus.
   3. The patient should be able to respond to physical stimulus.
   4. The use of an oral airway is helpful in maintaining respiration.

3. American Society of Anesthesiologists (ASA) standard II for continual monitoring includes which of the following?

   1. Temperature
   2. Oxygenation
   3. Circulation
   4. Ventilation

4. The physiologic response to electroconvulsive therapy (ECT) can include which of the following?

   1. Tachycardia
   2. Bradycardia
   3. Hypertension
   4. Decrease in cerebral blood flow

5. Which of the following statements regarding dental surgery is/are TRUE?

   1. Ketamine and midazolam can be given intravenously, intramuscularly, or orally.

2. Laryngospasm is not a postoperative complication.
3. Tracheal intubation may be required.
4. Ketamine always abolishes upper airway reflexes.

6. Anesthetic considerations for ECT include which of the following?

   1. Etomidate is associated with a shorter duration of seizures.
   2. The anesthetic agent need not provide for amnesia.
   3. Propofol may result in longer duration of seizures compared with barbiturates.
   4. Succinylcholine is most commonly used as a muscle relaxant.

7. Which of the following statements regarding external-beam radiation treatment is/are TRUE?

   1. The patient needs to be immobile.
   2. Sedation is preferred to general anesthesia in children.
   3. The anesthesiologist should leave the treatment room.
   4. Patients require a deep level of anesthesia for this procedure.

8. Which of the following statements concerning magnetic resonance imaging is/are TRUE?

   1. The pulse oximeter may cause tissue burn.
   2. Anesthesia equipment can be made of aluminum or nonmagnetic steel.
   3. The technique is contraindicated in the presence of a pacemaker, an intracranial aneurysm clip, or an intravascular wire.
   4. There is no dangerous ionizing radiation.

9. Which of the following statements regarding radiological contrast material is/are TRUE?

   1. The use of newer low-osmolarity nonionic agents has been associated with an increased incidence of anaphylactic reaction.

2. Patients should be fluid restricted because of the large volume load presented by the contrast agent.
3. Prophylaxis with diphenhydramine or methylprednisolone should be administered in all patients.
4. The incidence of severe reaction to contrast media is 0.04%.

10. Which of the following statements regarding cardioversion is/are TRUE?

1. Invasive monitoring is rarely required.
2. Etomidate provides a more stable electrocardiogram tracing than thiopental.
3. In general, patients do not require intubation.
4. Propofol produces less hypotension than etomidate.

ANSWERS

1. **E.** The ASA developed a standard to apply to anesthesia remote locations. Before commencing an anesthetic, it is vital to confirm the presence and proper functioning of all equipment an anesthesiologist would expect in the operating room. This includes a central oxygen supply, spare oxygen cylinders, wall suction, overhead lighting, gas scavenging systems, and electrical outlets. (See page 1331: General Principles.)

2. **A.** Conscious sedation is a state in which the patient is calm and relaxed, yet able to respond to verbal or physical stimulation. The patient is able to maintain both a patent airway and protective airway reflexes during this minimally depressed level of consciousness. (See page 1331: General Principles.)

3. **E.** The ASA basic standards of monitoring should be adhered to in any location where anesthesia or sedation is being performed. Standard I requires a qualified anesthesia provider to be present in the room throughout the conduct of anesthesia. Standard II calls for continual evaluation of the patient's oxygenation, ventilation, circulation and temperature. The degree of invasive monitoring that should be used will depend on the patient's status and the procedure being undertaken. (See page 1331: General Principles.)

4. **A.** A minimum seizure duration of 25 seconds is recommended to ensure adequate antidepressant efficacy. The cardiovascular response includes increased cerebral blood flow and intracranial pressure. Generalized autonomic nervous system stimulation results in an initial 10 to 15 seconds of bradycardia and occasional asystole, followed by a more prominent sympathetic response of hypertension and tachycardia. Occasional cardiac dysrhythmias, myocardial ischemia, infarction, or neurologic vascular event may be precipitated. (See page 1340: Electroconvulsive Therapy.)

5. **B.** Ketamine is a useful induction agent. It may be used alone or in combination with atropine and midazolam by an intravenous, oral, intramuscular, rectal, or intranasal route. Ketamine is also advantageous in that, in standard doses, it does not abolish upper airway reflexes. Tracheal intubation, often via the nasal route, is required to protect the airway, although recently the laryngeal mask airway has been used successfully for adults and children undergoing dental surgery. The immediate postoperative complications include, bleeding, airway obstruction, and laryngospasm. (See page 1341: Dental Surgery.)

6. **D.** The anesthetic goals for a patient undergoing ECT include amnesia, airway management, prevention of bodily injury from seizures, control of hemodynamic changes, and a smooth and rapid emergence. Etomidate is associated with seizures of longer duration. Propofol is effective for ECT, and its effect on outcome is similar to that of barbiturates. Several investigators have found that propofol tends to result in seizures of shorter duration. Muscle relaxants are needed to prevent injury to the patient during the grand mal seizure. Succinylcholine is most commonly used because of its rapid onset and short duration. (See page 1340: Electroconvulsive Therapy.)

7. **B.** Because the radiation dose is so high, all medical personnel must leave the room during the actual treatment. Direct observation of the patient is not possible. Closed-circuit television and microphones are used. The need for patient immobility is a primary reason anesthesia is required for these procedures; it is difficult for children to keep completely still when only sedation is administered. If sedation is attempted, airway management problems increase, and the recovery period is greatly prolonged. General anesthesia offers several advantages over conscious sedation. Because there is no surgical stimulation, patients can be maintained at light levels of anesthesia; emergence and recovery can then be rapid. (See page 1334: Radiology and Radiation Therapy.)

8. **E.** Magnetic resonance imaging is noninvasive and produces no ionizing radiation. There are no reports of harm from tissue contact with the magnetic field itself. Several types of physiologic monitors, oxygen-powered ventilators, laryngoscopic

equipment, and anesthesia machines can be used within the magnetic resonance imaging suite. Most of the equipment differs in that it is made of aluminum or nonferromagnetic material. Absolute and relative contraindications for magnetic resonance imaging scanning include patients with cardiac pacemakers near the site of scanning, intracranial aneurysm clip, or intravascular wires. (See page 1337: Magnetic Resonance Imaging.)

9. **D.** Contrast media are eliminated via the kidneys, and thus contrast-induced nephropathy is a concern. Adequate hydration, careful monitoring of urine output, and the use of low-osmolarity contrast media help to reduce the risk of contrast-induced nephropathy. The overall incidence of adverse drug reactions with nonionic contrast media is reported to be 3.13%, and the incidence of severe reactions is 0.04%. Patients receiving contrast agents usually diurese large volumes of urine because of the osmotic load of the dye. Adequate hydration of these patients should be ensured to prevent worsening of pre-existing hypovolemia or azotemia. For patients with a history of reactions to dyes, and/or for those patients for whom a dye reaction is anticipated, it is beneficial to treat them prophylactically with diphenhydramine and/or steroids. (See page 1334: Radiology and Radiation Therapy.)

10. **B.** Cardioversion is a brief but distressing procedure that usually is performed after a small bolus of intravenous induction agent. Invasive monitoring is rarely required. Propofol produces more hypotension than etomidate. Etomidate causes a high incidence of myoclonus that can render interpretation of the electrocardiogram difficult. In general, patients do not require intubation for cardioversion unless there is a risk of aspiration. (See page 1339: Cardioversion.)

CHAPTER 52 ■ OFFICE-BASED ANESTHESIA

For all questions, choose A if 1, 2, and 3 are correct; B if 1 and 3; C if 2 and 4; D if 4; E if all.

1. Which of the following statements regarding injuries during office-based anesthesia is/are TRUE?

   1. Most occur intraoperatively.
   2. The second most common incidence is in the recovery room.
   3. Fifty percent of injuries have a respiratory cause.
   4. Injuries after discharge account for <10% of the injuries.

2. Which of the following statements regarding patient selection for office-based anesthesia is/are TRUE?

   1. The surgeon's office staff can arrange the surgery for patients with American Society of Anesthesiologists (ASA) status I and II.
   2. Close monitoring of oxygen saturation in an intensive care setting may be required postoperatively for patients with obstructive sleep apnea.
   3. Preoperative anesthesia consultation should be obtained for ASA status IV patients.
   4. A preoperative history and physical should be obtained within 6 months of the date of surgery.

3. Which of the following statements regarding office-based anesthesia is/are TRUE?

   1. Continuous heart rate monitoring is required.
   2. The ability for continuous electrocardiographic (ECG) monitoring is needed.
   3. Monitoring of oxygen saturation is required.
   4. At least 12 bottles of dantrolene should be available.

4. Which of the following contribute(s) to the mortality rate in liposuction procedures?

   1. Pulmonary embolism
   2. Abdominal perforation

3. Fat embolism
4. Anesthetic "causes"

5. Epidural and spinal anesthesia for liposuction is discouraged in office-based anesthesia because of possible:

   1. vasodilatation
   2. fluid overload
   3. hypotension
   4. paralysis

6. Which of the following statements regarding office-based gastrointestinal endoscopy is/are TRUE?

   1. Endotracheal intubation is often required.
   2. General anesthesia is usually required.
   3. Colonoscopy does not cause cardiac dysrhythmia.
   4. Hypotension may be caused by colonoscopy.

7. Which of the following ophthalmic and otorhinolaryngologic procedures is/are suitable for office-based anesthesia?

   1. Cataract extraction
   2. Ocular plastic
   3. Lacrimal duct probing
   4. Endoscopic sinus surgery

8. Which of the following statements regarding the use of ketamine for office-based analgesia is/are TRUE?

   1. It functions as an analgesic.
   2. It is not associated with nausea and vomiting.
   3. It can be used as an induction agent.
   4. It may decrease the risk of aspiration.

9. All of the following statements regarding postoperative nausea and vomiting in office-based anesthesia are true EXCEPT:

   1. Opioids cause nausea and vomiting.
   2. Dexamethasone potentiates the effects of antiemetics.

3. Adequate hydration can decrease postoperative nausea and vomiting.

4. Routine prophylaxis using dexamethasone is advantageous.

ANSWERS

---

1. **B.** Injuries during office-based procedures occur throughout the perioperative period, and are multifactorial in origin. Most occur intraoperatively, whereas 14% occur in the postanesthesia care unit, and 21% occur after discharge. Fifty percent of injuries are respiratory and included airway obstruction, bronchospasm, inadequate oxygenation and ventilation, and unrecognized esophageal intubation. The second most common events are drug related. (See page 1346: Office Safety.)

2. **A.** Guidelines change. As of this writing, the patient should have a preoperative history and physical examination recorded within 30 days of the procedure, including all pertinent laboratory tests and any medically indicated specialist consultations. If the patient is an ASA status I or II, the surgeon's office can arrange the surgery as per office protocol. However, if a patient has a significant comorbid condition, a preoperative anesthesiology consultation should be obtained before scheduling a patient for office surgery. Morbidly obese patients and patients with obstructive sleep apnea present unique challenges. It has been recommended that an observational unit with close monitoring of oxygen saturation or an intensive care unit setting be used for postoperative monitoring of patients with obstructive sleep apnea. (See page 1347: Patient Selection.)

3. **E.** Perioperative monitoring should adhere to the standards for basic anesthetic monitoring. These standards include continuous monitoring of heart rate and oxygen saturation, intermittent noninvasive blood pressure monitoring, and the capacity for both temperature and continuous ECG monitoring. The office-based anesthesiologist should be prepared to begin the initial treatment of malignant hyperthermia, which requires having at least 12 bottles of dantrolene. (See page 1348: Office Selection.)

4. **E.** Mortality related to liposuction is secondary to pulmonary embolism, abdominal viscous perforation, anesthesia-related "causes," fat embolism, infection, and hemorrhage. (See page 1350: Specific Procedures: Liposuction.)

5. **A.** Epidural and spinal anesthesia in an office setting is discouraged because of the possibility of vasodilatation, hypotension, and fluid overload. (See page 1350: Specific Procedures: Liposuction.)

6. **D.** Upper gastrointestinal procedures rarely require endotracheal intubation because the stomach is emptied under direct visualization. The procedure can be accomplished with sedation using midazolam and small doses of propofol. Colonoscopy is painful secondary to insertion and manipulation of the endoscope, and it may be associated with cardiovascular effects, including dysrhythmia, bradycardia, hypotension, hypertension, myocardial infarction, and death. (See page 1351: Gastrointestinal Endoscopy.)

7. **E.** Ophthalmologic procedures suitable for the office include cataract extraction, lacrimal duct probing, and ocular plastics. Topical anesthesia or periorbital and retrobulbar blocks are frequently used to provide analgesia. Otolaryngology procedures acceptable for an office setting include endoscopic sinus surgery, septoplasty, and myringotomy. (See page 1352: Ophthalmology/Otolaryngology.)

8. **E.** Ketamine, a phencyclidine derivative, functions as both an anesthetic and an analgesic. It does not depress respiration and will increase laryngeal reflexes, thus decreasing the risk of aspiration. It is not associated with nausea and vomiting; however, ketamine can increase secretions and can cause hallucinations. (See page 1353: Anesthetic Agents.)

9. **D.** Opioid analgesics are commonly associated with nausea, vomiting, sedation, dysphoria, pruritus, constipation, urinary retention, and respiratory depression. Dexamethasone has been shown to improve the efficacy of both serotonin (5-HT$_3$) antagonists as well as dopamine antagonists. Routine prophylaxis use of this medication however, has not shown any advantage over symptomatic treatment. Ensuring adequate hydration is an intervention that may be useful in the prevention of postoperative nausea and vomiting. (See page 1354: Postanesthesia Care Unit.)

CHAPTER 53 ■ ANESTHESIA FOR ORGAN TRANSPLANTATION

For questions 1 to 7, choose the best answer.

1. Which of the following statements concerning transplant immunology is FALSE?

   A. Transplant recipients who are not seropositive for cytomegalovirus (CMV) should receive CMV-negative blood.
   B. Interleukin-2 (IL-2) is involved in T-cell activation.
   C. Calcineurin enhances transcription of IL-2.
   D. The major blood group antigens are not potent transplant antigens.
   E. T lymphocytes play a major role in the immune response to a transplanted organ.

2. Which of the following statements concerning renal transplantation is FALSE?

   A. Cadaveric grafts can be safely transplanted after 24 hours of cold ischemia time.
   B. Intraoperative administration of insulin has not been formally studied for improving outcome, but it likely is helpful in diabetic patients with elevated glucose concentrations.
   C. Regional anesthesia for kidney transplantation has limited use.
   D. Inhaled anesthetic techniques are better at preserving (graft) renal flow than intravenous techniques.
   E. Patients undergoing cadaveric transplants are more prone to pulmonary edema.

3. Which of the following is not a major anesthetic consideration during liver transplantation?

   A. Hypothermia
   B. Hypovolemia
   C. Hypocalcemia
   D. Metabolic alkalosis
   E. Reperfusion syndrome

4. Which of the following statements concerning organ transplantation in children is FALSE?

   A. Children are susceptible to lymphoproliferative malignancy as a consequence of immunosuppressive therapy.
   B. Children have a lower rate of successful renal transplantation than adults.
   C. Small children receiving large grafts may have respiratory compromise with abdominal closure.
   D. Hyperacute rejection does not occur because of the immaturity of the immune system and the absence of antibodies to various antigens.
   E. ABO incompatible transplantation is contraindicated in the pediatric population.

5. The maximum tolerable cold ischemia time for a kidney that is being transported for transplantation is _____ hour(s)?

   A. 1
   B. 3
   C. 12
   D. 36
   E. 60

6. Which of the following is not a contraindication for a heart transplant?

   A. Significant atherosclerosis
   B. Intrinsic renal disease
   C. Forced expiratory volume in 1 second (FEV_1) <50%
   D. Severe irreversible pulmonary hypertension
   E. Ischemic cardiomyopathy

7. Which of the following statements concerning lung transplantation is TRUE?

   A. Diabetes and hypertension are contraindications to lung transplantation.
   B. The age limit for single lung transplantation is 55 years.

C. Left-side endobronchial double-lumen tubes typically are preferred for right as well as left transplants.
D. Patients are not screened for malignancy.
E. Hepatitis B and hepatitis C are not contraindications to lung transplantation.

For questions 8 to 20, choose A if 1, 2, and 3 are correct; B if 1 and 3; C if 2 and 4; D if 4; and E if all.

8. Which of the following statements concerning glucocorticoids is/are TRUE?

    1. They produce glucose intolerance.
    2. They can cause hypertension.
    3. They can cause weight gain.
    4. They facilitate cytotoxic T-cell expansion.

9. Which of the following statements concerning azathioprine is/are TRUE?

    1. Cardiac arrest and upper airway edema have been reported complications.
    2. Pancytopenia is a side effect.
    3. The S phase of the cell cycle is affected.
    4. The M phase of the cell cycle is affected.

10. Which of the following statements concerning cyclosporine is/are TRUE?

    1. It may exacerbate risk factors for coronary artery disease.
    2. It is nephrotoxic.
    3. It may cause hypertension.
    4. It may induce ischemic vascular disease.

11. Which of the following statements concerning monoclonal and polyclonal antibodies is/are TRUE?

    1. OKT3 antibody does not affect T cells.
    2. OKT3 may cause generalized weakness, fever, chills, and hypotension.
    3. Antilymphocyte globulin administration is not specific for lymphocytes.
    4. They contain human constant regions in the immunoglobulin.

12. Which of the following statements concerning the recipient during renal transplantation is/are TRUE?

    1. Once the first anastomosis is started, diuresis is initiated with mannitol and furosemide.
    2. Nonsteroidal anti-inflammatory agents may be used in renal transplant recipients.
    3. Recipient iliac artery and vein are usually used for graft vascularization.
    4. The donor should be kept relatively volume depleted to minimize the kidney's work of filtration.

13. Which of the following statements accurately describe the anhepatic stage of orthotopic liver transplantation?

    1. Venovenous bypass from the portal and femoral veins to the axillary vein may be instituted to minimize intra-abdominal venous congestion.
    2. Most patients can be managed without venovenous bypass.
    3. Venovenous bypass improves venous return.
    4. Venous return falls by 50 to 60% with complete caval clamping.

14. Which of the following may be seen upon unclamping the new liver after vascular anastomosis?

    1. Hypotension
    2. Bradycardia
    3. T-wave elevation
    4. Ventricular arrhythmias

15. Which of the following may be effective therapy for the patient with severe, irreversible pulmonary hypertension?

    1. Heterotopic heart transplant
    2. Orthotopic heart transplant
    3. Heart-lung transplant
    4. Left ventricular assist device

16. Which of the following statements concerning heart transplantation is/are TRUE?

    1. The pulmonary artery catheter is withdrawn from the surgical field before caval cannulation.
    2. In the classic approach to transplantation, none of the native heart remains.
    3. Isoproterenol is used frequently to increase graft heart rate.
    4. Prostacyclin infusion is often indicated to decrease systemic vascular resistance selectively.

17. Which of the following statements about patients after cardiac transplantation is/are TRUE?

    1. The transplanted heart is able to compensate in a reflex manner for hemodynamic changes induced by neuraxial anesthesia.
    2. Isoproterenol is the mainstay of chronotropic therapy in these patients.
    3. The alpha-effects of epinephrine and norepinephrine are exaggerated in heart transplant recipients.
    4. The transplanted heart is relatively resistant to indirect-acting agents such as ephedrine.

18. Which of the following statements concerning electrical conduction and autonomic sensitivity in the heart after transplantation is/are TRUE?

    1. The basal rate of the donor atria tends to be less than that of the native atria.
    2. Digoxin does not increase the refractory period of the atrioventricular node.
    3. Denervation results in significant slowing of resting ventricular conduction.
    4. Atropine has minimal effect on heart rate.

19. Which of the following statements about heart-lung and lung transplant is/are TRUE?

    1. Hepatitis B and hepatitis C are absolute contraindications for lung transplantation.
    2. Single-lung transplantations can be performed without cardiopulmonary bypass (CPB).
    3. During one-lung ventilation, clamping of the nondependent pulmonary artery may improve oxygenation.

    4. Heart-lung transplantation is not effective for the patient with Eisenmenger syndrome.

20. Which of the following is/are likely to be required during the anhepatic stage of liver transplantation?

    1. Positive end-expiratory pressure
    2. Insulin
    3. Calcium
    4. Potassium

ANSWERS

---

1. **D.** The antigens on the tissue's cell surface induce an immunologic reaction. T lymphocytes play a primary role in the immune response and allograft destruction. The major blood group antigens (ABO) are particularly potent transplant antigens. Calcineurin enhances transcription of T-cell IL-2. "Humanized" antibodies are both directed against a portion of the IL-2 receptor and work by blocking IL-2–mediated T-cell activation. Because recipients will be immunosuppressed, a diagnosis of occult infection (e.g., tuberculosis) should be excluded. For the same reason, it is standard to order CMV-negative blood for transfusion for seronegative recipients. (See page 1361: Immunosuppressive Drugs; and page 1362: Renal Transplantation.)

2. **D.** Cadaveric grafts can be safely transplanted after 24 hours of cold ischemia time, and up to 36 hours, thus allowing scheduling of preoperative dialysis. In general, concerns over uremic platelet dysfunction and residual heparin from preoperative dialysis have limited the use of regional anesthesia for kidney transplantation. The major anesthetic consideration is maintenance of renal blood flow. No data are available to determine whether inhaled or intravenous techniques are better at preserving (graft) renal flow. For patients with diabetes, intraoperative administration of insulin to normalize blood glucose has not been formally studied for improving outcome. However, recent studies in patients in intensive care units suggest that outcome is significantly improved when glucose is tightly controlled. Therefore, optimal management of glucose (80–110 mg/dL) seems a reasonable anesthetic goal during renal transplantation. (See page 1362: Renal Transplantation.)

3. **D.** Loss of ascitic fluid and persistent bleeding may lead to hypovolemia and associated oliguria during liver transplantation. Metabolic acidosis may result from poor perfusion; it tends to persist in the absence of hepatic metabolic function. Rapid blood replacement may cause citrate-induced hypocalcemia.

Preparation of fluid-warming units, gas circuit humidifiers, warming blankets, and nonconductive wraps for the head and extremities is essential for optimal preservation of normothermia. Sodium bicarbonate and calcium are given just before unclamping to counteract the effects of potassium on the heart. The original descriptions of reperfusion syndrome emphasized (often severe) hypotension and bradycardia with portal reperfusion. (See page 1364: Liver Transplantation.)

4. **E.** Immunosuppressed children, as well as adults, are susceptible to lymphoproliferative malignancies. Although ABO incompatible transplantation is contraindicated in the adult population, it is more successful in pediatric recipients. Hyperacute rejection does not occur because of the immaturity of the immune system and the absence of antibodies to various antigens, including blood group antigens. Pediatric renal transplantation is associated with somewhat lower rates of success than adult transplantation, with vascular thromboses of the grafts more common in young children. Small children receiving large grafts may have respiratory compromise with abdominal closure. (See page 1361: Immunosuppressive Drugs, and page 1362: Renal Transplantation.)

5. **D.** A cadaver allograft may be transplanted semielectively because the tolerable ischemic time for kidneys is up to 36 hours. (See page 1362: Renal Transplantation: Preoperative Considerations.)

6. **E.** Pulmonary hypertension is associated with increased perioperative mortality, so severe, irreversible pulmonary hypertension is a contraindication to cardiac transplant. Other contraindications to cardiac transplantation include significant noncardiac diseases. Because immunosuppressive agents have renal and hepatic side effects, the presence of intrinsic renal or hepatic disease increases the perioperative risk of organ dysfunction or failure. Patients with FEV_1 <50%

predicted despite optimal management of congestive heart failure are at increased risk for ventilatory failure and respiratory infections after the transplant procedure. The presence of significant atherosclerosis is a contraindication because of the increased perioperative morbidity and mortality of atheroembolic phenomena. The most common diagnoses leading to cardiac transplantation are ischemic and idiopathic dilated cardiomyopathies. (See page 1370: Heart Transplantation.)

7. **C.** Because the right upper lobe bronchial orifice is relatively close to the origin of the main bronchus, left-sided endobronchial double-lumen tubes have been recommended for both right and left single-lung transplants, as well as for the bilateral operation. As for other transplants, patients are screened for malignancy (e.g., mammography, Pap test, colonoscopy). Systemic disease processes such as diabetes and hypertension are not considered contraindications, as long as they are clinically stable and medically optimized Absolute contraindications are significant dysfunction of other organs, human immunodeficiency virus (HIV) infection, chronic hepatitis B or C, and malignancy (other than basal cell or squamous cell skin carcinoma). Recommended age limits are as follows: heart-lung transplant, 55 years; double-lung transplant, 60 years; single-lung transplant, 65 years. (See page 1367: Lung Transplantation.)

8. **A.** Corticosteroids disrupt expression of many cytokines in T cells, antigen-presenting cells, and macrophages. Well-known side effects are hypertension, diabetes, hyperlipidemia, weight gain (including cushingoid features), and gastrointestinal ulceration. (See page 1362 : Calcineurin Inhibitors.)

9. **A.** Azathioprine is hydrolyzed in blood to 6-mercaptopurine, a purine analog and metabolite with the ability to incorporate into DNA during the S phase of the cell cycle. Because DNA synthesis is a necessary prerequisite to mitosis, azathioprine exerts an antiproliferative effect. Azathioprine's major side effect is repression of bone marrow cell cycling, which can cause pancytopenia. Cardiac arrest and severe upper airway edema are rare complications. The intravenous dose is about half the oral dose. (See page 1362: Azathioprine.)

10. **E.** Complications of cyclosporine use include hypertension (often requiring therapy), hyperlipidemia, ischemic vascular disease (including in heart recipients), diabetes, and nephrotoxicity. Ischemic cardiac disease is the leading cause of death in kidney transplant recipients, in part because of the underlying disease that preceded transplantation, but the use of calcineurin inhibitors can exacerbate risk factors for coronary artery disease. (See page 1362: Calcineurin Inhibitors.)

11. **C.** Antilymphocyte globulin is a polyclonal antibody that seems to diminish the availability of activated T lymphocytes and T-cell proliferation. OKT3 antibody is directed against a component of the T-cell receptor complex and affects immunosuppression by blocking T-cell function. Acute administration of OKT3 in awake patients (especially first administration) may result in generalized weakness, fever, chills and some hypotension. More severe hypotension, bronchospasm, and pulmonary edema have been reported. (See page 1361: Immunosuppressive Drugs.)

12. **B.** The recipient iliac artery and vein are used for graft vascularization. Once the first anastomosis is started, a diuresis is initiated (mannitol and furosemide are often both given). The major anesthetic consideration is maintenance of renal blood flow. No data are available to determine whether inhaled or intravenous techniques are better at preserving (graft) renal flow. Therefore, typical hemodynamic goals during transplantation are systolic pressure >90 mm Hg, mean systemic pressure >60 mm Hg, and central venous pressure >10 mm Hg. These goals are usually achieved without use of vasopressors, by using isotonic fluids and adjusting anesthetic doses. (See page 1362: Renal Transplantation.)

13. **E.** During the anhepatic stage, many centers employ venovenous bypass from the portal and femoral veins extracorporeally to the axillary vein. This helps to avoid drastic falls in venous return and relieves venous congestion in the lower body, bowel, and kidneys. With complete vena cava cross-clamp, venous return falls by 50 to 60%, often resulting in hypotension. Most patients can be managed without venovenous bypass by using some volume loading. (See page 1364: Liver Transplantation.)

14. **E.** The original descriptions of reperfusion syndrome emphasized (often severe) hypotension and bradycardia with portal reperfusion. Now with flushing techniques that precede reperfusion, and changes in preservation solution, bradycardia is uncommon. Typically, reperfusion is associated with hypotension (further drop of already low systemic vascular resistance and increase in cardiac output), which may or may not require treatment. Portal unclamping can result in a rise in serum potassium. T waves can become elevated following unclamping. Ventricular arrhythmias, bradyarrhythmias, and severe hypotension can also occur. (See page 1364: Liver Transplantation.)

15. **D.** Pulmonary hypertension is associated with increased perioperative mortality, so severe, irreversible pulmonary hypertension is a contraindication to transplantation. These patients may be candidates for left ventricular assist device insertion as definitive therapy or as a bridge to

transplantation. Totally implantable artificial hearts are not currently used because of technical issues. Heterotopic heart transplantation has been virtually abandoned. Bilateral sequential lung transplant has largely replaced heart-lung transplantation, combined with advances in the pharmacologic management of pulmonary hypertension and right ventricular failure. (See page 1370: Heart Transplantation; and page 1370: Heart-Lung Transplant.)

16. **B.**   During heart transplantation, a long sterile sheath should cover the pulmonary artery catheter so that it may be pulled back before caval cannulation. The recipient heart is excised, except for the left atrial tissue encompassing the pulmonary veins. In the classic approach, the atria are transected at the grooves. Isoproterenol is used frequently for its direct effects on cardiac beta-receptors, to increase graft heart rate. Use of temporary epicardial pacing is sometimes needed until isoproterenol has had adequate time to reach maximal effect. Therapy for graft right-sided heart failure is similar to therapy for right-sided heart failure in other cardiac cases. The goals are to improve contractility and to decrease pulmonary vascular resistance. If intravenous agents are not adequate to wean the patient from CPB, inhaled nitric oxide and inhaled prostacyclin (Iloprost) have been shown to be beneficial in this population. (See page 1370: Heart Transplantation.)

17. **C.**   The transplanted heart cannot respond to indirect-acting agents, such as ephedrine, or to peripheral attempts to induce hemodynamic changes, such as carotid massage, Valsalva maneuver, or laryngoscopy. Beta-effects of epinephrine and norepinephrine are exaggerated in heart transplant recipients (versus alpha effects). Isoproterenol is the mainstay of chronotropic therapy in these patients. The denervated heart does not compensate in reflex fashion for hemodynamic changes induced by regional anesthetics. (See page 1372: Anesthetic Management of the Transplant Patient for Nontransplant Surgery and page 1373: Heart Transplant Recipients.)

18. **C.**   The electrocardiogram of the heart after transplantation may contain both donor and native P waves. Because the sinus node normally is under continual vagal influence, the rate of the native atria tends to be less than that of the donor atria, especially with parasympathetic activation (e.g., visceral traction). In contrast to effects on the sinuatrial node, denervation generally does not alter the atrioventricular nodal conduction time or affect ventricular conduction. Drugs that act indirectly on the heart will fail to produce their typical effects after denervation. Atropine is not vagolytic in the denervated heart. Digoxin still causes its direct inotropic effect but does not increase the refractory period of the atrioventricular node, because this effect of digoxin is mediated vagally. (See page 1372: Anesthesia Management of the Transplant Patient for Non-Transplant Surgery.)

19. **A.**   Primary pulmonary hypertension (PPH) and pulmonary hypertension associated with Eisenmenger syndrome are the most common indications for heart-lung transplant. CPB is indicated during lung transplantation if adequate oxygenation cannot be maintained despite ventilatory and pharmacologic maneuvers or pulmonary artery clamping by the surgeon. The inability to ventilate and the development of right ventricular dysfunction are also indications for CPB. Absolute contraindications are significant dysfunction of other organs, HIV infection, chronic hepatitis B or C, and malignancy (other than basal cell or squamous cell skin carcinoma). (See page 1370: Heart-Lung Transplant (Adult and Pediatric); and page 1367: Lung Transplantation.)

20. **A.**   During the anhepatic stage, the need for vigorous retraction under the diaphragm often worsens hypoxemia; positive end-expiratory pressure may be helpful. Citrate intoxication as a result of rapid infusion may necessitate the need to administer calcium. Hyperkalemia may require treatment with insulin. (See page 1364: Liver Transplantation.)

SECTION VI ■ POSTANESTHESIA AND CONSULTANT PRACTICE

CHAPTER 54 ■ POSTOPERATIVE RECOVERY

1. The greatest postanesthesia care unit (PACU) cost is for:

   A. disposable items
   B. antiemetics
   C. routine diagnostic testing
   D. staffing
   E. respiratory therapy

2. Postoperative patient triage decisions should be based on:

   A. ambulatory versus inpatient status
   B. potential for postoperative complications
   C. age
   D. American Society of Anesthesiologists (ASA) classification
   E. insurance coverage

3. Disadvantages of intramuscular opioid administration (compared with intravenous administration) include all of the following EXCEPT:

   A. unpredictable uptake
   B. larger dose requirements
   C. shortened onset
   D. pain on administration
   E. risk of hematoma formation

4. Which of the following statements regarding epidural opioid analgesia is FALSE?

   A. Serotonin antagonists may be used to treat side effects.
   B. It may improve outcome after urologic procedures.
   C. The addition of clonidine enhances analgesia.
   D. It is a useful technique for controlling pain after gastroplasty surgery.
   E. Delayed respiratory depression results from vascular uptake.

5. All of the following are causes of hypotension in the PACU EXCEPT:

   A. myocardial ischemia
   B. blood pressure cuff with a narrow width
   C. rewarming of a hypothermic patient
   D. addisonian crisis
   E. furosemide therapy

6. Which of the following is not an important sign or symptom of hypotension in the postoperative period?

   A. Hypercarbia
   B. Metabolic acidosis
   C. Mental confusion
   D. Nausea
   E. Angina

7. Which of the following is not an example of relative hypovolemia?

   A. Vasovagal stimulation
   B. Epidural analgesia
   C. Pregnancy
   D. Positive-pressure ventilation
   E. Hemorrhage

8. Which of the following statements concerning postoperative bradycardia is TRUE?

   A. Most bradycardias are benign and are secondary to autonomic imbalance.
   B. Nodal rhythm is common and is best treated with an alpha-adrenergic agonist.
   C. Idioventricular rhythms are usually benign.
   D. Idioventricular rhythms usually respond well to atropine.
   E. Cardiac pacing is rarely effective for bradyarrhythmia.

9. Which of the following statements concerning the postoperative appearance of atrial premature contractions is TRUE?

   A. The cause is most frequently a structural injury to the mitral valve.

B. The P wave is usually normal.

C. Usually, there is a compensatory pause.

D. There can be wide QRS complexes; however, they resemble normal QRS complexes in general shape.

E. Generally, they result in hemodynamic compromise requiring urgent treatment.

10. Choose the TRUE statement regarding perioperative carbon monoxide poisoning.

   A. Cyanosis is the most reliable sign.

   B. PaO_2 is usually low.

   C. The risk is greatest for patients anesthetized outside the operating room.

   D. Symptoms of nausea, vomiting, and headache in the PACU are specific for carbon monoxide poisoning.

   E. Carbon monoxide irreversibly binds to hemoglobin.

11. Choose the TRUE statement regarding hypoxemia in the PACU.

   A. Hypoxemia rarely occurs after regional anesthesia.

   B. Children with adenotonsillar hypotrophy are at risk of hypoxemia.

   C. The incidence of hypoxemia in postoperative patients breathing room air in the PACU is low.

   D. The cost of providing supplemental oxygen is prohibitive.

   E. Use of oxygen prevents hypoxemia.

12. Which of the following is not a cause of hyponatremia?

   A. Intravenous administration of excess free water

   B. Use of sodium-free irrigating solutions

   C. Excess use of salt-wasting diuretics such as furosemide

   D. Syndrome of inappropriate antidiuretic hormone secretion

   E. Prolonged attempts of induction of labor with oxytocin

13. Which of the following statements concerning postoperative nausea and vomiting is FALSE?

   A. The incidence is increased in patients with a history of motion sickness.

   B. The incidence is increased following surgery involving manipulation of extraocular muscles.

   C. The incidence is greater after general anesthesia than after regional anesthesia.

   D. The incidence is greater with halothane than with isoflurane anesthesia.

   E. The incidence is greater with opioid than with pure inhalation anesthesia.

14. Which of the following induction agents has the lowest incidence of perioperative nausea and vomiting?

   A. Thiopental

   B. Methohexital

   C. Etomidate

   D. Propofol

   E. Ketamine

15. Which of the following agents administered intravenously is not an appropriate treatment for nausea and vomiting?

   A. Metoclopramide

   B. Scopolamine

   C. Ondansetron

   D. Ephedrine

   E. Propofol

16. Choose the correct statement regarding adjuncts used for postoperative analgesia.

   A. Rofecoxib administration provides a secondary cardioprotective benefit.

   B. Ketorolac administration may decrease cardiac ischemic events.

   C. Ibuprofen and acetaminophen are ineffective when they are administered orally before surgery.

   D. Agonist–antagonist analgesics are the best adjuncts to supplement analgesia.

   E. The use of clonidine is limited by bradycardia.

For questions 17 to 41, choose A if 1, 2, and 3 are correct; B if 1 and 3; C if 2 and 4; D if 4; and E if all.

17. The level of postoperative care a patient requires is determined by:

   1. underlying illness

   2. duration and complexity of anesthesia and surgery

   3. risk of postoperative complications

   4. the inhalation anesthetic used

18. Upon arrival in PACU, each patient assessment should include:

   1. heart rhythm

   2. temperature

   3. ventilatory rate

   4. skin color

19. Which of the following statements concerning postoperative pain management is/are TRUE?

   1. Appropriate postoperative pain management will help to control hypertension and tachycardia.

   2. A tachycardic patient with low blood pressure should be treated aggressively with opioids.

   3. Sufficient analgesia is the desired end point, even if large doses of opioids are necessary.

   4. Agonist–antagonist analgesics are of significant value in treating a patient with opioid tolerance.

20. Discharge criteria for the PACU include:

   1. observation for at least 60 minutes after the last intravenous opioid is administered

   2. achieving of normal body temperature

3. monitoring of oxygen saturation for 45 minutes after discontinuation of supplemental oxygen
4. the presence of airway reflexes to prevent aspiration

21. Which of the following statements concerning the treatment of postoperative hypotension is/are TRUE?

1. Definitive therapy should be directed at the specific abnormality that reduces systemic blood pressure.
2. A 20 to 30% reduction in systolic blood pressure usually requires treatment.
3. Hypovolemia is the most common cause of postoperative hypotension.
4. If intravenous fluid administration of 300 to 500 mL does not improve hypotension, a second similar bolus should be instituted immediately.

22. Which of the following statements concerning patients with pre-existing hypertension who subsequently develop postoperative hypertension is/are TRUE?

1. They have no increased risk of morbidity.
2. They should have blood pressure normalized within 1 to 2 minutes.
3. Increased systemic vascular resistance should be treated with potent vasodilators.
4. Treatment should be directed toward the cause of increased sympathetic nervous system activity.

23. Postoperative hypertension should be treated if:

1. The patient develops angina.
2. The patient is having large amounts of postoperative bleeding.
3. The patient had a cerebral aneurysm clipping.
4. The diastolic blood pressure is 10% above baseline.

24. Which of the following statements concerning postoperative tachycardia is/are TRUE?

1. Sinus tachycardia is nearly always associated with physiologic increases in sympathetic nervous system activity.
2. The treatment of choice for sinus tachycardia is digoxin.
3. Rapid atrial fibrillation accompanied by serious hypotension is best treated by direct current cardioversion.
4. Postoperative ventricular tachycardia is most likely caused by hypokalemia.

25. Choose the TRUE statement(s) regarding postoperative ventricular ectopy.

1. Premature ventricular contractions are usually the result of life-threatening conditions.
2. Patients with preoperative premature ventricular contractions commonly experience them in the PACU.
3. Premature ventricular contractions usually require medical intervention.

4. The preoperative presence of premature ventricular contractions usually is not predictive of an unfavorable postoperative outcome.

26. Which of the following statements concerning upper airway edema is/are TRUE?

1. It often leads to complete obstruction of the airway.
2. It may necessitate emergency endotracheal intubation.
3. It should be treated with emergency jet ventilation as soon as possible.
4. It may be exacerbated by laryngoscopy.

27. Which of the following can be used to treat postoperative wheezing?

1. Intravenous aminophylline
2. Intramuscular terbutaline
3. Ipratropium bromide
4. Intravenous epinephrine infusion

28. Select the medications(s) known to potentiate neuromuscular relaxation.

1. Diltiazem (Cardizem)
2. Intravenous phenytoin (Dilantin)
3. Digoxin
4. Furosemide

29. Which of the following tests reliably predict recovery of airway protective reflexes?

1. A negative inspiratory pressure of <-25 cm H_2O
2. Sustained head lift for 10 seconds
3. Return of train-of-four response to preoperative levels
4. None of the above

30. Pulmonary dead space increases with:

1. pulmonary embolism
2. endotracheal intubation
3. pulmonary hypotension
4. pneumothorax

31. Increased CO_2 production in the PACU can be caused by:

1. shivering
2. infection
3. malignant hyperthermia
4. hyperalimentation

32. Which of the following usually are effective treatments for postoperative hypoxemia?

1. Incentive spirometry
2. Intermittent positive-pressure breathing techniques
3. Continuous positive airway pressure by mask
4. Endotracheal intubation without continuous positive airway pressure

33. Which of the following can worsen ventilation–perfusion matching?

1. An increase in pulmonary artery pressure
2. A decrease in pulmonary artery pressure
3. Impaired hypoxic pulmonary vasoconstrictive reflex
4. An increase in the percentage of inspired oxygen

34. Aspiration of gastric contents:

   1. typically results in bacterial tracheal bronchitis
   2. can rapidly progress to acute respiratory distress syndrome and pulmonary edema
   3. is much more likely to occur in elderly patients, even if they have no coexisting disease
   4. often causes an increase in pulmonary dead space

35. Patients who aspirate a large amount of gastric contents:

   1. should be intubated and undergo suctioning before the administration of positive-pressure ventilation
   2. should have tracheal pH ascertained and bicarbonate solutions instilled to increase the pH in the trachea to >7.4
   3. should be observed for 24 to 48 hours with serial temperature, white blood cell count, chest radiograph, and arterial blood gas measurements
   4. should receive prophylactic antibiotics

36. Treatment of patients with significant aspiration and resultant hypoxemia includes:

   1. the administration of furosemide
   2. the administration of high-dose steroids
   3. aggressive fluid restriction
   4. positive end-expiratory pressure mechanical ventilation

37. Risk factors for corneal abrasion include:

   1. pediatric patients
   2. head or neck surgery

3. supine positioning
4. long surgical time

38. Which of the following statements concerning hypothermia and shivering in the PACU is/are TRUE?

   1. Severe shivering can increase CO_2 production by >200%.
   2. Myocardial ischemia and ventilatory failure can occur secondary to severe shivering.
   3. Intensity of shivering can be accentuated by inhalation anesthetic–related tremor.
   4. Meperidine is an effective treatment for postoperative shivering.

39. The probable cause(s) for prolonged unresponsiveness after anesthesia is/are:

   1. pseudocholinesterase deficiency
   2. hypoglycemia
   3. hypothermia
   4. residual inhalation anesthetic

40. Hearing impairment after anesthesia and surgery:

   1. is a rare event
   2. occurs in 8 to 16% of patients after dural puncture for spinal anesthesia.
   3. is never bilateral
   4. is often related to disruption of the round window or tympanic membrane rupture.

41. Regarding medications for prophylaxis and treatment of postoperative nausea and vomiting, guidelines from the ASA endorse the use of:

   1. serotonin blocking agents
   2. dexamethasone
   3. multiple antiemetic agents
   4. prophylaxis for all patient receiving general anesthesia

---

ANSWERS

1. **D.** The greatest PACU cost is for staffing. The mix of nursing staff (e.g., amount of training, experience, salaries and benefit levels), the number of patients per caregiver, and the duration of PACU stay all determine an overall personnel cost per admission. Routine postoperative diagnostic testing increases costs for securing and processing tests, as well as for professional interpretation. Use of routine therapies such as oxygen, antiemetic therapy, and respiratory therapy increases the expenditure per patient for drugs and disposable items and can add to the staffing resources required per patient. (See page 1380: Assessing the Value of Postanesthesia Care.)

2. **B.** Patients must be carefully evaluated to determine which level of postoperative care is most appropriate. Triage should be based on clinical condition and the potential for complications that require intervention. Alternatives to PACU care must be employed in a nondiscriminatory fashion. Triage should not be based on age, ASA classification, ambulatory versus inpatient status, or type of insurance. A wide margin of safety and applicable PACU standards should be preserved when appropriate. (See page 1380: Selecting the Appropriate Level of Postoperative Care.)

3. **C.** Disadvantages of the intramuscular route include larger dose requirements, delayed onset, and unpredictable uptake in hypothermic patients. The

risk of hematoma formation is also a consideration in anticoagulated patients. (See page 1381: Postoperative Pain Management.)

4. **E.** Epidural opioid analgesia is effective after thoracic and abdominal procedures. It helps to wean patients with obesity or chronic obstructive pulmonary disease from mechanical ventilation. Immediate and delayed ventilatory depression can occur, related to vascular uptake and cephalad spread in cerebrospinal fluid, respectively. Nausea and pruritus are troubling side effects. Nausea resolves with antiemetics, whereas pruritus often responds to naloxone infusion. Epidural analgesia may also improve surgical outcomes after orthopaedic and urologic procedures. Addition of local anesthetic or clonidine enhances analgesia and decreases the risk of side effects from epidural opioids. (See page 1381: Postoperative Pain Management.)

5. **B.** A blood pressure cuff that is too large yields a falsely low value. Hypothermic patients can sometimes experience hypotension during the rewarming period. Postoperative myocardial ischemia is often initiated in high-risk patients by tachycardia or hypotension. Hypotension caused by ischemic ventricular dysfunction can quickly cause irreversible infarction. Rarely, hypotension reflects steroid deficiency in patients in whom adrenal function is suppressed by exogenous steroid use. Furosemide therapy may precipitate hypotension by producing hypovolemia. (See page 1383: Cardiovascular Complications.)

6. **A.** Systemic hypotension is a common postoperative complication that can cause hypoperfusion of organ systems. The resulting tissue hypoxia promotes inefficient anaerobic metabolism and accumulation of lactic acid. During hypotension, the sympathetic nervous system preferentially delivers blood flow to the brain, heart, and kidneys. Symptoms of hypotension referable to these organ symptoms indicate exhaustion of compensatory mechanisms. These include mental confusion, disorientation, loss of consciousness, nausea, angina, and reduced urine output. (See page 1383: Postoperative Hypotension.)

7. **E.** A reduction in circulating intravascular volume is the definition of absolute hypovolemia. Relative hypovolemia is characterized by a normal intravascular volume. It may result from a decrease in endogenous sympathetic nervous system activity, as can occur with vasovagal stimulation or with blockade of the sympathetic nervous system. Impedance of venous return by compression of thoracic veins secondary to positive-pressure ventilation or from compression of the vena cava by a gravid uterus also can result in decreased venous return. These are forms of relative hypovolemia. (See page 1384: Hypovolemia.)

8. **A.** Factors that increase parasympathetic nervous system activity or decrease sympathetic nervous system activity reduce supraventricular pacemaker rates and promote sinus bradycardia. Frequently, this causes emergence of a nodal pacemaker in the lower atrioventricular node or the bundle of His. Nodal rhythms usually are benign unless a low ventricular rate or lack of coordinated atrial contraction reduces cardiac output and blood pressure. If hypotension occurs, atropine or beta-stimulating medications usually can restore sinus rhythm. Idioventricular bradycardia is life-threatening and seldom generates adequate cardiac output. Atropine will not increase ventricular pacemaker rates because the ventricle lacks significant parasympathetic nervous system innervation. Epinephrine, isoproterenol, and cardiac pacing will accelerate the ventricular rate. (See page 1387: Bradycardia.)

9. **D.** An aberrant impulse arising in the atrium, atrioventricular node, or upper bundle of His generates an atrial premature contraction that typically has an early but otherwise normal QRS complex that often is not preceded by a P wave. In postoperative patients, atrial premature contractions usually appear with increased central nervous system activity and seldom cause hemodynamic compromise. If a supraventricular impulse enters the ventricular conduction system where all pathways have recovered excitability, asynchronous ventricular depolarization will generate wide high-amplitude electrocardiogram complexes that are difficult to distinguish from true premature ventricular contractions. These aberrantly conducted premature supraventricular depolarizations are sometimes preceded by an abnormal P wave and often exhibit a noncompensatory pause. The aberrant QRS complex often resembles normal complexes in general shape; increased sympathetic nervous system activity usually is responsible. (See page 1388: Premature Contractions.)

10. **C.** Carbon monoxide reversibly binds to hemoglobin with 200 times the affinity of oxygen, thus creating carboxyhemoglobin, which impedes both the binding of oxygen and the dissociation of oxygen from oxyhemoglobin. The overall risk of exposure to carbon monoxide is estimated as 0.26%, but the risk increases to 0.46% for the first cases of the days and to 2.9% for first cases performed in peripheral anesthetizing locations. Symptoms of moderate carbon monoxide exposure such as headache, nausea, vomiting, irritability, and altered visual or motor skills are nonspecific and common during recovery. Carbon monoxide seldom causes cyanosis. A pulse oximeter interprets carboxyhemoglobin as oxyhemoglobin, so SpO_2 reads falsely high. The PaO_2 is often high, although SpO_2 is low and metabolic acidemia is significant. (See page 1393: Carbon Monoxide Poisoning.)

11. **B.**   The incidence of hypoxemia in postoperative patients is high. In one study of PACU patients placed on room air, 30% of patients younger than 1 year old, 20% of those 1 to 3 years old, 14% of those 3 to 14 years old, and 7.8% of adults had hemoglobin saturations fall to <90%. Perioperative hypoxemia occurs more frequently in children with respiratory infections or chronic adenotonsillar hypertrophy. Hypoxemia occurs frequently after regional anesthesia. Use of oxygen neither consistently prevents hypoxemia nor addresses underlying causes. The cost of supplemental oxygen is minimal, the inconvenience to patients is minor, and the overall risk is small. (See page 1393: Supplemental Oxygen.)

12. **C.**   Postoperative hyponatremia occurs when excess free water is infused during surgery or sodium-free irrigating solution is absorbed by prostatic sinuses during transurethral prostate resection. Free-water retention can also be caused by inappropriate antidiuretic hormone secretion or prolonged induction of labor with oxytocin. Therapy for hyponatremia includes administration of normal saline and intravenous furosemide to promote renal wasting of free water in excess of sodium. (See page 1397: Hyponatremia.)

13. **D.**   Nausea and vomiting are common problems in the PACU; the incidence varies with the surgical procedure and the anesthetic technique. Multiple factors have been recognized that increase the incidence of postoperative nausea and vomiting. The incidence seems to be lower after regional rather than general anesthesia, although this difference narrows when intrathecal opioids are included to control postoperative pain. The incidence of nausea does not appear to differ among inhalation anesthetics but is increased if opioids are used intraoperatively. (See page 1397: Nausea and Vomiting.)

14. **D.**   Induction with barbiturate agents such as thiopental or methohexital seem less likely to cause postoperative nausea and vomiting than induction with etomidate or ketamine. Propofol appears to have the lowest overall incidence of postoperative nausea and vomiting and may possess an antiemetic effect. (See page 1397: Nausea and Vomiting.)

15. **B.**   Many agents are useful for postoperative nausea and vomiting in the PACU and work by various mechanisms. Using intravenous scopolamine as an antiemetic causes unacceptable psychogenic reactions during recovery. Although transdermal scopolamine may have some prophylactic benefit, its low efficacy and tendency to cause visual disturbances make it a poor substitute for other agents. Metoclopramide, ondansetron, ephedrine, and propofol all have been used effectively in the PACU setting. (See page 1397: Nausea and Vomiting.)

16. **B.**   Perioperative oral or intravenous administration of COX-2 inhibitors offers promising adjuvant therapy to augment postoperative analgesia. Unfortunately, recent concerns about negative cardiac side effects of these agents led to the withdrawal of rofecoxib and clouded the overall appropriateness of this approach. Ibuprofen and acetaminophen are effective when administered orally before surgery. The antiplatelet properties of ketorolac may decrease cardiac ischemic events in patients with coronary artery disease. Agonist–antagonist analgesics offer little advantage. The use of clonidine to supplement analgesia is effective but can be limited by hypotension. (See page 1381: Postoperative Pain Management.)

17. **A.**   For both ambulatory and inpatient surgery, the level of postoperative care a patient requires is determined by the degree of the underlying illness, the duration and complexity of the anesthesia and surgery, and the risk of postoperative complications. Using a less intensive postanesthesia setting for selected patients can reduce the cost for a surgical procedure and can allow the facility to divert scarce PACU resources to patients with greater needs. (See page 1380: Selecting the Appropriate Level of Postoperative Care.)

18. **E.**   Every patient admitted to a PACU should have heart rate and rhythm, systemic blood pressure, and ventilatory rate recorded. Assessment every 5 minutes for the first 15 minutes and every 15 thereafter is a prudent minimum. Temperature should be documented at least on admission and discharge, along with level of consciousness, airway patency, and skin color. (See page 1381: Admission to the Postanesthesia Care Unit.)

19. **B.**   Relief of surgical pain with minimal side effects is a primary goal in PACU care. Improving patient comfort and relief of pain reduces sympathetic nervous system response, thereby helping to control postoperative hypertension and tachycardia. Analgesics can precipitate hypotension in hypovolemic patients who rely on sympathetic activity for cardiovascular homeostasis. Such is the case in a tachycardic patient with normal or low blood pressure. Sufficient analgesia is the desired clinical end point for all patients even if large doses of opioids are necessary. Agonist–antagonist analgesics are thought to offer little advantage over regular opioids in those with opioid tolerance. (See page 1381: Postoperative Pain Management.)

20. **D.**   Before discharge from the PACU, each patient should be sufficiently oriented to assess his or her physical condition and to summon assistance upon discharge. Airway reflexes and motor function must be adequate to prevent aspiration. Blood pressure, heart rate, and indices of peripheral perfusion should be relatively constant for at least 15 minutes.

Achieving normal body temperature is not an absolute requirement. Patients should be observed for at least 15 minutes after the last intravenous opioid or sedative is administered. Oxygen saturation should be monitored for 15 minutes after discontinuation of supplemental oxygen to detect hypoxemia. (See page 1383: Discharge Criteria.)

21. **A.**   Generally, 20 to 30% reductions in systolic blood pressure and/or symptoms of vital-organ hypoperfusion are indications for treatment of hypotension. The most common cause of postoperative hypotension is hypovolemia, and treatment should thus begin with fluid administration. If hypotension is spurious or is caused by reduced systemic vascular resistance or ischemia, the amount of fluid infused while these diagnoses are established is usually inconsequential. Definitive therapy, however, should be directed at the specific abnormality that is reducing the systemic blood pressure. If fluid administration of 300 to 500 mL does not improve hypotension, myocardial dysfunction should be considered. (See page 1386: Treatment of Postoperative Hypotension.)

22. **D.**   A moderate elevation in systemic blood pressure is common in the postoperative period. However, significant hypertension (defined as 20–30% above the baseline level) does increase the risk of morbidity and should be evaluated and treated. Patients with pre-existing hypertension often have exaggerated postoperative blood pressure responses. This is frequently the result of enhanced sympathetic nervous system activity, and measures aimed at treatment of this sympathetic nervous system activity are usually indicated. Blood pressure should not be reduced below preoperative levels because lower than normal systemic pressures may promote vital-organ hypoperfusion in patients with chronic hypertension. Potent vasodilators, such as nitroprusside or nitroglycerin, are reserved only for refractory or profound hypertension. (See page 1386: Postoperative Hypertension.)

23. **A.**   Indications for treatment of postoperative hypertension include a systolic or diastolic pressure 20 to 30% above baseline, signs or symptoms of complications (headache, bleeding, ocular changes, angina, ST segment depression), or an unusual risk of morbidity (increased intracranial pressure, mitral regurgitation, open eye injury). (See page 1386: Postoperative Hypertension.)

24. **B.**   Postoperative sinus tachycardia nearly always is associated with physiologic increases in sympathetic nervous system activity. Sinus tachycardia usually is harmless but can decrease diastolic filling time and precipitate myocardial ischemia. Beta-blockade is useful to control the rate, whereas digoxin usually is ineffective unless ventricular failure is the underlying cause of the tachycardia. Sudden onset of atrial fibrillation can generate ventricular rates in excess of 150 beats/minute and can result in hypotension. In the presence of serious hypotension, direct current cardioversion should be used to convert fibrillation to sinus rhythm. Postoperative ventricular tachycardia or fibrillation almost always reflects severe myocardial ischemia, systemic acidemia, or hypoxemia. (See page 1388: Tachycardia.)

25. **C.**   Ventricular ectopy that exists preoperatively usually reappears in the PACU, with somewhat decreased frequency. Ectopy does not usually predict postoperative outcome. In postoperative patients, abnormal ventricular complexes are almost always benign and seldom require treatment. Most premature ventricular contractions are caused by nonthreatening conditions. (See page 1388: Premature Contractions.)

26. **C.**   Acute extrinsic upper airway compression must be relieved if possible. If the obstruction is fixed, emergency tracheal intubation may become necessary. However, airway manipulation is fraught with danger. Even minor trauma from intubation attempts can convert a partially obstructed airway into a totally obstructed airway. Complete obstruction from airway edema is rare. Edema is often resolved by nebulized racemic epinephrine. Small doses of corticosteroid have also been effective. An acute airway emergency can be precipitated if tracheal intubation or facemask ventilation cannot be accomplished. In this case, cricothyroidotomy and emergency jet ventilation would be the treatment of choice. However, this should be attempted after endotracheal intubation has failed. (See page 1389: Increased Airway Resistance.)

27. **E.**   The treatment of small airway resistance is directed at an underlying etiology. Patients often respond well to their existing regimen of albuterol or other inhaler. Intramuscular or sublingual terbutaline can be added. If ventilation is still compromised or is unduly labored, an aminophylline loading dose and maintenance infusion may be administered. Bronchospasm resistant to beta-sympathomimetic medication may improve with an anticholinergic medication such as atropine or ipratropium. If bronchospasm is life-threatening, an intravenous epinephrine infusion usually yields profound bronchodilation. (See page 1389: Increased Airway Resistance.)

28. **C.**   Medications that potentiate neuromuscular relaxation include some antibiotics, furosemide, propranolol, and acutely administered (intravenous) phenytoin. Conversely, long-term phenytoin use increases the dose requirements for nondepolarizing neuromuscular blocking agents. (See page 1390: Neuromuscular and Skeletal Problems.)

29. **D.**   Forced vital capacity of 10 to 12 mL/kg and an inspiratory pressure of <-25 cm H_2O imply that the strength of ventilatory muscles is adequate to sustain

ventilation. The ability to sustain head elevation in a supine position is a rough index of muscular recovery. Tactile train-of-four assessment accurately assesses the ability to ventilate. However, none of these clinical end points reliably predicts recovery of airway protective reflexes. (See page 1390: Neuromuscular and Skeletal Problems.)

30. **B.** Any decrease in pulmonary blood flow, as would be caused by pulmonary embolism or pulmonary hypotension, will cause an increase in physiologic dead space. Upper airway dead space (anatomic dead space) has been shown to be reduced by approximately 75% after endotracheal intubation and almost eliminated by tracheostomy. Pneumothorax is a cause of shunt and does not affect dead space. (See page 1391: Increased Dead Space).

31. **E.** In the PACU, metabolic rate and CO_2 production can increase by as much as 40%. Shivering, high work of breathing, infection, sympathetic nervous system activity, and rapid carbohydrate metabolism during intravenous hyperalimentation also accelerate CO_2 production. Malignant hyperthermia generates CO_2 production many times greater than normal. (See page 1391: Increased Carbon Dioxide Production.)

32. **B.** In the PACU, conservative measures to improve lung volume often produce lasting improvements in oxygenation. Incentive spirometry and mask continuous positive airway pressure both increase functional residual capacity and improve ventilation–perfusion matching, resulting in improved oxygenation. Intermittent positive-pressure breathing techniques probably are not effective. Endotracheal intubation without continuous positive airway pressure results in a progressive reduction of functional residual capacity and ventilation–perfusion mismatching that may actually worsen arterial hypoxemia. (See page 1392: Distribution of Ventilation.)

33. **E.** Increased pulmonary artery pressure may interfere with ventilation–perfusion matching by increasing blood flow to less dependent (and less ventilated) portions of the lung as well as by increasing flow through the bronchial circulation and pulmonary arterial venous anastomoses. Reduction in pulmonary artery pressures can also change ventilation–perfusion matching by compromising perfusion to the nondependent lung. Inhalation anesthetics, nitroprusside, and other medications impair hypoxic pulmonary vasoconstriction; this partially explains the increase in the alveolar-arterial oxygen gradient associated with general anesthetics. The effects of anesthetics on hypoxic pulmonary vasoconstriction persist into the recovery period. An increased inspired O_2 fraction can interfere with ventilation–perfusion matching in patients with acute lung disease, perhaps resulting from interference with hypoxic pulmonary vasoconstriction or promotion of reabsorption

atelectasis. (See page 1392: Distribution of Perfusion.)

34. **C.** Aspiration of gastric contents during vomiting or regurgitation causes chemical pneumonitis that is characterized initially by diffuse bronchospasm, hypoxemia, and atelectasis. This can rapidly progress to acute respiratory distress syndrome and pulmonary edema. Occlusion or destruction of the pulmonary microvasculature often is evident, resulting in increased pulmonary vascular resistance and increased dead space. Bacterial infection rarely results. Advancing age, in the absence of coexisting disease, is not a risk factor for aspiration. (See page 1393: Perioperative Aspiration.)

35. **B.** Patients who aspirate a large amount of gastric contents should be observed for 24 to 48 hours for the development of aspiration pneumonitis. Observation includes serial temperature checks, white blood cell counts with differential chest radiographs, and blood gas determinations. Fluffy infiltrates may appear on the chest radiograph within 24 hours of the event. If a large aspiration has occurred, the trachea should be intubated, and suctioning should be performed before institution of positive-pressure ventilation (to avoid widely disseminating any aspirated material into the distal airways). Instillation of saline or alkalotic solutions is not recommended. Bacterial infection does not necessarily follow aspiration, and prophylactic antibiotics are thus not recommended. In fact, they may promote colonization by resistant organisms. (See page 1393: Perioperative Aspiration.)

36. **D.** If significant aspiration causes hypoxemia, increased airway resistance, consolidation, or pulmonary edema, then institution of supplemental oxygen, continuous positive airway pressure, or mechanical ventilation with positive end-expiratory pressure may be necessary. Pulmonary edema is usually secondary to increased capillary permeability and should not be treated with diuretics. Hypovolemia from fluid losses into the lung can necessitate aggressive fluid infusion. High-dose steroids yield little improvement of long-term outcome after aspiration. (See page 1393: Perioperative Aspiration.)

37. **C.** Corneal abrasions occur more frequently in elderly patients, after long cases, with lateral or prone positioning, and after head or neck surgery. (See page 1399: Ocular Injuries and Visual Changes.)

38. **E.** Postoperative shivering is uncomfortable and increases the risk of accidental trauma. Moreover, severe shivering can increase oxygen consumption and CO_2 production by 200 to 300%. This increases cardiac output and minute ventilation; myocardial ischemia or ventilatory failure can result. The intensity of postoperative shivering is sometimes accentuated by inhalation anesthetic–related tremors. Meperidine is a particularly effective treatment for

postoperative shivering. (See page 1400: Hypothermia and Shivering.)

39. E. Residual sedation from inhalation anesthetics is a frequent cause of prolonged unconsciousness, particularly after long procedures, in obese patients, or when high inspired concentrations are continued through the end of surgery. Profound residual neuromuscular paralysis can mimic unconsciousness by precluding any motor response to stimuli. This may occur after gross overdose, if reversal agents are omitted in patients with unrecognized neuromuscular disease, or in patients with phase II blockade (caused by either excessive succinylcholine administration or pseudocholinesterase deficiency). Hypothermia ($<33°C$) impairs consciousness and increases the depressant effect of medications. A serum glucose level should be evaluated to rule out hypoglycemia. (See page 1400: Persistent Sedation.)

40. C. Hearing impairment after anesthesia and surgery is relatively common. Although impairment is often subclinical, patients sometimes experience decreased auditory acuity, tinnitus, or roaring. The incidence of detectable hearing impairment is particularly high after dural puncture for spinal anesthesia (8–16%), and it varies with needle size, needle type, and patient age. Impairment can be unilateral or bilateral and usually resolves spontaneously. Hearing loss is often related to disruption of the round window or tympanic membrane rupture. (See page 1399: Hearing Impairment.)

41. A. Guidelines on postoperative care from the ASA endorse the use of serotonin blocking agents and dexamethasone and multiple agent therapy. These antiemetics have different sites of action, so combination therapy may generate better results by simultaneously treating two or more precipitating factors, although their effects appear merely additive rather than synergistic. Prophylaxis should be used only in patients at medium or high risk of emesis. (See page 1397: Nausea and Vomiting.)

CHAPTER 55 ▪ MANAGEMENT OF ACUTE POSTOPERATIVE PAIN

For questions 1 to 7, choose the best answer.

1. Which of the following statements concerning nerve fiber classification is TRUE?

   A. Approximately 50 to 80% of type C fibers transmit nociceptive impulses.
   B. Class C fibers are thinly myelinated.
   C. Class A fibers are less excitable than those in class B.
   D. Class B fibers are unmyelinated.
   E. Class A gamma fibers mediate nociceptive impulses.

2. All of the following substances may attenuate nociceptive impulses when acting peripherally or in the spinal cord EXCEPT:

   A. gamma-aminobutyric acid (GABA)
   B. neostigmine
   C. cholinergic agonists
   D. substance P
   E. enkephalins

3. Which of the following statements concerning nociception is FALSE?

   A. The sense organs for pain are free nerve endings.
   B. Nociceptors may be exteroceptors.
   C. Nociceptors exhibit high response thresholds and persistent discharge to suprathreshold stimuli.
   D. Peripheral afferent fibers transmitting pain signals have their cell bodies in the dorsal root ganglion.
   E. Overstimulation of pressure receptors results in the sensation of pain.

4. The circulating levels of which of the following hormones is not increased postoperatively?

   A. Insulin
   B. Glucagon
   C. Antidiuretic hormone
   D. Angiotensin II
   E. Cortisol

5. Which of the following statements concerning the analgesia provided by intrathecal clonidine is FALSE?

   A. It affects alpha-receptors in the dorsal horn.
   B. It produces analgesia in a dose-dependent fashion.
   C. It interacts synergistically with opioids and local anesthetics.
   D. At low doses, it causes hypotension and bradycardia. At high doses, blood pressure normalizes.
   E. It produces respiratory depression comparable to that produced by morphine.

6. Which of the following statements is FALSE?

   A. Intra-articular bupivacaine provides effective analgesia following arthroscopy.
   B. Penile blocks should be performed with dilute, epinephrine-containing local anesthetic solutions.
   C. Local anesthetics inhibit sodium channels and keep the membrane in its polarized state.
   D. Advantages of local anesthetic infiltration include simplicity and lack of effect on the patient's general sensorium.
   E. Intercostal nerve blocks should be performed beneath the inferior border of the rib.

7. Stimulation of which receptor produces miosis and sedation?

   A. Mu
   B. Kappa
   C. Delta
   D. Sigma
   E. Epsilon

For questions 8 to 20, choose A if 1, 2, and 3 are correct; B if 1 and 3; C if 2 and 4; D if 4; and E if all.

8. Which of the following statements concerning modulation of nociception is/are TRUE?

   1. Peripheral nociceptors are sensitized by local tissue mediators of injury.
   2. The "windup" phenomenon refers to temporal summation of action potentials in dorsal horn neurons.
   3. The "windup" phenomenon results in a persistence of action potentials for up to 60 seconds after the discontinuation of the stimulus
   4. Long-term potentiation refers to more permanent changes in the second-order neurons as a consequence of "windup."

9. Surgical stress leads to:

   1. coronary vasoconstriction that may result in severe myocardial ischemia
   2. reflex inhibition of urinary bladder tone resulting in retention and subsequent urinary tract infections
   3. increased skeletal muscle tension leading to a decrease in total lung compliance
   4. decreased platelet adhesiveness and increased fibrinolysis leading to a bleeding tendency

10. Which of the following statements concerning attenuation of the surgical stress response is/are TRUE?

    1. An intravenous anesthetic technique with 10 to 30 μg/kg of fentanyl is effective at preventing the stress response.
    2. Epidural anesthesia attenuates postoperative hypercoagulability.
    3. Any beneficial effects of epidural anesthesia on stress mitigation are greatest in low-risk patients.
    4. Outcome improvement requires the intraoperative initiation of central neuraxial blockade followed by postoperative continuation of this modality.

11. With regard to intramuscular administration of analgesics:

    1. Onset is more rapid than with oral administration.
    2. Absorption depends upon the potency of the agent.
    3. There is potential for delayed respiratory depression.
    4. It provides more effective analgesia than intravenous administration.

12. Tramadol:

    1. increases production of serotonin
    2. has less potential for substance abuse than morphine
    3. is approximately half as potent an analgesic as morphine
    4. inhibits norepinephrine reuptake

13. Cyclo-oxygenase exists as two separate isomers: COX-1 and COX-2. Which of the following is/are TRUE regarding these isomers?

    1. COX-2 is predominately found in the brain, kidney, and prostate.
    2. COX-1 is found in platelets.
    3. COX-1 primarily regulates renal, gastric, and vascular homeostasis.
    4. Inflammatory cytokines induce the expression of the COX-2 enzyme that generates the prostaglandins involved in pain.

14. Regarding spasm of the sphincter of Oddi following morphine administration:

    1. The effect can last 24 hours after a single therapeutic dose.
    2. Low doses of naloxone can be used to reverse the effect.
    3. It is a less frequent problem with partial agonist–antagonists than with pure agonists.
    4. Vasodilating agents can relieve the spasm.

15. Regarding the transepithelial administration of fentanyl:

    1. Nausea and vomiting remain common side effects.
    2. First-pass metabolism is less problematic than after oral administration.
    3. The fentanyl patch should be applied several hours before emergence from anesthesia.
    4. Unpredictable drug absorption makes titration difficult.

16. Which of the following statements concerning patient-controlled analgesia (PCA) is/are TRUE?

    1. Less total drug is used compared with more traditional methods.
    2. Only the patient should initiate a PCA bolus dose.
    3. The system compensates for pharmacodynamic variability.
    4. Elderly and debilitated patients are ideally suited for this system.

17. Which of the following statements concerning intrathecal bolus injections of opioids is/are TRUE?

    1. Compared with epidural opioid administration, respiratory depression is rare.
    2. The incidence of side effects is less than with epidural administration.
    3. The problem of titratability is overcome.
    4. Onset is directly related to the lipid solubility of the agent.

18. Which of the following statements concerning epidural anesthesia with opioids is/are TRUE?

    1. Compared with fentanyl, morphine produces a more segmental block.
    2. Hydromorphone produces longer lasting analgesia than morphine.

3. Fentanyl may provide adequate analgesia after thoracotomy if it is infused at the L3–L4 level.
4. Hydromorphone has a reduced incidence of pruritus and nausea compared with morphine.

19. Which of the following statements concerning caudal blocks is/are TRUE?

1. They are technically easier in adults than in children.
2. The caudal block is usually placed with the pediatric patient in the lateral position.

3. The caudal needle should pierce the sacral cornua.
4. Compared with a lumbar puncture, larger volumes of local anesthetic generally are required.

20. Regarding pediatric acute pain management:

1. Evaluation of pain intensity is easier than in the adult population.
2. Morphine exhibits a shorter half-life in newborns as a result of cytochrome P450 induction.
3. Decreased total body water content of children increases the risk of respiratory depression.
4. Morphine exhibits a higher fraction of free drug in neonates than in adults.

ANSWERS

1. **A.** Class A fibers are large, fast-conducting, myelinated fibers that exhibit a lower threshold (higher excitability) than neurons in either class B or class C. Nociceptive stimuli are carried through A delta or C fibers, with 50 to 80% of class C fibers carrying pain impulses. Fibers of class C are either thinly myelinated or unmyelinated and thus have slow conduction velocities (0.5–2.0 m/second). Class B fibers are lightly myelinated. (See page 1405: Fundamental Concepts.)

2. **D.** Modulation of the nociceptive impulse occurs at several sites in the pathway between the receptor and the sensory cortex. Neurotransmitter substances can modulate transmission in the dorsal horn, as can spinal reflexes. Inhibitory substances in the regulation of afferent transmission include the enkephalins, P-endorphin, GABA, norepinephrine, and possibly somatostatin. Recent work has shown that muscarinic pathways modulate nociceptive pathways and produce analgesia; cholinergic agonists and neostigmine have such effects. Substance P release in the region of the dorsal horn enhances the pain sensation. (See page 1407: Modulation of Nociception.)

3. **E.** Nociceptors are free nerve endings and are found in nearly every region of the body. They are classified into exteroceptors (which receive stimuli from skin surfaces) and interoceptors (which receive stimuli from deeper structures). Nociceptors exhibit high response thresholds and persistent discharge to suprathreshold stimuli. Nociceptors are specific for pain; pain is not produced by overstimulation of other receptors. Peripheral afferent fibers transmitting pain signals, so-called first-order neurons, have their cell bodies in the dorsal root ganglion. They send projections into the dorsal horn and other areas of the spinal cord. In the spinal cord, a synapse occurs with a second-order neuron that can be a nociceptive-specific neuron or a wide dynamic-range neuron. (See page 1405: Nociception.)

4. **A.** The surgical stress response to pain includes a rise in the level of circulating catecholamines, cortisol, angiotensin II, glucagon, growth hormone, and antidiuretic hormone, as well as a fall in levels of anabolic hormones (testosterone and insulin). The overall metabolic effects are gluconeogenesis, hyperglycemia, a negative nitrogen balance, and sodium and water retention. The magnitude of the neuroendocrine and cytokine response to surgery correlates with the degree of tissue injury and with overall outcome. (See page 1410: Pathophysiology of Pain.)

5. **E.** Alpha$_2$-agonists (e.g., clonidine) produce analgesia when they bind to the alpha$_2$-receptors in the dorsal horn of the spinal cord. They modulate pain sensation in a manner similar to that of the opioids and act synergistically with opioids and local anesthetics to produce analgesia. The synergism is nonlinear. Hypotension and bradycardia can occur with epidurally administered clonidine, probably as a result of inhibition of the preganglionic sympathetic fibers. This effect is most predominant at lower doses, presumably because at higher doses systemic vasoconstriction overrides the central hypotensive effect. The alpha$_2$-agonists produce minimal respiratory depression compared with the opioids. (See page 1426: Selection of Analgesics.)

6. **B.** Epinephrine-containing solutions should not be used for penile blocks because vasoconstriction and ischemic necrosis of the skin can result. Local anesthetics exert their neuronal blocking effect by inhibiting sodium channels and keep the membrane in its polarized state. Advantages of local anesthetic infiltration include simplicity and the lack of change

in the patient's general sensorium. Intra-articular administration of 100 mg of bupivacaine provides effective analgesia while maintaining serum concentrations below toxic levels. Intercostal nerve blocks are performed beneath the inferior aspect of the rib to deliver drug near the neurovascular bundle. Conversely, intrapleural catheters should be inserted over the superior aspect of the rib. (See page 1429: Peripheral Nerve Blocks.)

7. **B.** The enkephalins and opiates have affinity and activity at the mu_2-receptor, which mediates supraspinal analgesia, prolactin release, and euphoria. Opiate-selective mu_2-receptors appear to mediate respiratory depression and physical dependence. Delta- and kappa-receptors are at least partially responsible for spinal analgesia. Miosis and sedation are a result of kappa-receptor activity, whereas sigma activity can produce dysphoria and hallucinations. (See page 1416: Opioid Analgesics.)

8. **E.** Peripheral nociceptors are sensitized by local tissue mediators of injury. Neuroplasticity is a functional change in spinal cord processing secondary to efferent impulses. The "windup" phenomenon refers to the temporal summation of the number and duration of action potentials in the dorsal horn neurons. The windup phenomenon results in a persistence of action potentials for up to 60 seconds after the discontinuation of the stimulus. Long-term potentiation refers to more permanent changes in the second-order neurons as a consequence of windup. (See page 1407: Neuroplasticity: The Dynamic Modulation of Neural Impulses.)

9. **A.** Surgical stress and pain result in consistent metabolic, cardiovascular, urologic, hematologic, and gastrointestinal responses. Catecholamines from sympathetic nerve endings and the adrenal medulla, together with other endocrine responses to stress, result in hypertension and tachycardia; this response can lead to myocardial ischemia. Pain-induced increases in skeletal muscle tension can lead to a decrease in total lung compliance, splinting, and hypoventilation. Postoperatively, pain-induced paralytic ileus may result. Stress may also cause reflex inhibition of urinary bladder tone, resulting in retention and subsequent urinary tract infections. Surgical stress results in a hypercoagulable state with increased platelet adhesiveness and diminished fibrinolysis. Therefore, thromboembolic effects are more likely to occur postoperatively, and preventive measures should be instituted. (See page 1410: Components of Surgical Stress Response.)

10. **C.** General anesthesia, with inhalation or intravenous agents, does not effectively attenuate the perioperative neuroendocrine stress response. High-dose narcotic (e.g., fentanyl 50 μg/kg) and deep inhalation anesthetics suppress some, but not all, aspects of the perioperative response. Studies have shown a beneficial effect of central neuraxial techniques on the cortisol response to surgery if all afferent pathways from the surgical site are blocked. The beneficial effects of epidural anesthesia on the surgical stress response appears to be greatest in patients at high risk of complications who undergo high-risk procedures. In addition, epidural anesthesia using local anesthetics with or with out opioids enhances fibrinolytic activity, hastens the return of antithrombin III to normal levels, and attenuates the postoperative increase in platelet activity. Outcome improvement requires the intraoperative initiation of central neuraxial blockade followed by postoperative continuation of this modality. (See page 1412: Influence of Anesthesia on the Surgical Stress Response and Outcome.)

11. **B.** Intramuscular administration of analgesics results in a faster onset than oral administration. Potency of the agent is not related to absorption. Plasma levels are less consistently maintained. There is, however, the potential for delayed respiratory depression. (See page 1420: Routes of Analgesic Delivery: Intramuscular.)

12. **C.** Tramadol, an analog of codeine, has a weak affinity for the mu_1-receptor and also inhibits norepinephrine and serotonin reuptake. It is approximately one-tenth as potent an analgesic as morphine but has less of a respiratory depressant effect and less potential for substance abuse. (See page 1416: Opioid Analgesics.)

13. **E.** COX-1 is found in most tissues, especially platelets, vascular endothelial cells, and collecting tubules. COX-2 is generally undetectable in most tissues except the brain and kidney. The COX-1 enzyme primarily produces prostaglandins that regulate renal, gastric, and vascular homeostasis. Inflammatory cytokines induce the expression of the COX-2 enzyme that generates the prostaglandins involved in pain. (See page 1413: Pharmacology of Postoperative Pain Management.)

14. **E.** The effect of morphine on the sphincter of Oddi can last 24 hours after a single therapeutic dose. Low doses of naloxone can be used to reverse the effect. This problem is less frequent with partial agonist–antagonists than with pure agonists. Vasodilating agents can relieve the spasm. (See page 1418: Adverse Effects.)

15. **E.** The delivery of opioid agents, such as fentanyl, by the transepithelial route decreases the degree of first-pass metabolism. However, the usual side effects of opioids (e.g., nausea, vomiting, constipation, sedation, and respiratory depression) remain troublesome. As with the oral route, unpredictable drug absorption makes it difficult to titrate drug delivery. For optimal effects, the fentanyl patch should be applied several hours before emergence from anesthesia. (See page 1420: Transepithelial.)

16. **A.** PCA has been shown to provide superior analgesia with less total drug use, less sedation, and a quicker return to physical activity than more traditional methods of opioid analgesic delivery. The patient selects the frequency of intravenous analgesic administration; thus, the system incorporates a feedback control. The dose delivered more closely matches the patient's requirements and therefore compensates for pharmacodynamic variability. The PCA device requires patient understanding and cooperation; therefore, it is not well suited for many elderly and debilitated patients. Only the patient should initiate a PCA bolus dose. Ideally, an agent used via PCA should be highly efficacious and have a rapid onset of action, a moderate duration of effect, and a large therapeutic window. Unfortunately, morphine and meperidine, the agents most frequently used in this technique, are less than ideal. (See page 1433: Patient-Controlled Analgesia.)

17. **D.** Intrathecal opioids provide long-lasting analgesia after a single dose. Onset of analgesia is directly related to lipid solubility, whereas duration of action is greater with hydrophilic agents. However, in common with other intermittent administration techniques, titratability is a problem. Respiratory depression is a greater risk than with epidural opioid administration, because of rostral spread of the opioid. There is a higher incidence of side effects than with epidural administration. (See page 1422: Central Neuraxial Analgesia.)

18. **D.** Various opioids, including agonist–antagonist agents, can be used via the epidural route. Lipophilic agents, such as fentanyl, tend to provide a greater segmental analgesic effect; therefore, the epidural catheter should be sited in a position to cover the dermatomes included in the surgical field. Morphine is more hydrophilic and thus can be infused at a lower lumbar level and still provide analgesia for upper abdominal and thoracic procedures. Hydromorphone is more lipid soluble than morphine and therefore has a shorter duration of action than morphine when administered epidurally. Hydromorphone also has less incidence of pruritus and nausea compared with morphine. A mixed agonist–antagonist such as butorphanol can be used to provide epidural analgesia; it tends to produce less respiratory depression but more somnolence. (See page 1422: Central Neuraxial Analgesia.)

19. **C.** Caudal blockade is usually performed with the pediatric patient in the lateral position. The needle is introduced through the skin and sacrococcygeal ligament before it is advanced through the sacral hiatus. A caudal block is easier to perform in children because the sacral cornua, which flank the sacral hiatus, are easier to palpate. Because the dura ends at the level of S2–S3 and a caudal block is performed through the sacral hiatus at the S5 level, dural puncture rarely occurs. Larger volumes of local anesthetic typically are required for a caudal than for a lumbar puncture. (See page 1428: Caudal.)

20. **D.** Assessment of the degree of pain often is more difficult in children because of their poor communication ability and their emotional responses. Neonates tend to have immature hepatic function, lower plasma protein levels, and impaired protein binding, all of which increase the fraction of unbound drug. This is offset, to a certain extent, by their higher total body water content and the increased cardiac output. Morphine has a longer half-life in infants younger than 1 month of age, which is attributable to immature glucuronidation pathways. (See page 1433: Special Considerations in Pediatric Acute Pain Management.)

CHAPTER 56 ■ CHRONIC PAIN MANAGEMENT

For questions 1 to 3, choose the best answer.

1. Wide dynamic-range neurons are located in which of the following dorsal horn layers?

   A. I
   B. II
   C. III
   D. IV
   E. V

2. "Windup" phenomenon involves which of the following nerve fibers?

   A. A beta
   B. B
   C. A delta
   D. C
   E. A gamma

3. _____ is a condition in which the individual intentionally creates signs that are intended to lead a physician to suspect a medical or surgical disorder.

   A. Somatization
   B. Malingering
   C. Depressive disorder
   D. Hypochondriasis
   E. Factitious disorder

For questions 4 to 13, choose A if 1, 2, and 3 are correct; B if 1 and 3; C if 2 and 4; D if 4; and E if all.

4. Mechano-heat nociceptors do not respond to:

   1. light touch
   2. pressure
   3. warm temperature
   4. intense stimulation

5. Which of the following is/are chemical mediators that are released following injury?

   1. Substance P
   2. Serotonin
   3. Bradykinin
   4. Histamine

6. Which of the following is/are considered excitatory amino acids?

   1. Arginine
   2. Aspartate
   3. Valine
   4. Glutamate

7. Which of the following statements regarding chronic regional pain syndrome is/are TRUE?

   1. Trauma commonly occurs before the development of this syndrome.
   2. The affected limb is usually warm early in the disease process.
   3. The venous catecholamine level in the affected limb is not increased.
   4. Sympathetic activity can stimulate mechano-sensitive afferents.

8. Which of the following statements concerning complex regional pain syndrome (CRPS) is/are TRUE?

   1. Fractures and sprains commonly occur before the development of CRPS type I.
   2. Causalgia is also known as CRPS type II.
   3. The pain associated with CRPS is usually burning in quality.
   4. CRPS type I is almost always associated with a major nerve trunk injury.

9. Which of the following statements regarding herpes zoster is/are TRUE?

   1. A thoracic dermatome is most commonly involved.
   2. Steroids reduce incidence of postherpetic neuralgia.
   3. Antiviral agents are only effective in the treatment of the acute phase.

4. A local anesthetic block is effective in long-term management of postherpetic neuralgia.

10. Which of the following statements regarding tricyclic antidepressants is/are TRUE?

   1. Xerostomia is a common side effect.
   2. Sleep pattern improvement is usually prompt after initiation of these drugs.
   3. The antidepressant effects are typically delayed.
   4. They reduce reuptake of norepinephrine.

11. Which of the following is/are considered to be side effects of intraspinal opioid administration?

   1. Nausea
   2. Urinary retention
   3. Pruritus
   4. Diarrhea

12. Which of the following statements concerning the difference between phenol and alcohol when used in neurolytic blocks is/are TRUE?

1. Phenol takes 15 minutes for neurolysis, whereas the neurolytic effect of alcohol is immediate.
2. Phenol usually does not produce pain on injection.
3. Intrathecal alcohol is hypobaric, whereas phenol is hyperbaric.
4. Phenol is approximately twice as effective as alcohol.

13. Which of the following statements concerning celiac plexus block is/are TRUE?

   1. Needles are placed just anterior to the body of L1.
   2. Injections are performed with 5 mL of 50% alcohol.
   3. Orthostatic hypotension is a potential side effect.
   4. Approximately 50% of patients with upper abdominal cancer experience good to excellent pain relief.

ANSWERS

1. **E.** Two groups of cells in the dorsal horn respond to noxious stimulation. One group, located mainly in lamina I, responds exclusively to noxious stimulation. Most of these cells, termed nociceptive specific, have relatively limited receptive fields confined to some fraction of a dermatome. The second group of cells, termed wide dynamic-range neurons, can be activated by either tactile or noxious stimuli. Most of these cells are located in lamina V. (See page 1444: Dorsal Horn Mechanisms.)

2. **D.** The "windup" phenomenon involves C fibers. (See page 1444: Activation of the Dorsal Horn Projection System.)

3. **E.** Factitious disorders (Munchausen syndrome) present with reporting of symptoms and the intentional creation of signs that are intended to lead a physician to suspect a medical or surgical disorder. The motivation of this behavior is to copy the role of a patient. The reasons for this goal are poorly understood. (See page 1449: Psychologic Mechanisms.)

4. **A.** Most cutaneous nociceptors respond both to intense mechanical stimulation and to high temperature and are termed mechano-heat nociceptors. They do not respond to low-threshold mechanical stimulation (light touch, pressure) or to warm temperatures below the noxious range. (See page 1442: Cutaneous Nociceptors.)

5. **E.** Numerous chemical mediators are released following injury. These substances include bradykinin, serotonin, prostaglandins, leukotrienes, histamine, and substance P. Bradykinin, which is released locally following tissue injury, is capable of evoking pain on intradermal injection. (See page 1442: Cutaneous Nociceptors.)

6. **C.** There is considerable evidence that excitatory amino acids such as glutamate and aspartate are the principal neurotransmitters responsible for activation of dorsal horn neurons following noxious stimulation. (See page 1444: Activation of Dorsal Horn Projection System.)

7. **E.** Following trauma, surgery, and certain illness, a syndrome of pain, hyperalgesia, autonomic dysfunction, and dystrophy, known as complex regional pain syndrome (CRPS), can occur. Early in the course of the syndrome, the affected limb is usually warm and erythematous. Microneurographic recording studies have failed to demonstrate alterations in sympathetic outflow in the affected limb, and venous catecholamine levels in the affected limb are not elevated. There is considerable evidence that sympathetic fibers are in direct contact with mechanoreceptors and that sympathetic activity can sensitize mechano-sensitive afferents. (See page 1448: Sympathetically Maintained Pain.)

8. **A.** Common antecedents to the development of CRPS include crush injury, lacerations, fractures, sprains, and burns. The pain is usually burning in quality and is often accompanied by diffuse tenderness and pain on light touch. The hand and foot are commonly the major sites of pain. The term causalgia, which has been used to indicate a specific syndrome of burning pain and autonomic dysfunction associated with major nerve trunk injury, has been replaced by the term CRPS type II. (See page 1456: Complex Regional Pain Syndromes.)

9. **B.** Herpes zoster most commonly involves the thoracic and the trigeminal dermatomes, with the ophthalmic division of the trigeminal nerve being second most common. Antiviral agents have been advocated for management of acute stage of the disease. Corticosteroids have enjoyed some popularity for the treatment of pain form acute herpes zoster; however, studies have failed to demonstrate a reduction of incidence in postherpetic neuralgia. There is substantial evidence that local anesthetic blocks are ineffective in the management of postherpetic neuralgia; at best, they provide very temporary relief. (See page 1458: Herpes Zoster.)

10. **E.** The most popular explanation for the analgesic property of tricyclic antidepressants is a reuptake inhibition of serotonin and norepinephrine, which increases the level of these inhibitory neurotransmitters in the brainstem and spinal cord. Although the antidepressant and pain-relieving effects are often delayed in onset, the improvement in sleep patterns provided by these drugs usually occurs promptly, often with the initial dose. The common antimuscarinic side effects of tricyclics include xerostomia, impaired visual accommodation, urinary retention, and constipation. (See page 1460: Adjuvant Analgesics.)

11. **A.** The use of intraspinal opioids in patients who had not previously been receiving systemic opioids is associated with nausea, vomiting, urinary retention, pruritus, and respiratory depression. (See page 1462: Intraspinal Opioids.)

12. **A.** Alcohol and phenol are the agents most commonly used for the prolonged interruption of neural function. There is relatively little difference in overall efficacy between these agents. Phenol produces no pain on injection, has an initial anesthetic effect, and takes about 15 minutes to exert its neurolytic effect. Alcohol causes significant pain on injection and produces neurolysis promptly. When used for intrathecal neurolysis, alcohol is hypobaric, whereas phenol is usually hyperbaric. (See page 1463: Neurolytic Block.)

13. **B.** Thompson et al. reported that 94% of 97 patients who underwent celiac plexus block for pain of upper abdominal cancer had good to excellent pain relief. Injections were performed with 50 mL of 50% alcohol: 10 patients experienced transient orthostatic hypotension, and one patient had partial motor loss in one leg. The classical technique for percutaneous injection of the celiac plexus involves bilateral placement of the block needle just anterior to the body of L1 and posterior to the aorta and diaphragmatic crura. (See page 1463: Neurolytic Block.)

CHAPTER 57 ■ ANESTHESIA AND CRITICAL CARE MEDICINE

1. According to a recent study examining the transfusion threshold in the critically ill, barring any extenuating circumstances (active bleeding, early shock, active neurologic injury, or acute myocardial infarction), the transfusion threshold should be which of the values below?

    A. 10 g/dL
    B. 9 g/dL
    C. 8 g/dL
    D. 7 g/dL
    E. 6 g/dL

For questions 2 to 13, choose A if 1, 2, and 3 are correct; B if 1 and 3; C if 2 and 4; D if 4; and E if all.

2. Which of the following statements regarding acute respiratory distress syndrome is/are TRUE?

    1. Pulmonary injury is not the only trigger for the syndrome.
    2. The mortality rate is approximately 50%.
    3. Positive end-expiratory pressure (PEEP) is a useful adjunct in maintaining oxygenation.
    4. Late in the syndrome, increasing inspired O_2 resolves the hypoxia more effectively than PEEP.

3. Which of the following statements is/are TRUE regarding tissue plasminogen activator (t-PA) administration in patients suffering an embolic cerebral occlusion?

    1. The t-PA must be administered within 12 hours of the onset of symptoms.
    2. It reduces mortality.
    3. Intra-arterial administration is more effective than peripheral administration.
    4. Patients should not be treated with any other anticoagulants after receiving t-PA.

4. Patients with chronic obstructive pulmonary disease (COPD) are at increased risk of developing auto PEEP while intubated. Which of the following strategies help prevent the development of auto PEEP?

    1. Reducing tidal volumes to 6 to 8 mL/kg
    2. Permissive hypercapnia and resultant respiratory acidosis
    3. Prolonged expiratory phase of ventilation
    4. Limiting inspired O_2 concentration

5. Which of the following statements regarding glucose management in the critically ill is/are TRUE?

    1. Tight control reduces the risk of infection.
    2. The goal of therapy should be to keep the glucose level below 110 g/dL.
    3. Patients in the intensive care unit (ICU) may have elevated blood glucose levels because of total parenteral nutrition (TPN) or steroid administration.
    4. Elevated blood glucose levels in traumatic brain-injury (TBI) patients are expected and do not require intervention.

6. Which of the following statements is/are TRUE regarding propofol sedation of the TBI patient.

    1. Propofol improves cerebral O_2 balance better than benzodiazepines.
    2. Prolonged administration of high-dose propofol can produce lactic acidosis and death.
    3. Propofol can decrease cerebral perfusion pressure (CPP) because of hemodynamic instability.
    4. Propofol improves mortality resulting from improved intracranial pressure (ICP) regulation.

7. Following a subarachnoid hemorrhage (SAH) and successful clipping of the aneurysm, a patient at day 7 following the initial bleed develops cerebral ischemic symptoms. Which of the following is/are TRUE

regarding delayed ischemic neurologic deficits (DINDs)?

1. It occurs in about one-third of all patients with SAH.
2. Oral nimodipine can be used for prophylaxis.
3. Transcranial Doppler is the diagnostic modality used to identify and quantify cerebral vasospasm.
4. Hypervolemic, hypertensive therapy improves mortality in symptomatic individuals.

8. Which of the following statements is/are TRUE regarding splanchnic resuscitation?

1. Intestinal villi, because of their countercurrent circulation, are very vulnerable to septic shock–mediated alterations in perfusion.
2. Metabolic acidosis will not occur if there are sufficient levels of O_2 delivery.
3. Intramucosal pH and P_{CO_2} can be used to assess the splanchnic metabolic rate.
4. Insufficient splenic circulation can result in thrombocytopenia.

9. Which of the following statements is/are TRUE regarding norepinephrine administration to individuals in shock?

1. Its effects are mediated through alpha- and beta-receptors.
2. In volume-resuscitated hypotensive individuals, norepinephrine improves renal perfusion.
3. Norepinephrine produces a reduction in lactate levels by improving perfusion pressure through an increase in systemic vascular resistance (SVR) and by increasing O_2 consumption.
4. Norepinephrine should be administered at the first sign of septic shock because early intervention can prevent profound septic shock.

10. Which of the following statements regarding vasopressin use in patients suffering from shock is/are TRUE?

1. It significantly increases SVR.
2. It significantly increases heart rate (HR).
3. In patients with hepatorenal syndromes, vasopressin improves urinary output.
4. It produces a significant increase in pulmonary vascular resistance (PVR).

11. Ventilator-associated pneumonia (VAP) occurs in patients who are intubated and ventilated in the ICU. Which of the following statements is/are TRUE regarding VAP?

1. Early onset VAP is associated with organisms such as *Haemophilus influenzae*, *Streptococcus pneumoniae*, and methicillin-sensitive *Staphylococcus aureus*.
2. Strict hand washings and head-up position reduce the incidence.
3. Late-onset VAP carries a higher risk of mortality than early-onset VAP.
4. Acid suppression therapy helps reduce the incidence of VAP.

12. Which of the following statements is/are TRUE regarding dexmedetomidine?

1. It is an alpha$_2$-adrenergic receptor agonist.
2. It has some analgesic effects.
3. It produces sedation without inducing unresponsiveness.
4. It produces a dose-dependent reduction of responses.

13. Which of the following statements is/are TRUE regarding nutritional supplementation in the ICU?

1. Gastric feeding should be started within 48 hours of ICU admission.
2. Postpyloric positioning of feeding tubes reduces the risk of pneumonia.
3. Enteral and parenteral feedings are both equally efficient.
4. Raising the head of the bed to 30 to 40 degrees helps reduce aspiration.

ANSWERS

1. **D.** A recent study examined critically ill patients and found that patients transfused at 7 g/dL hemoglobin level had no higher mortality level than those patients transfused at a 10 g/dL threshold. (See page 1489: Anemia and Transfusion Therapy in Critical Illness.)

2. **A.** Acute respiratory distress syndrome is a syndrome that arises from various underlying physiologic perturbations, such as sepsis, trauma, hypotension, and amniotic fluid embolism. The syndrome arises from a loss in pulmonary endothelium integrity, which results in leakage of plasma and red blood corpuscles into the alveoli. Leukoaggregation on the endothelial surface and proliferation of type II pneumocytes also occur. The white blood cells produce prostaglandin products, complement, free radicals, and digestive enzymes, which add to the injury of the alveoli. The signs and symptoms arise from pulmonary consolidation, which leads to shunt. There is a large increase in the arterial-alveolar (A-a) gradient for O_2, and the patient will complain of dyspnea and be tachypneic with increased work of breathing. Initially, increased

inspired O_2 will improve oxygenation, but as the shunt fraction increases and the work of breathing overwhelms the patient, positive-pressure ventilation will have to be instituted. PEEP pressure is the mainstay of treatment to improve oxygenation. Because the disease process is one of shunt, PEEP helps recruit nonventilated alveoli and thereby reduces the A-a gradient. PEEP also reduces pulmonary water and decreases the work of breathing. Fluid management is also very important, as one should attempt to reduce the Starling forces, which increase pulmonary fluid, while maintaining sufficient preload to prevent hypotension. Acute respiratory distress syndrome resolves if time is provided for the lungs to heal themselves. (See page 1484: Acute Respiratory Failure and Clinical Manifestations.)

3. **D.**   t-PA must be administered within 3 hours of the symptoms of cerebral occlusion to be effective. Its administration does not reduce mortality, but it does improve neurologic outcome. It can be administered peripherally or via direct arterial injection; however, direct arterial injection has yet to be proven more effective than peripheral administration. Once t-PA has been administered, no other anticoagulants can be administered as it increases the risk of cerebral bleeding and increases mortality. (See page 1478: Acute Ischemic Stroke.)

4. **A.**   To reduce the occurrence of auto PEEP, one should limit tidal volume to 6 to 8 mL/kg. The expiratory phase of ventilation should be made as long as possible to facilitate alveolar emptying. Both the foregoing strategies may result in insufficient ventilation, and respiratory acidosis may occur. This produces minimal physiologic effects and should be tolerated. O_2 concentration in the inspired mixture does not affect auto PEEP. (See page 1484: Principles of Mechanical Ventilation.)

5. **A.**   Increased blood glucose levels in critically ill patients result from diabetes, TPN, and steroid administration as well as from stroke or trauma to the central nervous system. For all cases, the elevated blood glucose levels result in increased risk of infection, increased mortality, multisystem organ failure, renal failure, and other end-organ damage. An elevated glucose level in patients with brain trauma is a harbinger of a poor outcome and should be treated to reduce mortality and morbidity. (See page 1487: Glucose Management in Critical Illness.)

6. **A.**   Propofol is an ideal drug for sedating patients with TBI. It produces a rapidly reversible sedation that reduces cerebral metabolic demand and coupled blood flow. This, in turn, results in a reduction of ICP, which improves CPP. In inadequately resuscitated individuals, propofol can produce hypotension, which would result in a worsening of CPP. Prolonged high-dose administration of propofol (>80 mg/kg per

minute and >24 hours) can produce lactic acidosis and death. Sedation-mediated alterations in CPP and reduced cerebral O_2 requirements have not produced a reduction in mortality. (See page 1476: Traumatic Brain Injury.)

7. **A.**   Patients with SAH face a one in three chance of developing DINDs. They typically occur 3 days out from the initial hemorrhage, peak at 7 to 10 days, and resolve over day 10 to 14 after the SAH. Prophylaxis can be accomplished through the administration of nimodipine for up to 3 weeks. Transcranial Doppler is used to identify and quantify the degree of cerebral vasospasm. Hypertensive hypervolemic therapy has not been shown to improve mortality in symptomatic patients. (See page 1477: Subarachnoid Hemorrhage.)

8. **A.**   In shock states, circulation is altered because of vasodilation and altered hemodynamics resulting in abnormalities in circulation. Intestinal villi have a countercurrent flow, which makes them susceptible to low flow states. These alterations result in insufficient blood flow to the intestinal mucosa, which produces localized acidosis. This flow can be indirectly measured (intramucosal pH and PCO_2), and hemodynamic therapy can be altered to improve splanchnic oxygenation. Despite sufficient O_2 delivery, septic shock can result in inadequate tissue delivery of O_2 because of decreased cellular O_2 extraction. Decreased splanchnic circulation does not cause thrombocytopenia. (See page 1481: Septic Shock.)

9. **A.**   Norepinephrine's effects are mediated through alpha- and beta-receptors. Norepinephrine produces an increase in systolic blood pressure with variable effects on CO and HR. In septic individuals, norepinephrine increases SVR, which improves splanchnic blood flow and decreases lactate levels. Similarly, in patients who are septic and euvolemic, norepinephrine increases renal blood flow. In all cases, norepinephrine should not be administered to improve hemodynamics before fluid administration has been attempted. (See page 1482: Management of Septic Shock with Vasopressors/Inotropes.)

10. **B.**   Vasopressin administration results in significant increase in systemic blood pressure with little or no effect on CO, HR, or PVR. At low doses, it does not affect renal blood flow, and in hepatorenal syndrome, it increases urinary output. (See page 1482: Management of Septic Shock with Vasopressors/Inotropes.)

11. **A.**   VAP occurs typically in two forms: early, which is a low-mortality form; and late, a high-mortality form. The early form of VAP is caused by *Haemophilus influenzae, Streptococcus pneumoniae,* and methicillin-sensitive *Staphylococcus aureus.* Late-onset VAP is associated with virulent organisms

such as methicillin-resistant *S. aureus*, *Pseudomonas aeruginosa*, and *Acinetobacter*. Late-onset VAP has a high mortality rate, whereas early-onset VAP has almost no mortality rate. Precaution through hand washing and head-up position can reduce its incidence. Acid suppression therapy increases the risk of VAP because of bacterial overgrowth. (See page 1491: Ventilator-Associated Pneumonia.)

12. **A.**   Dexmedetomidine is an alpha$_2$-adrenergic receptor agonist like clonidine, which produces sedation and mild analgesia. It does not produce respiratory depression. The sedation it creates allows the patient to be responsive when stimulated. The drug is expensive and is currently recommended only for 24 hours. (See page 1490: Sedation of the Critically Ill Patient.)

13. **D.**   Enteral nutrition should be started as early as possible after admission in the ICU. Early feeding (within 4 hours) resulted in less organ dysfunction than delayed (36 hours) initiation. Parenteral nutrition is inferior to enteral nutrition. Patients who receive enteral nutrition have a lower infection risk and reduced translocation and nitrogen imbalance as compared with patients receiving parenteral nutrition. The location of the feeding tube does not affect mortality, ICU length of stay, or development of pneumonia. Elevating the head of the head of the bed can reduce aspiration. (See page 1489: Nutrition in the Critically Ill Patient.)

CHAPTER 58 ■ CARDIOPULMONARY RESUSCITATION

1. Which of the following statements is FALSE?

   A. Cardiovascular mortality in the United States is approximately 50%.
   B. Optimum outcome from ventricular fibrillation is obtained if ventilation and chest compressions are initiated within 4 minutes.
   C. In the operating room, cardiac arrest occurs approximately seven times for every 10,000 anesthetics.
   D. The highest rate of survival following out-of-operating room cardiovascular arrest occurs in patients cared for in the intensive care unit (ICU).
   E. Optimum outcome from ventricular fibrillation is obtained if defibrillation is applied within 8 minutes.

2. All of the following are correct EXCEPT:

   A. There are two levels of cardiopulmonary resuscitation (CPR) care, basic life support and advanced cardiac life support.
   B. The guidelines for CPR care in the United States are developed by the American Heart Association's National Conference on CPR.
   C. "Do not resuscitate" orders are automatically suspended when patients consent for surgery.
   D. Patients in cardiac arrest can receive all forms of therapy except those specifically stated in their "do not resuscitate" orders.
   E. Changes to CPR protocols are based on the most current scientific literature.

3. Considering basic life support, all the following statements are true EXCEPT:

   A. Techniques for airway support should take precedence.
   B. In case of choking, aggressive maneuvers are not indicated if the coughing mechanism is intact.

   C. Performing mouth-to-mouth ventilation could harm the patient considering its low O_2 concentration.
   D. Both the cardiac pump and thoracic pump mechanisms are responsible for the blood flow during CPR.
   E. During CPR, the brain and the heart receive the most of the blood flow.

4. Which of the following doses is not correct?

   A. Sodium bicarbonate: 1 mEq/kg, with 0.5 mEq/kg every 10 minutes PRN
   B. Atropine: 1.0 mg, repeated every 3 to 5 minutes to a total of 0.04 mg/kg
   C. Epinephrine: 1.0 mg, repeated every 3 to 5 minutes
   D. Amiodarone: 1,000-mg intravenous bolus, with 500 mg PRN to total daily dose of 4 g
   E. Calcium chloride 2–4 mg/kg

5. All of the following statements regarding patient ventilation during cardiac arrest are true EXCEPT:

   A. Mouth-to-mouth ventilation is sufficient to maintain viability.
   B. During rescue breathing without an endotracheal tube, volumes of 2 L should be given quickly (i.e., <1 second).
   C. Studies have shown that cricoid pressure can prevent gastric insufflation and gastric distention.
   D. Current recommendations for rescue breathing are two breaths every 15 compressions during single rescuer.
   E. During rescue breathing with an endotracheal tube, breaths should be given at a steady continuous rate without a pause in chest compressions.

6. All the following statements regarding the adequacy of circulation are correct EXCEPT:

A. Myocardial perfusion correlates with diastolic pressure, whereas the pulse pressure correlates with systolic pressure.

B. A minimum blood flow of 15 mL/100 g myocardium per minute is necessary for successful resuscitation.

C. The critical coronary perfusion pressure is associated with a diastolic pressure of ≥ 40 mm Hg.

D. The end-tidal carbon dioxide ($ETCO_2$) during CPR is an accurate measure of tissue perfusion.

E. Ten to 15 minutes after administration of bicarbonate, $ETCO_2$ will return to previous baseline.

7. Which of the following statements is TRUE?

A. According to advanced cardiac life support protocol, medication administration is key to survival in patients in cardiac arrest.

B. Epinephrine, lidocaine, atropine, and sodium bicarbonate can all be given through the endotracheal tube.

C. The efficacy of epinephrine use for cardiac arrest results from its strong beta-adrenergic stimulus.

D. Of all the medications currently used in advanced cardiac life support, only epinephrine is acknowledged as being helpful.

E. A possible postresuscitation complication of epinephrine is hypotension.

For questions 8 to 11, choose A if 1, 2, and 3 are correct; B if 1 and 3; C if 2 and 4; D if 4; and E if all.

8. Which of the following statements is/are TRUE?

1. The recommended first step in airway management for cardiac arrest is the head-tilt–chin-lift or jaw-thrust maneuver.

2. Endotracheal intubation is the most definitive airway control method and limits the risk of aspiration.

3. A complication of abdominal thrust includes spleen or liver laceration.

4. Signs of total airway obstruction include rasping or wheezing respirations.

9. Regarding the mechanism and physiology of CPR, which of the following statements is/are TRUE?

1. The cardiac pump mechanism assumes that sternal compression increases intraventricular pressure.

2. The thoracic pump mechanism assumes that sternal compression increases intrathoracic pressures in all cardiac chambers equally.

3. Abdominal compression or ventilation with chest compression increases arterial pressure.

4. Chest wall compliance influences the mechanism of blood flow during CPR.

10. Which of the following statements concerning defibrillation is/are TRUE?

1. The most important determinant of failure to resuscitate a patient with ventricular fibrillation is the duration of ventricular fibrillation.

2. Defibrillation is significantly more successful if epinephrine is given immediately before application of current.

3. Defibrillation occurs via current passing through a critical mass of myocardium, causing simultaneous myofibril depolarization, with the primary determinant of energy delivery being transthoracic impedance.

4. Because of large body size, adult patients in cardiac arrest respond better to initial energy levels of >300 J.

11. Which of the following statements is/are TRUE?

1. Children usually experience cardiac arrest primarily because of intrinsic cardiac dysfunction.

2. When indicated, standard defibrillation energy levels in children are 2 J/kg, and these are doubled if defibrillation fails.

3. To prevent postresuscitation cerebral hyperemic flow, mean blood pressure should be maintained at <90 mm Hg.

4. A high correlation exists in postresuscitation patients between neurologic function and creatinine kinase-BB levels in cerebrospinal fluid.

ANSWERS

1. **D.** Although cardiovascular mortality has declined since the mid-1960s, the leading cause of death is still cardiovascular disease, at a rate of nearly 50%. Prompt chest compressions and defibrillation (4 and 8 minutes, respectively) are the most important determinants of optimum survival following ventricular fibrillation. Cardiac arrest in the operating room occurs at a rate of seven of 10,000 anesthetics;

4.5 of 10,000 arrests are anesthesia related. Successful resuscitation occurs in approximately 90% of anesthesia-related arrests, leading to a small (0.4 of 10,000) anesthetic mortality rate. Within the hospital, the operating room is the location where CPR has the highest rate of success. Outside the operating suite, the best initial resuscitation rates are found in the ICU, whereas the best survival rates are for patients who experience cardiac arrest in the emergency department. (See page 1500: Scope of the Problem.)

2. **C.** Basic life support and advanced cardiac life support are the two forms of CPR. Guidelines are periodically updated for CPR by the American Health Association's National Conference on CPR in accordance with the latest scientific evidence in CPR therapy. Although they can be uncomfortable for anesthesia and surgical caregivers, "do not resuscitate" orders can be maintained throughout surgery. However, therapies that the patient wishes *not to receive* need to be clearly delineated in the order, and care excluding these specific items can be rendered by appropriate personnel. (See page 1500: Organizing a Solution; and page 1501: Ethical Issues.)

3. **C.** Common practice is to approach a victim with the airway-breathing-circulation (ABC) sequence, although the circulation-airway-breathing (CAB) sequence has been used in some countries with comparable results. The signs of total airway obstruction are the lack of air movement despite respiratory efforts and the inability of the victim to speak or cough. Cyanosis, unconsciousness, and cardiac arrest follow quickly. Partial airway obstruction will result in rasping or wheezing respirations accompanied by coughing. If the victim has good air movement and is able to cough forcefully, no intervention is indicated. However, if the cough weakens or cyanosis develops, the patient must be treated as if there were complete obstruction. Mouth-to-mouth or mouth-to-nose ventilation is the most expeditious and effective method immediately available. Although inspired gas with this method will contain ~4% CO_2 and only ~17% O_2 (composition of exhaled air), it is sufficient to maintain viability. During the compression phase of the CPR, all intrathoracic structures are compressed equally by the rise in intrathoracic pressure caused by sternal depression, forcing blood out of the chest. Backward flow through the venous system is prevented by valves in the subclavian and internal jugular veins and by dynamic compression of the veins at the thoracic outlet by the increased intrathoracic pressure. Thicker, less compressible vessel walls prevent collapse on the arterial side, although arterial collapse will occur if intrathoracic pressure is significantly raised. These are thought to be the mainstay of events that belong to both the cardiac and thoracic pump mechanisms. Myocardial perfusion is 20 to 50% of normal, whereas cerebral perfusion is maintained at 50 to 90% of normal. Abdominal visceral and lower extremity flow is reduced to 5% of normal. (See page 1501: Basic Life Support.)

4. **D.** Correct doses include:

Sodium bicarbonate: 1 mEq/kg, with 0.5 mEq/kg every 10 minutes PRN

Atropine: 1.0 mg, repeated every 3 to 5 minutes to a total of 0.04 mg/kg

Epinephrine: 1.0 mg, repeated every 3 to 5 minutes

Amiodarone: 300-mg intravenous bolus, with 150 mg PRN to total daily dose of 2 g

Calcium chloride: 2 to 4 mg/kg of the 10% solution

Lidocaine: 1.5 mEq/kg with 0.5 to 1.5 mg/kg every 5 to 10 minutes to a total of 3 mg/kg

Routine use of sodium bicarbonate is not helpful. However, in cardiac arrest resulting from hyperkalemia, tricyclic antidepressant or phenobarbital overdose, or severe pre-existing metabolic acidosis, sodium bicarbonate may be indicated.

Although evidence is weak for its efficacy, atropine is given for pulseless electrical activity (PEA) and asystole. Atropine has few adverse side effects and may be helpful when prior chest compressions, oxygenation, and epinephrine have not resolved the situation.

Epinephrine remains the standard pharmacologic intervention for cardiac arrest. Studies comparing high-dose (3–5 mg) epinephrine with a standard dose (1 mg) have failed to show improved outcome in initial bolus dosing with high-dose epinephrine. However, it is beginning to appear that should initial therapy with standard-dose (1 mg) epinephrine fail, a second, higher dose (3–8 mg) should be considered.

Calcium chloride is indicated during cardiac arrest resulting from hyperkalemia, for hypocalcemia, or during calcium channel blocker toxicity. Calcium chloride is recommended because it produces higher and more consistent ionized calcium levels than other salts. Calcium gluconate contains one-third as much molecular calcium and requires gluconate metabolism in the liver.

Amiodarone is helpful at suppressing ectopic activity and aiding defibrillation when ventricular fibrillation is refractory to electrical countershock therapy. (See page 1510: Epinephrine Dose, Amiodarone, Lidocaine, Sodium Bicarbonate, Atropine, and Calcium.)

5. **B.** Mouth-to-mouth ventilation is effective at maintaining viability in victims of cardiac arrest despite a relatively low O_2 content (~17%). During rescue breathing without an endotracheal tube, care must be made to avoid insufflating the stomach. Large breaths (0.8–1.2 L) given over 1.5 to 2.0 seconds during pauses in chest compressions are effective for delivering proper tidal volumes without distending the stomach. The Sellick maneuver has also been shown to reduce or eliminate gastric insufflation, although two rescuers are often needed to accomplish this correctly. Ratios for breaths to compressions for one and two rescuers remain 2:15 and 1:5, respectively. After definitive airway management is achieved with

endotracheal intubation, interrupting chest compressions for breaths is unnecessary. In fact, circulation and subsequent oxygenation have been shown to improve with continuous chest compression. Pausing during mouth-to-mouth ventilations, however, is still necessary to reduce airway resistance, improve ventilation, and reduce gastric insufflation. (See page 1502: Ventilation; page 1502: Physiology of Ventilation During CPR; and page 1503: Techniques of Rescue Breathing.)

6. **E.** The adequacy of closed-chest compression is usually judged by palpation of a pulse in the carotid or femoral vessels. The palpable pulse primarily reflects systolic pressure. Cardiac output correlates better with mean pressure and coronary perfusion with diastolic pressure. In experimental models, a minimum blood flow of 15 to 20 mL/100 g per minute of myocardium has been shown to be necessary for successful resuscitation. During standard CPR, critical myocardial blood flow is associated with aortic diastolic pressure ≥ 40 mm Hg. $ETco_2$ also has been found to be an excellent noninvasive guide to the adequacy of closed-chest compressions. CO_2 excretion during CPR with an endotracheal tube in place is flow dependent rather than ventilation dependent. Sodium bicarbonate administration liberates CO_2 into the blood and causes a temporary increase in $ETco_2$. The elevation returns to baseline within 3 to 5 minutes of drug administration, and $ETco_2$ monitoring can again be used for monitoring effectiveness of closed-chest compressions. (See page 1505: Circulation: Assessing the Adequacy of Circulation during Cardiopulmonary Resuscitation.)

7. **D.** Although adjunctive medications such as bretylium, lidocaine, and atropine have been shown to be helpful to maintain rhythm once cardiac function returns, only epinephrine is acknowledged as being effective in regaining spontaneous cardiac function following cardiac arrest. Medication administration should be secondary to airway management, chest compressions, or defibrillation. Withholding these interventions to gain intravenous access and give medications is contraindicated. Although atropine, lidocaine, and epinephrine can be given via the endotracheal tube, sodium bicarbonate should not be given by this route. Medications given via the endotracheal tube should be in doses two to 2.5 times larger than intravenous doses and in volumes of 5 to 10 mL to ensure proper drug delivery and systemic effect.

Epinephrine's efficacy during cardiac arrest is related to its strong alpha-adrenergic properties. The alpha-adrenergic activity causes peripheral vasoconstriction, increased aortic diastolic pressure, and improved myocardial blood flow. Possible postresuscitation complications of epinephrine use are hypertension and tachyarrhythmias. Despite this, epinephrine is the vasopressor of choice in CPR, because of strong animal study evidence of its efficacy and extensive clinical experience with its use in humans. (See page 1509: Pharmacologic Therapy: Routes of Administration; and page 1509: Catecholamines and Vasopressors.)

8. **A.** The recommended first step in airway management of the unconscious victim is to perform the head-lift–chin-lift maneuver. This allows the tongue to move anterior to the posterior pharynx and creates a passage for airflow. The jaw-thrust maneuver (lifting the jaw forward with anterior force on the angle of the mandible) is also effective. Should CPR be required for a longer time, the most definitive means of airway management is endotracheal intubation. Should airway obstruction result from a foreign body, signs of total airway occlusion include lack of air movement despite respiratory efforts and inability to speak or cough. Abdominal thrusts are recommended to help dislodge the foreign body when total occlusion is present. Injury may occur with abdominal thrust, including liver or spleen laceration, gastric injury, or regurgitation. (See page 1501: Airway Management and Foreign Body Airway Obstruction.)

9. **E.** Although various techniques have been investigated regarding circulation during CPR, no theory or technique has shown improvements in survival over standard CPR. Thus, standard ventilation with chest compressions is still recommended as the most efficacious means of ventilatory support. Research continues regarding alternative means of circulation. The cardiac pump mechanism assumes that sternal compression increases intraventricular pressure, thus leading to mitral and tricuspid valve closure, causing forward blood flow as intrathoracic pressure increases. The thoracic pump mechanism assumes that sternal compressions increase intrathoracic pressures in all cardiac chambers equally, that the heart is merely a passive conduit, and that forward flow during increased intrathoracic pressure is the result of backflow prevention in the venous system by the valves in the subclavian and internal jugular veins that favors flow into nondistensible arteries (i.e., aorta and carotids). Evidence supporting the thoracic pump mechanism includes the observation that simultaneous abdominal compression or ventilation with chest compression increases arterial pressure and carotid blood flow compared with standard CPR. Factors that may influence the mechanism of blood flow during CPR include chest wall compliance and configuration, heart size, sternal compression force, and the duration of cardiac arrest. (See page 1503: Circulation; page 1503: Cardiac Pump Mechanism; and page 1503: Thoracic Pump Mechanism.)

10. **B.** Research continues to support the efficacy of immediate defibrillation. Decreasing time to defibrillation strongly correlates with survival. Defibrillation within 1 minute of fibrillation obviates the need for CPR. Although the amplitude of

fibrillation waves correlates with the success of defibrillation, and alpha-adrenergic agonists (e.g., epinephrine) increase fibrillation amplitude, little evidence supports increased success of defibrillation following epinephrine administration. On the contrary, defibrillation should not be delayed at all when indicated.

Defibrillation is the simultaneous depolarization of fibrillating myofibrils, thus providing an environment for more effective myocardial contraction and re-establishment of automatism. The average transthoracic impedance in human defibrillation is 70 to 80 ohm. Resistance is probably of little clinical significance when reasonably proper technique and high-energy (300 J) shocks are used. In fact, less myocardial damage, improved postdefibrillation rhythm, and improved ability to convert have been demonstrated with lower energy levels as the initial value (160–200 J). Only after failing to convert at low energy (200 J) should increasing levels of energy be used. (See page 1506: Electrical Pattern and Duration of Ventricular Fibrillation; page 1507: Defibrillators: Energy, Current, and Voltage; and page 1508: Adverse Effects and Energy Requirements.)

11. **C.** Cardiac arrest is less likely to be a sudden event and is more likely related to progressive deterioration of respiratory and circulatory function in the pediatric age group. Airway and ventilation problems lead to asystole and pulseless electrical activity (PEA) as the most common presenting rhythms. However, the consequences of myocardial and cerebral ischemia are the same as for the adult. Effective ventilation is especially critical because respiratory problems are frequently the cause of arrest. Mouth-to-mouth or mouth-to-nose and mouth (for infants) ventilation can be used as well as bag-valve mask devices until intubation is possible. Although defibrillation is less frequently necessary in children, the same principles apply as in the adult. However, the recommended starting energy is 2 J/kg, which is doubled if defibrillation is unsuccessful. Considerations for drug administration are the same as for the adult, except that the interosseous route in the anterior tibia provides an additional option in small children. The major factors contributing to mortality following successful resuscitation are progression of the primary disease and cerebral damage suffered as a result of the cardiac arrest. Because cerebral autoregulation of blood flow is severely attenuated, both prolonged hypertension and hypotension are associated with a worsened outcome. Therefore, mean arterial pressure should be maintained at 90 to 110 mm Hg. For the comatose survivor of CPR, the question of ultimate prognosis is important. Most patients who completely recover show rapid improvement within the first 48 hours. There is also a high correlation between severity of neurologic injury and the level of creatine kinase-BB found in the cerebrospinal fluid. (See page 1514: Pediatric Cardiopulmonary Resuscitation; page 1515: Postresuscitation Care; and page 1517: Prognosis.)

CHAPTER 59 ■ DISASTER PREPAREDNESS AND WEAPONS OF MASS DESTRUCTION

1. The United States federal agency in charge of organizing emergency assistance to state and local governments in the event of a disaster is:

   A. FEMA
   B. FDA
   C. National Guard
   D. JCAHO
   E. CDC

2. The initial response to any disaster situation occurs at what level of government?

   A. Local
   B. State
   C. Federal
   D. Judicial
   E. Executive

3. Which of the following statements regarding the National Pharmaceutical Stockpile is FALSE?

   A. It includes airway maintenance supplies.
   B. It was established by the Centers for Disease Control and Prevention (CDC).
   C. It is organized in two phases, the first phase involving distribution of prepackaged "push packages" with critical medical supplies and a second phase in which additional resources can be quickly mobilized if necessary.
   D. It includes certain antibiotics and chemical antidotes.
   E. It is controlled by the Federal Emergency Management Agency (FEMA).

4. The most common source of radiation injury comes from what type of disaster?

   A. Detonation of a nuclear bomb
   B. Terrorist attack
   C. Nuclear power plant accident
   D. Volcano eruption
   E. Earthquake

5. The American Academy of Pediatrics recommends that at least two tablets of potassium iodide be available for emergency use among which of the following populations?

   A. All children who live within 1 mile of a nuclear power facility
   B. All inhabitants who live within 1 mile of a nuclear power facility
   C. All children who live within 10 miles of a nuclear power facility
   D. All inhabitants who live within 10 miles of a nuclear power facility
   E. All individuals working in nuclear power facilities

6. Which of the following types of radiation exposure has the deepest penetrance?

   A. Alpha particles
   B. Beta particles
   C. Delta particles
   D. Gamma rays
   E. Sigma rays

7. Which of the following tissues are most sensitive to the effects of ionizing radiation?

   A. Lymphoid > gastrointestinal > reproductive > dermal > nervous system
   B. Dermal > gastrointestinal > lymphoid > reproductive > nervous system
   C. Lymphoid > reproductive > gastrointestinal > nervous system > dermal
   D. Lymphoid > dermal > reproductive > gastrointestinal > nervous system
   E. Nervous system > reproductive > lymphoid > dermal > gastrointestinal

8. The influenza virus typically associated with pandemics, including the Spanish flu of 1918, is of type:

   A. A
   B. B

C. C
D. D
E. E

9. Specific therapy for high-dose exposure to cyanide includes:

A. sodium thiosulfate
B. arsine
C. pralidoxime chloride
D. hyperbaric oxygen
E. pyridostigmine

For questions 10 through 12, choose A if 1, 2, and 3 are correct; B if 1 and 3; C if 2 and 4; D if 4; and E for all.

10. Which of the following statements regarding potential biological agents of terrorism is/are TRUE?

1. Smallpox transmission occurs mostly through aerosolized droplets.

2. The antibiotic treatment of choice for plague caused by *Yersinia pestis* is streptomycin.
3. *Bacillus anthracis* is a Gram-positive, spore-forming bacillus.
4. *Francisella tularensis* infection may present as a skin ulceration.

11. Which of the following is/are a unit used to measure radiation exposure?

1. Roentgen-equivalent-man (rem)
2. Sievert (Sv)
3. Gray (Gy)
4. Radiation absorbed dose (rad)

12. Which of the following is/are a Category A biological agent?

1. *Variola major*
2. *Clostridium botulinum*
3. *Bacillus anthracis*
4. *Vibrio cholerae*

ANSWERS

1. **A.** The Federal Emergency Management Agency (FEMA) provides management assistance to state and local governments in response to disaster. FEMA assists by distributing emergency relief to affected individuals and businesses, decontaminating affected areas, and helping to ensure public health safety. The Joint Commission on Accreditation of Healthcare Organizations (JCAHO) has made recommendations to help hospitals create emergency preparedness plans, but it is not part of the direct response to disaster management. The National Guard may be called upon to assist in disaster management but is not a lead agency by definition. The Center for Disease Control also has a role in disaster planning and response, specifically with the dissemination of necessary medical and surgical supplies to affected regions. However, the CDC does not take the lead in providing support to local and state governments when disaster occurs. The Food and Drug Administration (FDA) has no direct role in emergency planning or response. (See page 1525: Disaster Preparedness: Role of Government.)

2. **A.** The initial response to any disaster occurs at the local level. If the situation calls for resources beyond the capacity of local authorities, state emergency management resources and the National Guard may be mobilized through the governor's office. Federal authorities may also be called in should the situation warrant assistance beyond state control. (See page 1525: Disaster Preparedness: Role of Government.)

3. **E.** The National Pharmaceutical Stockpile was established by the CDC to ensure the rapid availability of medical supplies to facilitate emergency response in the event of a national disaster. The Stockpile contains specific antibiotics, chemical antidotes, life-support medications, intravenous administration supplies, and airway maintenance supplies, as well as other medical and surgical items. There are two phases to this program. The first is the provision of eight separate, yet identical, prepackaged caches of medical materials called 12-hour "push packages" that are deployed around the United States. The second involves mobilizing specific additional supplies from vendor management inventories (VMIs) capable of arriving within 24 to 36 hours of the initial request. FEMA does not have authority over the National Pharmaceutical Stockpile. (See page 1525: Disaster Preparedness: Role of Government.)

4. **C.** The disaster most likely to cause radiation injuries is contamination from a nuclear power plant or reactor. Although a terrorist attack or nuclear bomb detonation may also produce radiation causing human injury, these events are far less common. Neither volcano eruptions nor earthquakes typically involve radiation injury. (See page 1526: Nuclear Accidents.)

5. **D.** Because of the risk of exposure to ionizing radiation, the American Academy of Pediatrics recommends that at least two tablets of potassium iodide be readily available for all inhabitants within a

10-mile radius of a nuclear power facility. If taken soon enough, potassium iodide will protect the thyroid from the deleterious effects of radioactive iodine that may be released from an accident involving a nuclear power plant or nuclear reactor. (See page 1526: Nuclear Accidents.)

6. **D.** Of the choices listed, gamma rays have the deepest penetrance. In a nuclear accident, several types of radiation exposure may occur, including exposure to alpha and beta particles, as well as gamma rays and x-rays. These exposures are of various strengths. Human tissue can block alpha particles. In contrast, beta particles may be stopped by an aluminum shield, whereas gamma rays and x-rays are stopped only by a lead shield. Neither delta particles nor sigma rays are types of ionizing radiation. (See page 1526: Nuclear Accidents; page 1527: Table 59-6, Types of Radiation.)

7. **A.** Tissue sensitivity to the effects of ionizing radiation varies based on cellular turnover rate. In general, tissue with the highest turnover rate is most affected by exposure to ionizing radiation. From greatest to least, sensitivity of human tissue to ionizing radiation is as follows: lymphoid > gastrointestinal > reproductive > dermal > nervous system. (See page 1526: Nuclear Accidents.)

8. **A.** There were three large influenza pandemics in the twentieth century: one in 1918 during World War I, another in 1957 and 1958, and a third in 1968 and 1969. All of these pandemics were caused by antigenic shifts in the influenza type A virus. Major pandemics occur when a change in viral surface antigens occurs (antigenic shift) and naïve human hosts are exposed to a virus for which their immune systems have not made protective antibodies. Every year, influenza A vaccines are prepared in an attempt to predict the most likely combinations of viral surface antigens. However, because the behavior of the virus can be unpredictable, these vaccines are not 100% protective, and the risk of major outbreaks caused by unforeseen antigenic combinations is a persistent threat. (See page 1529: Biological Disasters.)

9. **A.** Cyanide ions are normally metabolized by the rhodanese liver enzyme in a sulfur-requiring step that leads to the formation of methemoglobin. In the setting of cyanide poisoning, sulfur stores are depleted, leading to enzymatic dysfunction. Treatment of cyanide poisoning therefore includes administration of sodium thiosulfate as a sulfur donor to regenerate enzymatic metabolism of cyanide ions. In the meantime, the patient may require tracheal intubation and mechanical ventilation, sodium bicarbonate to treat metabolic acidosis, and ionotropes and vasopressors for hemodynamic support. Arsine is one of the cyanogens that can cause cyanide toxicity, along with hydrogen cyanide, hydrocyanic acid, and cyanogen chloride. Hyperbaric oxygen may play a role in the management of carbon monoxide poisoning but is not indicated for cyanide poisoning. Pralidoxime chloride reactivates acetylcholinesterase and is used to counteract the muscarinic and nicotinic stimulant effects of nerve agents that inhibit acetylcholinesterase. Pyridostigmine is sometimes administered prophylactically in situations in which exposure to a nerve agent is anticipated because it binds to acetylcholinesterase and thereby protects it and allows for spontaneous enzyme regeneration. (See page 1535: Chemical: Blood Agents.)

10. **E.** Several types of biological agents carry the potential to be used as agents of terrorism. Smallpox is a highly infective virus most commonly transmitted via aerosolized droplets. Infection causes a prodrome of malaise, headache, and backache followed by the onset of high fever. As the fever subsides, smallpox lesions of multiple stages appear and are often particularly prominent on the face and distal extremities. Although not frequently fatal, smallpox is considered a biological threat because of its high infectivity and ability to cause significant and rapid morbidity. *Bacillus anthracis* is a Gram-positive spore-forming bacterium that causes three main types of infection: cutaneous, inhalation, and gastrointestinal. Anthrax spores are extremely resistant to destruction and may survive dormant in the soil for years. Inhalational anthrax is the most lethal form of infection, although far less common that the cutaneous form. In addition to supportive care, treatment should include ciprofloxacin or doxycycline. *Yersinia pestis* is a Gram-positive bacillus that causes plague. The treatment of choice is streptomycin, but chlorophenicol and tetracycline may also be used. *Francisella tularemia* is a Gram-negative rod that may be contracted by humans via direct contact with an infected animal (most common), ingestion of infected food, or inhalation of aerosolized bacteria. The bacteria invade the body via hair follicles or microabrasions of the skin. At the site of entry, swelling becomes visible, followed by the development of a necrotic ulcer with a black eschar. Alternatively, inhalation of tularemia may lead to the development of pneumonia. As with anthrax and plague, the treatment of tularemia includes streptomycin antibiotic therapy. (See page 1529: Biological Disasters.)

11. **E.** All of the units listed are measures of radiation exposure. Gray is the International System unit of measurement for the energy deposited by any type of radiation in joules per kilogram. Radiation absorbed dose also refers to the amount of energy deposited by any type of radiation to any tissue or other material, where 1 rad = 0.01 Gray. Roentgen-equivalent-man and sievert are used to quantify human exposure to radiation. The sievert is part of the International System of units and, like the gray, is measured in joules per kilogram. One sievert (1 Sv) is equivalent to 100 rem. (See page 1526: Nuclear Accidents; page 1527: Table 59-6, Types of Radiation.)

12. **A.**   Potential biological agents of warfare are classified into three categories based on degree of threat to national security: Categories A, B, and C. Category A agents are those with the greatest potential to cause harm as a result of relative ease of transmission and high mortality. *Bacillus anthracis* (anthrax), *Variola major* (smallpox), *Yersinia pestis* (plague), *Clostridium botulinum* (botulism), *Francisella tularensis* (tularemia), and the viruses that cause hemorrhagic fever (Ebola, Lassa, Marburg, Argentine) are the six agents currently listed in Category A. *Vibrio cholerae* (cholera) is a Category B agent. (See page 1529: Biological Disasters; page 1528: Table 59-7, Radiation Exposure Terms.)